Pediatric Pulmonology

THE REQUISITES IN PEDIATRICS

SERIES EDITOR   **Louis M. Bell,** M.D.
Patrick S. Pasquariello, Jr. Chair in General Pediatrics
Professor of Pediatrics
University of Pennsylvania School of Medicine
Chief, Division of General Pediatrics
Attending Physician, General Pediatrics and
   Infectious Diseases
The Children's Hospital of Philadelphia
Philadelphia, Pennsylvania

Pediatric Pulmonology

THE REQUISITES IN PEDIATRICS

Howard B. Panitch, M.D.
Associate Professor of Pediatrics
University of Pennsylvania School of Medicine
Director of Clinical Programs
Division of Pulmonary Medicine
The Children's Hospital of Philadelphia
Philadelphia, Pennsylvania

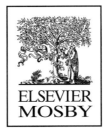

ELSEVIER
MOSBY

ELSEVIER
MOSBY

1600 John F. Kennedy Blvd.
Ste 1800
Philadelphia, PA 19103-2899

PEDIATRIC PULMONOLOGY
THE REQUISITES IN PEDIATRICS   ISBN 0-323-01909-9
Copyright © 2005, Mosby, Inc.

THE REQUISITES ™
THE REQUISITES
THE REQUISITES
THE REQUISITES
THE REQUISITES

THE REQUISITES is a proprietary trademark
of Mosby, Inc.

NOTICE

Knowledge and best practice in this field are constantly changing. As new research and experience broaden our knowledge, changes in practice, treatment and drug therapy may become necessary or appropriate. Readers are advised to check the most current information provided (i) on procedures featured or (ii) by the manufacturer of each product to be administered, to verify the recommended dose or formula, the method and duration of administration, and contraindications. It is the responsibility of the practitioner, relying on their own experience and knowledge of the patient, to make diagnoses, to determine dosages and the best treatment for each individual patient, and to take all appropriate safety precautions. To the fullest extent of the law, neither the Publisher nor the Editor assumes any liability for any injury and/or damage to persons or property arising out or related to any use of the material contained in this book.

The Publisher

Library of Congress Cataloging-in-Publication Data

Pediatric pulmonology : the requisites in pediatrics / [edited by] Howard Panitch.
    p. ; cm.
    ISBN 0-323-01909-9
    1. Lungs—Diseases. 2. Children—Diseases. 3. Pediatric respiratory diseases.
 I. Panitch, Howard.
    [DNLM: 1. Lung Diseases—Child. WS 280 P3668 2005]
 RJ431.P395 2005
 618.92′24–dc22

                                            2004052406

Acquisitions Editor: Anne Lenehan
Developmental Editor: Patrick M.N. Stone
Project Manager: Mary Stermel
Marketing Manager: Theresa Dudas

Printed in the United States of America

Last digit is the print number: 9   8   7   6   5   4   3   2   1

Working together to grow
libraries in developing countries

www.elsevier.com | www.bookaid.org | www.sabre.org

ELSEVIER   BOOK AID International   Sabre Foundation

To future caregivers of children with respiratory disease, and to our patients, who teach and inspire by their bravery and determination.

Contributors

Julian L. Allen, M.D.
Professor of Pediatrics
University of Pennsylvania School of Medicine
Chief, Division of Pulmonary Medicine
  and Cystic Fibrosis Center
Robert Gerard Morse Chair in
  Pulmonary Medicine
The Children's Hospital of Philadelphia
Philadelphia, Pennsylvania

Raanan Arens, M.D.
Associate Professor of Pediatrics
Division of Pulmonary Medicine
The Children's Hospital of Philadelphia
Philadelphia, Pennsylvania

Anita Bhandari, M.D.
Assistant Professor of Pediatrics
Division of Pulmonary Medicine
The Children's Hospital of Philadelphia
Philadelphia, Pennsylvania

Michael R. Bye, M.D.
Professor of Clinical Pediatrics
Columbia University College of Physicians
  and Surgeons
Acting Director, Pediatric Pulmonary Medicine
Morgan Stanley Children's Hospital of
  New York Presbyterian
New York, New York

Col. Charles W. Callahan, D.O.
Chief, Department of Pediatrics—Pediatric
  Pulmonology
Tripler Army Medical Center
Honolulu, Hawaii
Professor of Pediatrics
Uniformed University of the Health Sciences
Bethesda, Maryland

Russell G. Clayton, Sr., D.O.
Assistant Professor of Pediatrics
Division of Pulmonary Medicine
The Children's Hospital of Philadelphia
Philadelphia, Pennsylvania

Oscar H. Mayer, M.D.
Clinical Associate in Pediatrics
Division of Pulmonary Medicine
The Children's Hospital of Philadelphia
Philadelphia, Pennsylvania

Joshua P. Needleman, M.D.
Assistant Professor of Pediatrics
Albert Einstein College of Medicine
Section of Pediatric Respiratory Medicine
The Children's Hospital at Montefiore
Bronx, New York

Brian P. O'Sullivan, M.D.
Associate Professor of Pediatrics
University of Massachusetts Medical School
UMass Memorial Health Care
Worcester, Massachusetts

Howard B. Panitch, M.D.
Associate Professor of Pediatrics
University of Pennsylvania School of Medicine
Director of Clinical Programs
Division of Pulmonary Medicine
The Children's Hospital of Philadelphia
Philadelphia, Pennsylvania

Anand C. Patel, M.D.
Fellow, Pediatric Pulmonology
Department of Pediatrics
Division of Allergy and Pulmonary Medicine
St. Louis Children's Hospital/Washington University
  School of Medicine
St. Louis, Missouri

Clement L. Ren, M.D.
Associate Professor of Pediatrics
University of Rochester
Chief, Division of Pediatric Pulmonology
Golisano Children's Hospital at Strong
Rochester, New York

Gail L. Rodgers, M.D.
Associate Professor of Pediatrics
Section of Infectious Diseases
Drexel University College of Medicine
Attending Physician
St. Christopher's Hospital for Children
Philadelphia, Pennsylvania

Carlos Sabogal, M.D.
Pediatric Pulmonologist
Nemours Children's Clinic
Orlando, Florida

Thomas F. Scanlin, M.D.
Professor of Pediatrics
University of Pennsylvania School of Medicine
Director, Cystic Fibrosis Center
Division of Pulmonary Medicine
The Children's Hospital of Philadelphia
Philadelphia, Pennsylvania

Daniel V. Schidlow, M.D.
Professor and Chair
Department of Pediatrics
Drexel University College of Medicine
Chief Medical and Academic Officer
St. Christopher's Hospital for Children
Philadelphia, Pennsylvania

Jonathan Steinfeld, M.D.
Assistant Professor of Pediatrics
Department of Pediatrics
Drexel University School of Medicine
St. Christopher's Hospital for Children
Philadelphia, Pennsylvania

Isaac Talmaciu, M.D.
Pediatric Pulmonary and Allergy Associates
Plantation, Florida

Haviva Veler, M.D.
Pulmonary Fellow
Division of Pulmonary Medicine
The Children's Hospital of Philadelphia
Philadelphia, Pennsylvania

Judith A. Voynow, M.D.
Associate Professor of Pediatrics
Division of Pediatric Pulmonology
Duke University Medical Center
Durham, North Carolina

Daniel J. Weiner, M.D.
Assistant Professor
Department of Pediatrics
University of Pennsylvania School of Medicine
Attending Physician, Division of Pulmonary Medicine
Medical Director, Pulmonary Function Laboratory
The Children's Hospital of Philadelphia
Philadelphia, Pennsylvania

Foreword

As I review the fourth volume of **The Requisites in Pediatrics**, entitled *Pediatric Pulmonology*, two thoughts come to mind. First, a certain momentum is building as each new volume is published, adding substance and reality to the conceptual framework for this series. Recall that the goal of this series was to ask leading pediatric subspecialists to edit a book that would include the essential fund of pediatric knowledge in their subspecialty area. Each volume was to review the common pediatric conditions information that would guide primary care providers, resident physicians, nurse practitioners and students in the care of their patients. The editor and authors were asked to include information about appropriate referral to the specialist and to outline the laboratory testing that should be performed prior to the referral to assist the specialist in her or his search for the difficult diagnosis.

My second thought after reading *Pediatric Pulmonology*, edited by Howard Panitch, is how well this volume adheres to the vision for this series. The editor and authors have created a rare book, one that is both concise and thorough. Filled with radiographic images, tables, pathologic pictures and numerous illustrations, the information is accessible and practical.

There are 15 chapters in this volume, beginning with "Assessment and Approach to Common Problems" by Dr. Needleman and ending with "Viral Infections of the Respiratory Tract" by Dr. Bye. In between there are numerous examples of the combination of medical writing that is both "concise and thorough." For example, Chapter 2, "Noisy Breathing in Infants and Children" by Dr. Mayer is excellent. A common complaint in pediatrics, Dr. Mayer makes the important point that "with a focused

history and physical examination one should be able to come very close to a diagnosis before any evaluations are performed." He takes the reader through the logical approach to these patients.

Dr. Aren's Chapter 5, "Sleep-Disordered Breathing in Children" is a valuable contribution. He offers an excellent review of this important topic, particularly obstructive sleep apnea syndrome (OSAS) in children.

Another example of concise and thorough writing is the outstanding review of "Respiratory Failure in Children," Chapter 14, by Dr. Weiner. After reviewing normal respiratory physiology and the definition of hypoxia, he takes the reader to an understanding of respiratory failure and its causes and management. Non-traditional therapies to manage respiratory failure, such as prone positioning, negative pressure ventilation, high-frequency oscillatory ventilation, and liquid ventilation, are discussed.

After reviewing the newest volume in the **Requisites in Pediatrics** series, I congratulate Dr. Panitch and the authors for their wonderful contributions. We hope you enjoy *Pediatric Pulmonology*.

Louis M. Bell, M.D.
Patrick S. Pasquariello, Jr. Chair in General Pediatrics
Professor of Pediatrics
University of Pennsylvania School of Medicine
Chief, Division of General Pediatrics
Attending Physician, General Pediatrics
and Infectious Diseases
The Children's Hospital of Philadelphia
Philadelphia, Pennsylvania

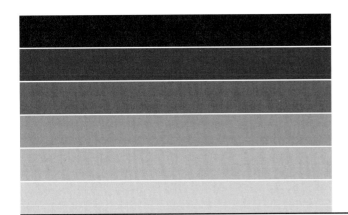

Preface

Pediatric pulmonology was recognized as a subspecialty of the American Board of Pediatrics less than two decades ago. Pediatric pulmonologists, however, have been caring for children with lung disease in the United States and around the world for much longer. Most pediatric pulmonary centers grew out of the teams of health care providers assembled to treat children with cystic fibrosis. A multidisciplinary approach was developed both to deliver care and also to study the pathophysiology of the disorder. Similar approaches have been developed to treat other pulmonary disorders like asthma, bronchopulmonary dysplasia, sleep-disordered breathing, and chronic respiratory failure. While such specialized teams, consisting of physicians, nurse specialists, nutritionists, social workers, physiotherapists, and other medical subspecialists have become indispensable for delivering care to children with chronic and complex respiratory disorders, the generalist remains at the forefront of diagnosis and management of children with respiratory disorders. Illnesses affecting the lung remain among the most common reasons for parents to seek medical care for their children.

Today, pediatric pulmonologists care for children with a variety of diseases that can be shared with other subspecialists: asthma with allergists, sleep disorders with neurologists, pneumonia with infectious disease specialists, respiratory failure with critical care physicians, to name a few. Pediatric Pulmonology combines respiratory embryology, physiology, and molecular biology in its approach to understanding and managing diseases, complementing those of other disciplines. It is that unique process that is highlighted in this volume.

Pediatric Pulmonology: The Requisites in Pediatrics is designed to provide students, residents, general practitioners and other non-physician health care providers with such an approach to a variety of respiratory disorders. The content emphasizes an orderly approach to the diagnosis and management of common respiratory conditions affecting infants, children, and adolescents. Whenever possible, disease manifestations are explained in terms of pathophysiologic alterations, which in turn are discussed in light of known underlying basic defects. Authors of each chapter endeavored to present practical information about their respective topics, including clinical pearls and indications for referral to a specialist.

Working with each of the authors on their chapters has been both a joy and a great learning experience. I hope the reader will experience the same enjoyment and sense of enlightenment in reading this work, and come away with a solid understanding of the requisites in pediatric pulmonology.

Howard B. Panitch, M.D.

Acknowledgments

I have many people to thank for completing this project. To begin, Drs. Louis Bell and Julian Allen gave me the opportunity to undertake and to fashion the contents of this volume. Thank you both for your guidance and words of encouragement. To the chapter authors, my friends and members of my "academic family tree," I am indebted to you for your enthusiasm and your willingness to put up with my innumerable queries and suggestions. Your love of the topics you wrote, and of your commitment both to caring for children with respiratory disease and to teaching others how to do so, shines through. I am indebted to Kathleen Sullivan, M.D., Ph.D., who helped to identify radiographic studies of patients with immunodeficiencies, and Avrum Pollock, M.D., who magnanimously provided publication-quality radiographs seen in several chapters.

Their contributions added critical visual reinforcements to the authors' texts, and were invaluable. To Kimberley Cox, Patrick Stone, Anne Lenehan, and others at Elsevier, thank you for keeping us on track and moving forward. This book would never have been completed without your gentle guidance. Thanks also to my mentors, Jules and Dan, who taught me that caring for one child can help the individual, but sharing wisdom and experience with others has a far greater effect on the health and welfare of our patients. You inspire by example, and I have been blessed to have you as my teachers. And finally, to Mary, Oren, and Becky, who put up with my preoccupations with this project on countless nights, weekends and vacations, thank you for your tolerance and patience. You are the loves of my life.

Contents

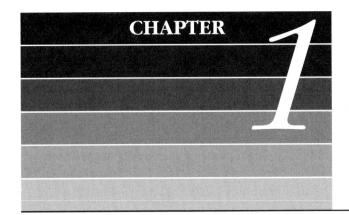

CHAPTER 1

Assessment and Approach to Common Problems

JOSHUA P. NEEDLEMAN, M.D.

Respiratory complaints are the most common reason for children to have sick visits and consultation with a physician. Recurrent or chronic respiratory problems are responsible for missed school, emergency room visits and hospitalizations in overwhelming numbers. Asthma alone is responsible for more than 10 million missed school days in the United States[1-3]. There is a large set of disease states and clinical problems that present with a limited variety of respiratory signs and symptoms. The challenge for the clinician is to isolate the pathophysiologic cause of the symptom and follow that path to diagnosis and eventual therapy. The object of this chapter will be to review the basic tools available to the clinician in the approach to common problems in pediatric pulmonology and the application of these tools to the most common clinical situations.

INVESTIGATIVE TECHNIQUES

History and Physical Examination

The history and physical examination continue to be the keystones of diagnosis and assessment of progress in respiratory disease. A careful respiratory history may require more than 30 minutes but is essential in determining the initial approach. In addition to the standard medical history that focuses on timing, duration and characterization of symptoms, there are aspects to the history of a chronic or recurrent respiratory problem that require extra emphasis.

- *Variation with time of day.* Do the symptoms vary between day and night? Are there certain times of the night that the symptoms are significantly worse? Some symptoms, such as those resulting from post-nasal drip or gastroesophageal reflux, are worse immediately upon lying down for bed due to positioning; others, related to airway inflammation, are worse in the middle of the night and early morning. Symptoms that are stress-induced or habitual will often keep the patient awake but will not awaken a sleeping patient.

- *Seasonal variation.* This is often quite helpful, especially with pre-school children in establishing exacerbating factors such as viral infection or potential allergens. It can help when planning a course of therapy with the family to have an idea if the symptoms are likely to be easier to control during the summer months or if they continue unabated.
- *Medication use and delivery devices.* In addition to the types of medications used and the clinical response observed, it is important to take careful note of exactly what type of delivery device is used for inhaled medications and to have the patient demonstrate his or her technique. Poor response to therapy is often a result of poor aerosol delivery and not incorrect therapy prescribed. If the patient uses a nebulizer, nebulizations should be supervised and given through a mouthpiece whenever possible. Patients with metered dose inhalers should all have spacers that are age-appropriate and they must demonstrate good technique in their use.
- *Exercise and activity limitations.* Many children with chronic or recurring respiratory problems have become acclimated to their disease states and will not report difficulty with activity or exercise unless pressed. Questions regarding the exact nature of exercise or gym class activity, the patient's level of participation, and after-school activities can yield valuable clues to the level of limitation.
- *Clarification of terminology.* Families will often use terms such as "wheezing," "croupy cough," and "distress" with a variety of meanings. It is obviously essential to be sure that the family and the clinician are communicating effectively[4].

The physical examination of the child with a persistent respiratory problem can also be time-consuming and require extra attention in certain areas. As young children are frequently anxious in medical settings, time and care are essential to acquiring accurate data. "Slapping a stethoscope" on the chest of a screaming toddler will, unfortunately, yield little useful information. As with the history, there are certain aspects worthy of extra emphasis.

- *Observation.* Observing the young child, whose shirt has been removed, from across the room yields insight into the baseline pattern of breathing. The inspiratory to expiratory ratio that is prolonged in obstructive disease, the presence or absence of retractions, the natural respiratory rate, and level of distress can all be determined this way.
- *Auscultation.* Carefully listening to all lung fields is essential to characterize abnormal breath sounds. Attention to variations in character of breath sounds across all lung fields, with notation of asymmetry, is critical. Auscultation of the chest at different lung volumes is important in order to comprehend the

pathology. After listening to tidal breathing, the patient must be encouraged to take deep inspirations and forced exhalations to reveal pathology in obstructed or partially collapsed airways. Small children who cannot comply with the forced exhalation maneuver should have the time-honored "squeeze the wheeze" technique applied. In this procedure, the clinician places his or her hands on the back and front of the chest with the stethoscope held in between the fingers. The chest is compressed, firmly yet gently, during exhalation to assist the patient in making a larger exhalation at a higher flow rate. Another result of this maneuver is that the subsequent inhalation will often be larger, and so a better assessment of inspiratory sounds can also be made.

- *Digital clubbing.* An often overlooked finding, the presence of clubbing can lead the clinician towards the diagnosis of a group of serious conditions (Table 1-1), and aid in following progress of patients with chronic chest disease.

Laboratory Evaluation

There are some basic laboratory tests that can be helpful in the initial approach to respiratory disease. Although there is no routine panel of tests for evaluation of respiratory problems, the history and physical examination will guide the clinician in effective use of the clinical laboratory. Some commonly utilized tests deserve extra discussion.

Table 1-1 Causes of Digital Clubbing

Conditions with chronic lung infection
    Cystic fibrosis
    Bronchiectasis
    Ciliary dyskinesia
    Lung abscess or empyema
Pulmonary conditions associated with hypoxemia
    Interstitial lung disease
    Pulmonary fibrosis
    Bronchopulmonary dysplasia
    Hypoventilation syndromes
        Congenital
        Severe obstructive sleep apnea
    Pulmonary hypertension
Pulmonary malignancy
Cardiac conditions
    Congenital cyanotic heart disease
    Bacterial endocarditis
Gastrointestinal conditions
    Liver disease
    Inflammatory bowel disease
Thyrotoxicosis
Familial (benign)

- *Quantitative sweat chloride.* This is a non-invasive, inexpensive, highly sensitive diagnostic test for cystic fibrosis (CF). A sweat test by pilocarpine iontophoresis should be performed at an accredited CF center as experience with proper collection technique and quality control is important. The sweat test should be considered in the evaluation of any patient with symptoms consistent with possible CF, or history of a sibling with CF.
- *Sputum culture.* Often overlooked in pediatrics, the sputum culture can be helpful in children who are old enough to expectorate their secretions successfully. Unusual isolates, such as *Pseudomonas*, should prompt further evaluation for underlying airway disease or immunodeficiency.
- *Arterial blood gas determination.* A measure of oxygen exchange and efficiency of ventilation, an arterial blood gas can prove valuable in evaluating potential hypoventilation syndromes, anxiety disorders, or potential shunting conditions. As arterial puncture is painful, it should be performed sparingly and with the use of topical anesthetic cream and intradermal lidocaine whenever possible. Transcutaneous pulse oximetry can provide a good measure of oxygen saturation and, therefore, an estimate of oxygen tension that can suffice for many patients. In addition, a venous bicarbonate level can provide an estimate of the degree of compensation for chronic hypoventilation in some patients.
- *Allergy testing.* RAST tests are available for specific allergens including fungi, dust mites and food proteins. These may be helpful in some patients, who report specific symptoms at certain times. Referral for skin testing is also an option for patients who appear to have a large allergic component to their symptoms.
- *Immunoglobulin levels.* Total IgE may be elevated in allergic problems and is part of the screening evaluation for allergic bronchopulmonary aspergillosis (ABPA). Quantitative immune globulins, including IgG subclasses, are part of the evaluation for immunodeficiency.

Pulmonary Function Testing

Pulmonary function testing includes a wide variety of procedures that aid in defining the underlying respiratory physiology and pathophysiology. Pulmonary function testing is useful in diagnosis of pulmonary disease, evaluating potential therapies, and monitoring progress of therapy. An understanding of the basic pulmonary function tests will lead to utilizing them effectively.

- *Spirometry.* The most commonly used pulmonary function test, spirometry consists of measures of forced expiratory flows. Spirometry can be used to detect obstructive lung disease and to estimate

whether the site of the obstruction is in the large or small airways. It can also be used to evaluate response to therapy, administration of bronchodilators (Figure 1-1). Many spirometers are portable, making them useful in diverse locations. With some instruction and patience, reliable data can be obtained from children as young as 5 or 6 years. Recently, children as young as 3 years of age have been shown to be able to perform spirometry reproducibly with careful coaching.

- *Measurements of lung volumes.* While spirometry measures air forced out of the lungs, the actual size of the lungs cannot be determined without measuring the air remaining at the end of exhalation. The measurement of lung volumes allows the diagnosis of restrictive lung disease and air trapping from obstructive lung disease to be made.

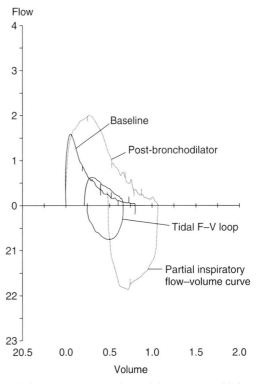

Figure 1-1 Spirometry performed by a 7-year-old boy with asthma. Flow is graphed on the ordinate and volume on the abscissa. Expiratory flow is above the baseline, while inspiratory flow is below it. Expired volumes progress left to right from the vital capacity to residual volume. The flow–volume loops are shown before and following bronchodilator administration (smaller and larger curves, respectively). The smaller loop represents a tidal volume breath. The baseline spirometry reveals marked airflow obstruction reflected in a concavity of the flow–volume loop towards the volume axis. There is an almost complete reversal of obstruction following the bronchodilator, with a significant increase in flow at all lung volumes. It is of note that the patient was asymptomatic and had a normal physical examination at baseline.

Lung volumes are measured by either gas dilution methods or in a plethysmographic box. Both techniques require equipment usually found only in pulmonary function laboratories and can be done in cooperative children as young as 7–8 years of age.

- *Bronchial provocation.* Bronchial provocation tests are used to provoke airway reactivity and aid in the diagnosis of asthma. Pulmonary function is measured at baseline and then at increasing doses of an inhaled bronchoconstrictor while lung function is measured serially. A reduction in pulmonary function of 20% or greater from baseline in response to the provocative agent is considered a positive sign of airway reactivity. Agents commonly used include methacholine, histamine, hypertonic saline and dry cold air.
- *Exercise testing.* As exercise limitation is a common complaint, exercise testing can be a valuable tool. In a formal exercise test, the subject performs spirometry and then exercises maximally on either a stationary bicycle or a treadmill. Oxygen consumption, carbon dioxide production, heart rate, oxygen saturation and blood pressure are all measured. Following exercise, spirometry is again measured serially for 20 minutes. Utilizing this test, the cause of the exercise limitation can be pinpointed. If there is a significant decline in lung function, for example, a diagnosis of exercise-induced asthma can be established. Non-pulmonary causes of exercise intolerance can be diagnosed as well.

Diagnostic Imaging

There are several important diagnostic imaging modalities available to the clinician in the initial approach to respiratory disease[5]. Diagnostic imaging can frequently establish a diagnosis, but is often just as useful to exclude unusual diagnoses and to allow the clinical impression to lead therapy. The most commonly used tests are reviewed below.

- *Chest radiographs.* Still the staple of evaluation of respiratory disease, the plain chest film is useful in excluding pneumonia, pneumothorax and thoracic tumors among other causes of symptoms. In addition to the presence of large lesions and infiltrations, the chest radiograph can demonstrate signs of inflammation and airflow obstruction such as peribronchial cuffing and hyperinflation. The plain film can demonstrate interstitial lung disease as well, which will lead the clinician to consider other possibilities.
- *Fluoroscopy.* Fluoroscopic evaluation of the airway can be useful in the diagnosis of large airway collapse. Although less sensitive than bronchoscopy, it is fast, does not require sedation and can be paired with an esophagram[6]. Fluoroscopy is also useful in detecting abnormal diaphragm function.

- *Esophagram.* A useful test for structural evaluation of the upper gastrointestinal tract in patients with gastroesophageal reflux, it is also helpful in the diagnosis of vascular anomalies that cause airway compression including vascular rings and slings.
- *Computed tomography (CT scan).* The CT scan provides a more detailed picture of the lungs with higher resolution than the standard chest radiograph. It is useful in the diagnosis of parenchymal problems such as interstitial lung disease, pneumonia and abscesses. The CT scan can also evaluate airway lesions including bronchiectasis, and pleural disease as well (Figure 1-2).
- *Magnetic resonance imaging and angiography (MRI/MRA).* While the CT scan provides a detailed image of the airways and lung parenchyma, MRI and MRA scans can provide the most detailed information about vascular structures in the chest. This can be useful in the evaluation of possible vascular anomalies that are compromising the airways.

Bronchoscopy

Visualization of the laryngeal structures, trachea and bronchi is useful in the evaluation of many respiratory symptoms[7]. When done while the patient is comfortable, sedated and breathing spontaneously, flexible bronchoscopy can yield valuable information about the structure of the airway and its function. In addition, flexible bronchoscopy affords the clinician the opportunity to sample distal airway secretions in the form of bronchoalveolar lavage fluid. Lavage fluid can be processed for cultures and for evidence of chronic aspiration or bleeding.

COMMON PROBLEMS IN PEDIATRIC PULMONARY MEDICINE

Cough

Cough is one of the most common symptoms for which patients present to their doctors[8]. The impact of cough on the quality of life for the patient and family cannot be overemphasized. In addition to discomfort and loss of sleep, a child with a chronic cough provokes worry and anxiety on the part of the entire family. While pursuing the diagnosis and appropriate treatment, the clinician must also be sensitive to the family's concerns and address them directly. This discussion will focus on the chronic cough, usually defined as a cough present for more than 6–8 weeks.

History and Physical Examination

The potential etiologies for a chronic cough are numerous (Table 1-2), and a careful history and physical

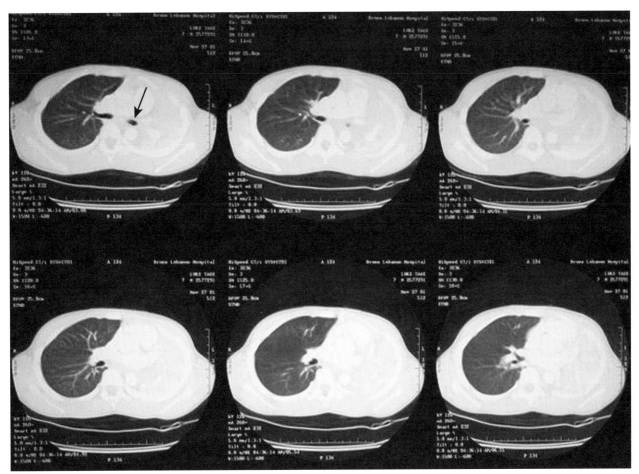

Figure 1-2   CT scan with contrast revealing obstruction of the left main bronchus and complete collapse of the left lung in a 9-year-old boy. The lumen of the left main bronchus can be seen just distal to the main carina in the left upper panel (arrow). As images are taken more caudally, the lumen of the airway disappears. The left lung is smaller than the right, suggesting central airway obstruction with atelectasis, and not a diffuse infiltrative process, as the cause of these findings. The patient had aspirated chewing gum while sleeping.

examination is the first step to narrowing the focus. Characterization of the cough, its timing and severity is important[9]. However, the quality of the cough (dry, wet, barky) often proves to be unhelpful, as patients may perceive the cough differently from a trained clinician. It is common, for example, for the parent of a child with sinusitis to say that the cough has "gone to his chest" despite the absence of any thoracic findings on examination.

The timing of the cough can be helpful in narrowing diagnostic options. Irritative coughs from post-nasal drip, sinusitis, or gastroesophageal reflux are often worse immediately upon lying down for sleep. Nocturnal cough is a major feature of asthma and often occurs in the middle of the night or early morning[10]. Cough following exercise or activity can also suggest an asthma component. The presence of any nocturnal symptoms would argue strongly against habit (psychogenic) cough[11].

The physical examination can prove helpful if positive findings are revealed, such as wheezing on forced exhalation suggesting asthma, or the presence of post-nasal drip in the hypopharynx. The presence of digital clubbing or nasal polyps would certainly raise the suspicion of CF. In many cases, however, the physical examination will prove to be unremarkable and leave the clinician with the list of diagnostic possibilities unaltered.

Laboratory Evaluation

A sweat test is the most commonly indicated test in the evaluation of the child with chronic cough. It should be considered in any child in whom the cause of the cough is not readily determined. As CF can present in a variety of ways, with variable severity, the sweat test should not be withheld because the patient is well-appearing[12]. Other laboratory tests that may be helpful in selected patients are allergy panels if there appears

Table 1-2 Causes of Chronic Cough in Children with Some Typical Features	
Upper respiratory tract irritation	
Post-nasal drip/rhinitis	Nasal congestion
	Throat clearing
	Complain of "tickle" in throat
	Worse on lying down
Sinusitis	Headaches
	Halitosis
	Worse on lying down
Gastroesophageal reflux	After feeds (especially infants)
	Worse on lying down
Swallowing dysfunction	Cough when eating or drinking
Infectious or postinfectious	
Respiratory syncytial virus (RSV)	Infants, seasonal
Chlamydia	Infants, history of eye discharge
Pertussis	May have missed immunization
Tuberculosis	Positive purified protein derivative (PPD)
Intrathoracic airway	
Tracheomalacia	Airway collapse on fluoroscopy/bronchoscopy
Bronchomalacia	Diagnosis by bronchoscopy
Foreign body	Sudden onset with choking episode
	Characteristic radiographic findings
Asthma	Responds to bronchodilators
	Worse with exercise or upper respiratory infections (URIs)
Gastroesophageal reflux	
Conditions with chronic infection	
Cystic fibrosis	Abnormal chest radiograph
	Gastrointestinal symptoms/poor growth
Primary ciliary dyskinesia	Sinusitis
	Otitis
Bronchiectasis	Purulent sputum, abnormal radiograph
Immunodeficiency	Recurrent infections
Medication-induced	
ACE inhibitors	Dry cough
Preservatives in inhaled medications	Temporal association
Habit cough	Not present while sleeping

to be an environmental or seasonal component, and an immunodeficiency investigation if a history of other infections is present.

Pulmonary Function Testing

The presence, on spirometry, of airflow obstruction that responds to bronchodilator inhalation confirms the presence of asthma in the child with a chronic cough. If initial spirometry is normal and the etiology of the cough is still in doubt, bronchial provocation may be indicated to further evaluate the possibility of asthma as a factor.

Diagnostic Imaging

A chest radiograph is often helpful in the evaluation of the child with chronic cough. Frequently unremarkable, it helps alleviate familial concerns, often unspoken, of tuberculosis or tumor as a cause of the symptoms. A radiograph that looks surprisingly "dirty" could suggest chronic inflammation or recurrent aspiration. If sinusitis is an etiologic possibility, a sinus CT scan is the modality of choice for making the diagnosis.

Bronchoscopy

Although infrequently indicated, when used judiciously bronchoscopy can add a great deal to the evaluation. It is the ideal method for diagnosis of large airway collapse and for sampling lower airway fluid for culture. The identification of lipid-laden macrophages provides circumstantial evidence that chronic aspiration may be playing a role in the symptoms.

When pursuing the cause and treatment of chronic cough in a child it is important to take the symptoms seriously and to be cognizant of their impact on the child and family. Evaluation of therapy is complicated by the fact that available treatments for post-nasal drip and gastroesophageal reflux are often only partially effective and that often a significant placebo effect exists. The clinician needs to remember, as well, that many patients can have more than one cause of cough at given times: the patient with asthma can develop sinusitis, for example. Patience in the evaluation and careful attention to the patient's complaints and reports will lead to a satisfactory conclusion.

Wheezing

A wheeze on auscultation is a musical, continuous sound that reflects increased airway narrowing at some point in the respiratory system. Although historically considered a sign of intrapulmonary disease, it has recently been shown that wheezing can occur with extrapulmonary obstruction as well[13]. The most common cause of wheezing is asthma, but careful consideration of alternative diagnoses will reveal additional problems as well (Table 1-3).

History and Physical Examination

The history is important with regard to timing and seasonal variation. Careful attention to diurnal variation in symptoms will help narrow the focus and allow the isolation of possible environmental factors. As previously stated, clarification of terminology can be critical, yet difficult; the word wheeze may have a different meaning to the patient versus the clinician.

The physical examination is vital if there are auscultatory findings. The clinician should try to provoke findings with forced exhalation maneuvers if they are absent. Wheezing can be categorized by phase of respiration (expiratory, inspiratory, or both) and by quality

Table 1-3   Causes of Recurrent or Chronic Wheezing in Children

	Features	Findings on Evaluation
Asthma	Worse with exercise or respiratory infections	Reversible obstruction on pulmonary function tests
	Responds to bronchodilators	Heterophonous wheeze
	Responds to steroids	Positive broncho-provocation
Tracheomalacia	Worse with activity	Homophonous wheeze
	Poor response to bronchodilators	Airway collapse on fluoroscopy
	Poor response to steroids	Collapsible trachea on bronchoscopy
Bronchomalacia	Worse with activity	Homophonous wheeze
	Poor response to bronchodilators	Collapsible bronchus on bronchoscopy
	Poor response to steroids	
Foreign body	Sudden onset in history	Differential breath sounds
		Differential hyperinflation or collapse on radiograph
Heart failure/pulmonary edema	Poor response to albuterol	Hepatomegaly
	Poor growth	Responds to diuresis
Bronchiolitis	Infant—viral infection	Positive viral studies
Vocal cord dysfunction	Poor response to all therapies	Pulmonary function tests: normal or with abnormal inspiratory loop
	Severe distress reported	Laryngoscopy: vocal cord adduction during inspiration
Cystic fibrosis	Poor growth, gastrointestinal symptoms	Positive sweat test
	Recurrent pneumonias	

of tone. A heterophonous wheeze, such as that heard in asthma or bronchiolitis, is diffuse and changes in tone and pitch as the stethoscope is moved across the chest. A homophonous wheeze, such as that heard in tracheomalacia or bronchomalacia, is uniform in tone and pitch throughout the thorax, although it may differ in amplitude regionally.

As in every evaluation, the presence of digital clubbing should raise suspicion that CF or some other chronic suppurative lung disease is present.

Laboratory Evaluation

The laboratory evaluation of the child with recurrent or chronic wheeze is usually limited and guided by suspicions raised on the physical examination. The most commonly ordered test is the sweat test to exclude CF. Additionally, allergy testing may be helpful in some cases. If ABPA is suspected then the appropriate serology can be obtained.

Pulmonary Function Testing

Whenever possible, pulmonary function should be obtained in children who are being evaluated for recurrent or chronic wheezing. The major constraint to obtaining spirometry is often the child's age. Infant pulmonary function testing exists but is still not available to most clinicians. All other children will have their evaluation enhanced by the presence of spirometry and additional lung function tests as indicated.

The demonstration of reversible airflow obstruction on spirometry is an important component in the establishment of a diagnosis of asthma. If there is no obstruction

documented, bronchial provocation may be considered next. Lung volumes are helpful in excluding restrictive disease. The patient with a great deal of distress, loud wheezing and non-obstructed pulmonary function tests on exhalation may have vocal cord dysfunction.

Diagnostic Imaging

The chest radiograph may reveal infiltration, collapse, or differential hyperinflation suggestive of a foreign body. Additional studies include an esophagram with fluoroscopy to look for large airway impingement or collapse, and a CT scan if the plain film suggests interstitial disease or bronchiectasis.

Bronchoscopy

When used judiciously the flexible bronchoscope can yield a wealth of information in the evaluation of chronic wheezing[7]. The larynx can be examined carefully and vocal motion assessed. Adduction of the vocal cords during inspiration in the awake or lightly sedated patient will confirm the diagnosis of vocal cord dysfunction (VCD). The trachea and bronchi can be assessed for malacia. Bronchoalveolar fluid can be sampled for signs of infection or aspiration.

Recurrent Pneumonia

The child with a history of more than one episode of pneumonia may require further evaluation. A single episode of pneumonia is usually not a cause for concern in a child, but more that one episode in a year, or three during childhood, should provoke further evaluation[14].

Table 1-4	Causes of Recurrent Radiographic Infiltration in Children
Asthma	Often right middle lobe
	May be atelectasis that is diagnosed as pneumonia
Cystic fibrosis	Sweat test positive
Primary ciliary dyskinesia	Chronic otitis, chronic purulent rhinitis, sinusitis
Bronchiectasis (idiopathic)	Seen on CT scan
Congenital pulmonary anomalies	
Cystic adenomatoid malformation	
Pulmonary sequestration	
Bronchogenic cyst	
Airway anomalies	Evaluated by bronchoscopy
Tracheomalacia	
Bronchomalacia	
Airway compression syndromes	
Immunodeficiency	Usually other infections as well and poor growth
Aspiration syndromes	Suggested by history, upper gastrointestinal and swallowing studies
Tracheo-esophageal fistula	
Dysphagia	
Gastroesophageal reflux	
Pulmonary hemosiderosis	Associated with anemia
Neuromuscular disease	Weak cough

Some studies have suggested that an underlying illness will be found as frequently as 80% of the time in these patients[15] (Table 1-4).

History and Physical Examination

The history is important to narrow the focus of the evaluation. Careful questioning for signs associated with asthma is important. Extrapulmonary symptoms are important to elicit, as they will suggest underlying diseases such as CF or immunodeficiency.

In addition to a careful respiratory examination, the physical examination should also look for extrapulmonary clues, such as digital clubbing, nasal polyps, or chronic purulent rhinorrhea, suggesting an underlying disease.

Laboratory Evaluation

A sweat test is, as previously noted, the test of choice for ruling out CF and should be considered in every evaluation of a child with recurrent pneumonia, especially when the area of involvement occurs in different locations. An immunodeficiency evaluation may be indicated as well.

Pulmonary Function Testing

Pulmonary function testing is helpful in the diagnosis of asthma, a common cause of recurrent radiographic findings in children. In addition, children with CF and other causes of bronchiectasis often have obstructive defects on their pulmonary function tests.

Diagnostic Imaging

Essential to the initial evaluation is the comparison of all radiographs obtained. Recurrent infiltrates or atelectasis in the same area suggest the possibility of an anatomic malformation, airway anomaly, or retained foreign body. This will guide the evaluation towards scrutiny of the airways, mediastinal structures, and lung parenchyma. Recurrent or persistent right middle lobe infiltration is common in children with asthma. Right upper lobe pneumonia with atelectasis is a frequent presenting finding in infants with CF.

CT scans can be valuable in the diagnosis of bronchiectasis and other parenchymal diseases. Congenital anomalies such as sequestrations or congenital cystic adenomatoid malformations that can become infected repeatedly can also be demonstrated on a CT scan with intravenous contrast. Swallowing studies and an esophagram may be indicated if dysphagia or reflux and aspiration are suspected.

Bronchoscopy

Bronchoscopy can be helpful in the diagnosis of retained foreign body, airway anomalies and in sampling bronchoalveolar fluid for microbiology studies[16]. Mucosal biopsies can also be taken to evaluate the cilia by electron microscopy. The lavage fluid, in addition to being cultured to detect possible infection, should be evaluated for hemosiderin-laden macrophages, as in the case of pulmonary hemosiderosis, and lipid-laden macrophages, which can be seen in large numbers in aspiration syndromes.

Exercise Limitation

A common complaint in the school-aged and adolescent patient is a limitation of activity or exercise. The initial challenge to the clinician is to determine whether

Table 1-5	Common Causes of Exercise Limitation in Children
Poor conditioning	Obesity
	Sedentary lifestyle
Respiratory disease	Exercise-induced asthma
	Restrictive lung disease
	Pulmonary fibrosis
	Chronic obstructive lung diseases
	Cystic fibrosis
	Bronchiectasis
	Emphysema
	Bronchopulmonary dysplasia
Cardiac disease	Cardiomyopathy
	Heart failure
	Pulmonary hypertension
Neuromuscular disease	Skeletal muscle weakness
	Respiratory muscle weakness
Systemic, chronic illness	Sickle cell disease
	Chronic metabolic acidosis
	Diabetes mellitus
Functional or psychogenic	Vocal cord dysfunction
	Anxiety reaction
	Poor effort

the symptoms represent pathology or merely poor conditioning or effort. The purpose of the initial evaluation is to localize the cause of the limitation to pulmonary disease, cardiac disease, musculoskeletal weakness, poor conditioning, or psychogenic causes[17] (Table 1-5).

History and Physical Examination

The history of the complaint will, as always, guide the course of the initial evaluation. Key features to establish in the history include:

- Timing of the problem with regard to exercise: does it happen at the start of exercise or after a period of intense exercise? Exercise-induced asthma usually manifests itself at the beginning of exercise, although it can also occur at the end of an exercise period. It is less likely to occur after a warm-up period, and usually self-resolves after 30–60 minutes[18].
- Past history of exercise. Has the patient been sedentary or athletic in the past? Is this a new problem or a long-standing one? If poor conditioning is a factor, it will often appear after a long hiatus from physical activity.
- Associated respiratory symptoms. The presence of cough, chest tightness or wheeze suggest that the problem is exercised-induced asthma.
- History of loss of consciousness or palpitations. The symptoms suggest a cardiac dysrhythmia and should prompt a cardiology evaluation.

The physical examination when performed at rest is often normal. All physical findings should be pursued, of course, but the patient may need to be stressed and exercised in order to produce both symptoms and physical findings.

Cardiology Evaluation

When suggested by the history and initial evaluation, a cardiac evaluation is indicated. This can include an electrocardiogram (ECG), an echocardiogram, a Holter monitor, and a stress test. The stress ECG can, ideally, be combined with measures of metabolism and pulmonary function in the cardiopulmonary exercise test.

Pulmonary Function Testing

Basic pulmonary function testing including spirometry with a bronchodilator challenge is often sufficient to establish a provisional diagnosis. If the patient demonstrates reversible airflow obstruction, it is likely that asthma is the cause of the exercise complaints and a trial of asthma therapy can be initiated.

If the initial pulmonary function testing is normal and the clinician suspects that the problem is asthma then two possible courses of action can follow: the patient can be given a therapeutic trial of asthma therapy or the evaluation can proceed with cardiopulmonary exercise testing. Cardiopulmonary exercise testing is indicated when the cause of the patient's exercise limitation is undetermined or the role of a known condition, such as asthma, in the patient's symptoms is unclear. Many patients who have asthma that is well controlled will also have poor conditioning and attribute their exercise symptoms to asthma instead of their lack of conditioning. These patients will often inappropriately limit their activity or increase their asthma therapy. Cardiopulmonary exercise testing can help tailor appropriate exercise regimens and programs for asthma control.

The role of exercise and play in a child's development and health should not be under-emphasized. Any limitation of a child or adolescent's activity level should be pursued and addressed. Careful attention to this aspect of the respiratory evaluation will have a large impact on the quality of life of many patients.

Chronic Stridor

Stridor, the harsh, coarse, grating sound with crowing quality, is indicative of extrathoracic airflow obstruction[19]. Stridor can be inspiratory or inspiratory and expiratory. Biphasic stridor implies a fixed airflow obstruction while a sound present only during inspiration is more likely to be from a dynamic extrathoracic lesion. While there are a number of possible causes of chronic stridor in infants and children (Table 1-6 and Chapter 2), a careful history and physical examination will differentiate the children who need aggressive evaluation from those who merely need observation.

Table 1-6 Causes of Chronic Stridor in Infants and Children

Nasal pharyngeal malformations	Often associated with dysmorphism or syndrome
Hypopharyngeal hypotonia	Worse with sleep
Laryngomalacia	Improved with sleep, prone position
Laryngeal web, cysts	Usually biphasic
Vocal cord paralysis	History of weak cry
Subglottic stenosis	Often history of intubation, usually biphasic
Subglottic hemangioma	Can be associated with other hemangiomas
Vascular malformation	Positive barium swallow
Foreign body aspiration	History can be positive
Esophageal foreign body	May have findings on chest radiograph
Gastroesophageal reflux	Can worsen laryngomalacia or cause laryngospasm
Hypocalcemia	Can cause tetany of vocal cords

History and Physical Examination

Specific issues to elucidate in the history include:

- *Timing of onset.* Has this problem been there since birth, such as laryngomalacia or a congenital stenosis, or did it arise after a traumatic event? Is there a history of choking or coughing preceding the development of stridor? Is there a history of behaviors, such as eating nuts or mouthing small objects, that would suggest a risk of possible foreign body aspiration[20,21]?
- *Relationship to feeding.* Both gastroesophageal reflux and primary aspiration can present with stridor[22,23], with timing of the respiratory noise during or soon after a meal.
- *Effect of position and sleep state on stridor.* Laryngomalacia is often better when the infant is in the prone position, is often worse with excitement or activity and is better with sleep. Hypopharyngeal hypotonia is often worse during sleep.
- *Observations of respiratory distress or apnea.* This can be critical in deciding which child should be observed and which needs an aggressive evaluation. Many children are noisy but are comfortable and are growing. Any report of poor growth, cessation of respiration, distress, or cyanosis would, obviously, require an in-depth evaluation.

When performing the physical examination, attention should be paid to the quality of the stridor and its phase. Stridor can be classified as inspiratory or biphasic. Some authors refer to the homophonous wheeze of intrathoracic, central airway obstruction as expiratory stridor. The stridor of laryngomalacia has softer, blowing quality than the harsh stridor of a fixed obstruction such as subglottic stenosis.

Diagnostic Imaging

Initial evaluation can begin with radiographs of the chest and soft tissues of the neck. This is helpful in cases with radio-opaque foreign bodies or retropharyngeal swelling. Some cases of subglottic narrowing will be apparent on the soft tissue neck films.

An esophagram is often the next study when considering the possibility of vascular compression of the airway[24]. In some situations CT scan reconstructions of the airway can provide information not obtained during bronchoscopy.

Bronchoscopy

Direct visualization of the airway is most often the key to diagnosis[25]. Ideally the patient will be comfortable and breathing spontaneously, allowing a dynamic evaluation of the respiratory system in motion. The airway should be evaluated completely from the opening of the nares to the trachea and bronchi. The presence of laryngomalacia does not exclude the possibility of pathology below the vocal cords, mandating a complete evaluation.

Polysomnography

Although not necessary for diagnosis, physiologic recordings of breathing patterns and oxygenation can be helpful in grading the severity of the airflow obstruction and in decision-making regarding intervention. The noisy breather who does not have hypoventilation or oxyhemoglobin desaturation is more likely to be one who can be watched carefully without intervention.

In summary, a wide variety of clinical entities present with a limited number of respiratory complaints. The challenge for the clinician is to determine the underlying pathophysiology and direct the evaluation and therapy appropriately. A careful history and physical examination will direct the clinician to a focused evaluation and the appropriate approach in the majority of cases.

MAJOR POINTS

1. A large number of clinical problems present with a limited variety of signs and symptoms.
2. A careful respiratory history will narrow the differential diagnosis and guide the evaluation.
3. The sweat test is the best test to rule out CF. Non-invasive and inexpensive, it should be considered in any patient with symptoms consistent with CF.
4. Pulmonary function testing can aid in the diagnosis and management of chronic respiratory conditions, providing information not obtainable through history or physical examination.
5. Flexible bronchoscopy, when used judiciously, can yield a great deal of information, especially with suspected central airway lesions.

REFERENCES

1. Taylor WR, Newacheck PW. Impact of childhood asthma on health. Pediatrics 90:657-662, 1992.

2. vonMutius E. The burden of childhood asthma. Arch Dis Child 82(Suppl II):ii2-ii5, 2000.

3. Maier WC, Arrighi HM, Morray B, Llewllyn C, Redding GJ. The impact of asthma and asthma-like illness in Seattle school children. J Clin Epidemiol 51:557-568, 1998.

4. Elphick HE, Sherlock P, Foxall G, Simpson EJ, Shiell NA, Primhak RA, Everard ML. Survey of respiratory sounds in infants. Arch Dis Child 84:35-39, 2001.

5. Harty MP, Kramer SS. Recent advances in pediatric pulmonary imaging. Curr Opin Pediatr 10:227-235, 1998.

6. Callahan CW. Primary tracheomalacia and gastroesophageal reflux in infants with cough. Clin Pediatr 37:725-732, 1998.

7. Schellhase DE, Fawcett DD, Shutze GE, Lensing SY, Tryka AF. Clinical utility of flexible bronchoscopy and bronchoalveolar lavage in young children with recurrent wheezing. J Pediatr 132:321-328, 1998.

8. Irwin RS, Madison JM. The diagnosis and treatment of cough. N Engl J Med 343:1715-1721,2000.

9. Schidlow DV. Cough in children. J Asthma 33:81-87, 1996.

10. Martin RJ, Banks-Schlegel S. Chronobiology of asthma. Am J Respir Crit Care Med 158:1002-1007, 1998.

11. Lokshin B, Lindren S, Weinberger M, Koviach J. Outcome of habit cough in children treated with a brief session of suggestion therapy. Ann Allergy 67:579-582, 1991.

12. Rosenstein BJ. What is a cystic fibrosis diagnosis? Clin Chest Med 19:423-441, 1998.

13. Newman KB, Mason UG, Schmaling KB. Clinical features of vocal cord dysfunction. Am J Respir Crit Care Med 152:1382-1386, 1995.

14. Owayed AF, Campbell DM, Wang EEL. Underlying causes of recurrent pneumonia in children. Arch Pediatr Adolesc Med 154:190-194, 2000.

15. Lodh R, Puranik M, Natch UC, Kabra SK. Recurrent pneumonia in children: clinical profile and underlying causes. Acta Pediatr 91:1170-1173, 2002.

16. Khan FW, Jones JM. Diagnosing bacterial respiratory infection by bronchoalveolar lavage. J Infect Dis 155:862-869, 1987.

17. Wasserman K, Hansen JE, Sue DY, Casaburi R. Pathophysiology of disorders limiting exercise. In: Principles of exercise testing, pp 95-114. Baltimore: Lippincott Williams and Wilkins, 1999.

18. McFadden ER, Gilbert IA. Exercised-induced asthma. N Engl J Med 330:1362-1367, 1994.

19. Friedman EM, Vastola AP, McGill TJ, Healy GB. Chronic pediatric stridor: etiology and outcome. Laryngoscope 100:227-280, 1990.

20. Virgilis D, Weinberger JM, Fisher D, Goldberg S, Picard E, Kerem E. Vocal cord paralysis secondary to impacted foreign bodies in young children. Pediatrics 107:e101, 2001.

21. Chan YL, Chang SS, Kao KL, Liao HC, Liaw SJ, Chiu TF, et al. Button battery ingestion: an analysis of 25 cases. Chang Gung Med J 25:169-174, 2002.

22. Sheikh S, Allen E, Shell R, Hruschak J, Iram D, Castile R, et al. Chronic aspiration without gastroesophageal reflux as a cause of chronic respiratory symptoms in neurologically normal infants. Chest 120:1190-1195, 2001.

23. Bibi H, Khvolis E, Shoseyov D, Ohaly M, Dor DB, London D, et al. The prevalence of gastroesophageal reflux in children with tracheomalacia and laryngomalacia. Chest 119:409-413, 2001.

24. Bove T, Demanet H, Casimir G, Viart P, Goldstein JP, Devaert FE. Tracheobronchial compression of vascular origin. Review of experience in infants and children. J Cardiovasc Surg 42:663-666, 2001.

25. Wood RE. The emerging role of flexible bronchoscopy in pediatrics. Clin Chest Med 22:311-317, 2001.

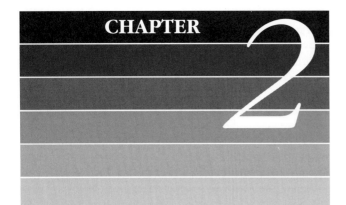

Noisy Breathing in Infants and Children

OSCAR H. MAYER, M.D.

Evaluating a child with noisy breathing can be challenging due to the wide range of potential causes of the noise. Obtaining a comprehensive history and physical examination is a critically important first step in assessing the child with noisy breathing, and often the diagnosis is evident afterwards and before any testing is performed.

Noisy breathing occurs as a result of turbulent airflow; therefore, airflow is necessary to produce noisy breathing. For example, a patient in status asthmaticus whose airflow is poor because of severe airway obstruction may only demonstrate very mild or even no wheezing. Clearly in this situation, a physical examination that includes a chest evaluation that is "clear to auscultation" would be a poor prognostic sign. The converse also holds, where improving aeration in a patient with an obstructive airway disease leads to more audible adventitious breath sounds, suggesting improvement rather than worsening. Therefore it is important to place findings from the physical examination within the proper paradigm.

HISTORY

It is helpful first to determine whether a condition is acute, chronic, or recurrent. If a condition is acute, its symptoms are present for less than 3 weeks. Acute symptoms can accompany a new episode of noisy breathing with no prior occurrence, or they may arise during a chronic or recurrent process as an exacerbation, as with asthma. Chronic conditions are present for over a month with baseline symptoms that never fully resolve or remit without therapy, such as with asthma. Recurrent conditions last through at least one treatment course and/or 2 weeks, but after treatment the symptoms completely resolve without the need for chronic intervention. Recurrent symptoms come back again after initial resolution of symptoms, but the intervening period between exacerbations should be free of symptoms. On occasion chronic or recurrent conditions will come to light during an acute exacerbation of symptoms. Initial onset of symptoms is also important to determine. Those that arise at birth or within the first 3–4 months of life often are associated with congenital lesions. Those that appear later are typically acquired.

After determining whether something is acute, chronic, or recurrent, one should then localize the lesion to the extra- or intrathoracic airway. This can often be accomplished by asking the patient or caregiver whether the noise occurs primarily during inspiration or expiration. Typically, inspiratory sounds are extrathoracic and expiratory sounds are intrathoracic. Noises that occur during both inspiration and exhalation, or biphasic sounds, usually represent a fixed intrathoracic or extrathoracic airway lesion. Less commonly, biphasic sounds can arise from two separate lesions, one residing in the intrathoracic and the other in the extrathoracic airway.

Response to previous therapies can yield important clues to the cause of a disorder. Resolution of symptoms after bronchodilator use, even if relief is partial or short-lived, reflects some component of reversibility of airway obstruction, which is a major component of asthma. Similarly, improvement with inhaled or systemic anti-inflammatory therapy would also be consistent with asthma or another inflammatory disease. The conditions or time of day when the symptoms are worst also provide important diagnostic clues. Asthma symptoms are often triggered by exercise, or environmental conditions such as hot or cold temperature or humid or dry air. Increased activity can also worsen symptoms in patients with dynamic obstruction such as laryngomalacia and those with fixed airway obstruction. Nocturnal symptoms are commonly seen with upper airway obstruction particularly from airway hypotonia or adenotonsillar hypertrophy. Patients with increased upper airway secretions from allergic rhinitis or sinusitis will demonstrate symptoms that are most prominent during the nighttime when they are recumbent.

An environmental history to evaluate home and community conditions is also important. Unrepaired water damage and excessive humidification can favor mold and dust mite growth that can increase symptoms in patients with allergic rhinitis or asthma. Patients who live in rural areas and in river basins can be exposed to a variety of endemic fungi to which they may develop a sensitivity.

Past medical history and previous medical interventions uncover pre-existing conditions and risk factors for acquired problems. Premature birth with the development of bronchopulmonary dysplasia, and prolonged invasive mechanical ventilation, can cause lung parenchymal and airway damage with airway smooth muscle hypertonia and hypersensitivity. Prior airway interventions, such as intubation for any period, can cause upper airway obstruction ranging from acute post-extubation inflammation and edema to fixed changes such as granulation tissue formation and subglottic stenosis. Many prior viral lower airway infections, such as those from respiratory syncytial, influenza, and parainfluenza viruses, can result in episodes of recurrent wheezing.

A thorough review of systems can pick up coincident conditions that may impact the respiratory system including those within the cardiac, gastrointestinal, and immune systems.

In performing a comprehensive history, one can significantly narrow the differential diagnosis before moving on to a physical examination and diagnostic testing.

PHYSICAL EXAMINATION

Observation should be the first and is perhaps the most important component of a physical examination.

How comfortably is the patient breathing? How well is the patient compensating for any difficulty that he or she may have? Is the chest wall motion symmetric? Is there evidence of asynchronous motion between the chest wall and abdomen (thoracoabdominal asynchrony)?

Common signs of respiratory difficulty that are evident on observation include alterations in respiratory rate and size of breath, accessory muscle use, and presence of retractions. The patient will adjust minute ventilation (the product of respiratory rate and tidal volume) in the most energy-efficient way, by increasing either depth of each breath, respiratory rate, or both, to satisfy the metabolic demands for oxygen and to remove the carbon dioxide produced during metabolic processes. However, the principal change in pattern will be an increase in the respiratory rate if the tidal volume is limited by a process that increases airway resistance or lowers respiratory system compliance (makes the lungs stiffer). This is evident in the tachypnea that is commonly seen in respiratory disease.

Accessory muscle use during inspiration (scalene and sternocleidomastoid muscles) and exhalation (rectus abdominus and lateral oblique muscles) is often seen with respiratory disease. Any process that stiffens the lungs (decreases compliance) or increases airway resistance will be reflected by retractions. In such cases, the increased negative intrathoracic pressure needed to produce inward airflow during inspiration causes intercostal, suprasternal, supraclavicular or sternal retractions. In obstructive airways disease there is commonly some component of air trapping after exhalation, which causes lung hyperinflation. This places the diaphragm in a more horizontal orientation at the end of exhalation, and at the onset of inspiration diaphragm contraction will be more in the horizontal plane and will cause inward motion of the inferior border of the ribcage with subcostal retractions (Figures 2-1, 2-2).

In perfectly healthy patients abdominal motion slightly leads chest wall motion through both inspiration and expiration, although this may be difficult to appreciate on physical examination. Asynchronous thoraco-abdominal motion (Figure 2-3) occurs when pulmonary mechanics are abnormal. Thoracoabdominal asynchrony is especially prominent in infants and young children whose chest walls are not stiff enough to withstand the increased intrathoracic pressure generated to overcome obstruction or low lung compliance.

If there are differential mechanics between the two sides of the chest, such as a unilateral increase in airways resistance resulting from a retained bronchial foreign body, there will be more airflow to the unaffected lung compared with the lung with the obstruction. This will cause asymmetric chest wall excursion between the two sides of the chest, with greater excursion occurring on

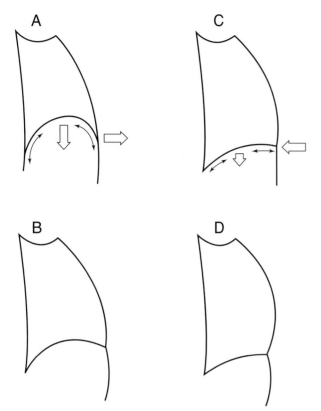

Figure 2-1 Subcostal retractions. In the normal situation (**A**) the diaphragm will contract inward and downward causing outward ribcage motion (**B**). In a patient with hyperinflation (**C**), the diaphragm will be in a more horizontal position and will cause primarily diaphragm contraction in the transverse plane and inward motion of the inferior rib cage (**D**).

the unaffected side. Similarly, unilateral diaphragm paralysis or paresis will cause diminished excursion of the affected side as well as a paradoxical *upward* inspiratory movement of the affected hemi-diaphragm, and the umbilicus

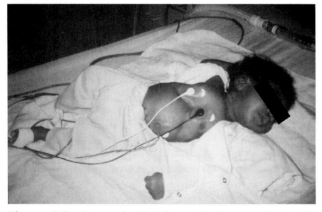

Figure 2-2 Six-month-old infant with laryngomalacia with marked lower costal and sternal retractions.

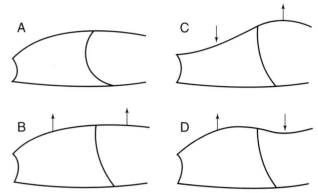

Figure 2-3 Thoracoabdominal motion. From end expiration (**A**) normal inspiration occurs with outward motion of the thorax and abdomen (**B**). Thoracoabdominal asynchrony can occur with outward abdominal and inward thoracic motion (**C**) or with outward thoracic and inward abdominal motion (**D**).

will swing to the affected side during inspiration as abdominal contents are drawn into the thoracic cavity ("belly dancer's" sign).

On auscultation one can evaluate other aspects of breathing not evident on inspection. During what phase of respiration is the sound heard? What are the characteristics of the sound? Is it continuous (wheeze if during expiration or stridor if during inspiration) or is it discontinuous (crackles)? Is the sound the loudest in one place or is it heard equally throughout the chest? At what point during a phase of respiration is the sound heard?

The phase of respiration in which the sound is heard is important since inspiratory sounds typically represent an extrathoracic obstruction, while expiratory sounds indicate an intrathoracic obstruction. Sounds heard in both inspiration and expiration are either from two separate lesions or the result of a "fixed" lesion, with the obstruction present during both inspiration and expiration. Sounds heard during only one phase of breathing are "dynamic" lesions, as the degree of obstruction varies with the respiratory phase.

Dynamic lesions exist because they accentuate airway caliber changes that normally occur as a result of phasic pressure differences across the airway wall. During inspiration intrapleural pressure becomes more negative, creating a pressure gradient from atmospheric pressure at the mouth to subatmospheric pressure in the alveoli. This gradient causes air to flow into the lungs. Pressure gradients, however, also develop across the airway wall especially during forceful inspiration (Figure 2-4). Thus, the *transmural* pressure in the extrathoracic airway (intraluminal pressure minus atmospheric pressure) favors narrowing of the airway during inspiration while the transmural pressure of the intrathoracic airway (intraluminal pressure minus pleural pressure) favors its

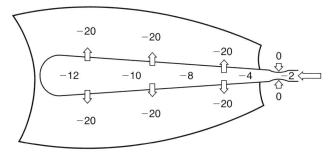

Figure 2-4 Forceful inspiration. Diaphragm contraction produces negative intrathoracic pressures and creates a gradient of decreasing pressure from the airway opening to the alveoli. The negative pressure in the airway creates pressure gradients favoring dilation of the intrathoracic airway and narrowing of the extrathoracic airway in regions that may be prone to collapse. The difference between the intrathoracic pressure (−20 cm H_2O) and the intra-alveolar pressure (−12 cm H_2O) is due to the inward elastic recoil of the lung. The numbers in the image reflect hypothetical pressures in cm H_2O.

expansion (Figure 2-4). Outward traction on the intraparenchymal airways by the expanding alveoli contributes to inspiratory dilation of the intrathoracic airways.

During exhalation, intrathoracic pressure becomes positive and creates a pressure gradient from high pressure in the alveoli to atmospheric pressure at the mouth (Figure 2-5). The positive pressure gradient results from the sum pressure of the elastic recoil of the lungs and chest wall, and any expiratory muscle activity. Airway resistance causes the airway pressure gradually to decrease as air travels proximally from smaller to larger airways. A point within the thorax exists where the intraluminal airway pressure will be equal to the intrathoracic pressure (Figure 2-5). This point is called the *equal pressure*

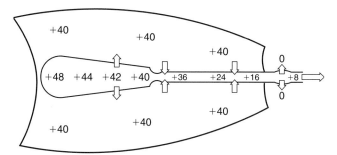

Figure 2-5 Forceful exhalation. The passive recoil of the lung is augmented by expiratory muscle activity to produce positive intrathoracic pressure and a gradient of decreasing pressures from alveoli to the airway opening. The gradient across the intrathoracic airway will maintain airway patency until the pressure in the airway is equal to the intrathoracic pressure, the equal pressure point (EPP). From the EPP to the thoracic inlet there is a gradient favoring airway narrowing. In contrast, in the extrathoracic airway the pressure gradient will favor dilation of the airway. The numbers in the image reflect hypothetical pressures in cm H_2O.

point and from that point to the thoracic inlet there is a gradient favoring airway collapse. Under normal circumstances, however, the equal pressure point occurs in the larger, more central airways that contain large amounts of cartilage in their walls to resist collapse. If, however, the central airway is collapsible (malacic) or if the equal pressure point moves to more distal airways because of increased peripheral airway resistance and a more rapid dissipation of pressure during exhalation, significant intrathoracic airway collapse can occur. In the extrathoracic airway, however, the intraluminal pressure will be greater than the surrounding atmospheric pressure favoring dilation of the extrathoracic airway (Figure 2-5).

After establishing the phase of respiration in which the sound is heard, the character of the sound is important to distinguish. Is the sound continuous or is it intermittent through inspiration, expiration, or both? Narrowing of the airway lumen causes turbulent airflow and produces continuous sounds. Such sounds can be heard in both phases of respiration, with "wheezing" used to describe an expiratory sound and "stridor" an inspiratory sound. The sound produced by wheezing is usually musical and that of stridor a "crowing" harsh noise; however, the stridor produced by laryngomalacia can be vibratory. Both wheezes and stridor can be of variable and multiple pitches. Intermittent sounds or crackles typically represent intraluminal obstruction of smaller airways either from narrowing or debris in the lumen, such as mucus or fluid. Crackles can occur during both inspiration and expiration. Crackles represent movement of air through an air–liquid interface, such as with air movement through airways secretions and equalization of airway pressure[1]. They also can be produced by sudden opening of closed airways[1]. Some have described crackles as sounding like crumpling Cellophane or separating Velcro.

The symmetry of the sound through the respiratory tract is important. Sounds that differ regionally in terms of pitch and composition of tones when heard throughout the respiratory tract (*heterophonous* sounds) are from multiple peripheral sites of obstruction. However, sounds that are symmetric in quality, or *homophonous*, represent a more central process.

The timing of the sounds within each phase of the respiratory cycle can help determine the severity of the obstruction. Since the caliber of the intrathoracic airways progressively narrows during exhalation, turbulent airflow and adventitious sounds will be produced earlier in airways with severe narrowing, whatever the cause. The earlier in the respiratory cycle the onset of the wheezing is, the more severe the airway obstruction. Abnormal breath sounds in milder obstructive airway disease will occur later in exhalation due to the greater amount of airway narrowing needed to cause turbulent airflow.

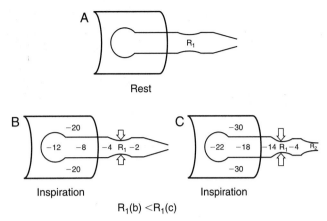

Figure 2-6 Extrathoracic airway resistances in series. With upper airway obstruction (R_1) (**A**) the negative intraluminal pressure during forceful inspiration will favor further airway narrowing in that airway segment (**B**). With added extrathoracic airway obstruction (R_2) closer to the airway opening, the pressure needed to overcome the higher airway resistance will increase (become more negative) and the initial site of obstruction (R_1) will narrow further (**C**).

Two separate areas of obstruction, such as the small airways in asthma and central airway in tracheomalacia, enhance each other's degree of obstruction by creating greater net resistance than either lesion would alone. This can occur both with extrathoracic obstruction during inspiration (Figure 2-6) and with intrathoracic obstruction during exhalation (Figure 2-7). When both peripheral and central airway obstruction coexist, the higher pleural pressure needed to overcome peripheral resistance

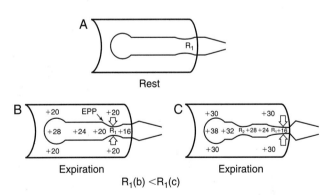

Figure 2-7 Intrathoracic airway resistances in series. With an intrathoracic obstruction (R_1) (**A**) the positive intrathoracic pressure during forceful expiration will favor airway narrowing past the equal pressure point (EPP) (**B**). With increased intrathoracic airway obstruction (R_2), the pressure needed to overcome the higher airway resistance will increase (more positive) and the initial site of obstruction (R_1) will narrow further (**C**). The extrathoracic airway will not narrow, and there will be a pressure gradient favoring dilation.

during exhalation will also compress the central airway and so will worsen the central airway obstruction. This is particularly likely in patients with collapsible airways, such as those with tracheomalacia and bronchomalacia. The converse also holds in that treating one site of airway obstruction can help to reduce the severity of another.

Since all respiratory noises require adequate flow to produce them, the most accurate physical examination of the respiratory system will occur when flow is increased to the point of flow limitation. Ideally, to reach this point the patient should inhale deeply to approximate total lung capacity and exhale forcefully to residual volume. To the extent the patient is unable to do this, the accuracy of the physical examination of the respiratory system decreases. With proper coaching during a physical examination, most cooperative children above the toddler age group can inhale and exhale deeply and forcefully. In infants and younger children, expiratory flow can be augmented by manually compressing the chest at the onset of expiration.

DIFFERENTIAL DIAGNOSIS OF NOISY BREATHING

With the information gleaned from a comprehensive history and physical examination, one can then create a more focused location-based differential diagnosis (Tables 2-1, 2-2). Causes of noisy breathing at each site can also be separated into acute and chronic problems.

Extrathoracic

The extrathoracic airway can be divided from proximal to distal into the nose, nasopharynx, oropharynx, hypopharynx, larynx/glottis, subglottis, and extrathoracic trachea (Table 2-1).

Nose/Nasopharynx
Acute

Nasal inflammation with turbinate edema and increased secretions can cause noisy breathing, especially in infants who are obligate nose-breathers. Because these conditions can cycle between different levels of severity within a short period of time, the character and loudness of the sounds produced can be quite variable. Retained foreign bodies are another important source of nasal obstruction and always need to be considered, especially in children of toddler age.

Chronic

Static conditions that cause noisy breathing result from fixed obstruction to nasal airflow. These include adenoidal enlargement (Figure 2-8) and less commonly nasal polyps. Uncommon congenital conditions include

Table 2-1   Differential Diagnosis of Noisy Breathing from Extrathoracic Airway Obstruction

Location	Acute	Chronic
Nose/nasopharynx	Nasal inflammation 　Nasal turbinate edema 　Nasal secretions 　　Allergic rhinitis 　　Upper respiratory infection 　　Maxillary sinusitis Foreign bodies	Adenoidal enlargement Nasal polyps 　Asthma 　Allergic rhinitis 　Cystic fibrosis Choanal stenosis Midface/maxillary hypoplasia 　Treacher-Collins syndrome 　Apert syndrome
Oropharynx	Infectious 　Peritonsillar abscess 　Retropharyngeal abscess 　Palatine tonsillitis	Adenotonsillar hypertrophy Macroglossia 　Down syndrome 　Beckwith–Wiedemann syndrome Micrognathia 　Pierre–Robin syndrome 　Moebius syndrome
Hypopharynx	Acute nose/nasopharyngeal/ 　oropharyngeal obstruction	Hypopharyngeal hypotonia 　Down syndrome 　Static encephalopathy 　Moebius syndrome 　Trigeminal, glossopharyngeal or vagus nerve injury Glossoptosis Obesity Neoplasia 　Lymphoma 　Lymphangioma
Larynx	Epiglottitis 　*Haemophilus influenzae* type B 　*Haemophilus* species (other than type B) 　*Staphylococcus aureus* 　Group A *Streptococcus* Laryngotracheobronchitis (croup) 　Parainfluenza types 1 and 3 　Respiratory syncytial virus 　Influenza Foreign bodies 　Large 　Irregular edges Laryngospasm	Laryngomalacia 　Primary/congenital 　Secondary 　　Chronic inflammation Papillomatosis 　Human papillomavirus Hemangioma Laryngeal granuloma Congenital 　Laryngeal cyst 　Laryngeal web 　Laryngocele
Glottis	Vocal cord paralysis/paresis 　Endotracheal intubation 　Trauma Vocal cord overuse injury 　Inflammation 　Polyps	Vocal cord dysfunction (paradoxic motion) Brainstem compression 　Structural 　　Chiari malformation 　　Dandy–Walker cyst 　Mass effect 　　Neoplasia 　　Hemorrhage Nerve injury 　Vagus nerve 　Glossopharyngeal nerve 　Recurrent laryngeal nerve Papillomatosis
Subglottis/ 　extrathoracic trachea	Endotracheal/tracheal intubation Laryngotracheobronchitis (croup) 　Parainfluenza types 1 and 3 　Respiratory syncytial virus 　Influenza Bacterial tracheitis 　*Staphylococcus aureus* 　*Haemophilus influenzae* 　*Streptococcus* species	Subglottic stenosis 　Congenital 　　Complete tracheal rings 　　Maldevelopment 　Secondary 　　Endotracheal/tracheal intubation Papillomatosis

Table 2-2   Differential Diagnosis of Noisy Breathing from Intrathoracic Airway Obstruction

Location	Acute	Chronic
Trachea		
Extrinsic compression	Uncommon	Cardiovascular
		Vascular anomaly (Table 2-3)
		Pulmonary artery
		Main/lobar bronchus compression (except right upper lobe bronchus)
		Cardiac
		Left main bronchus compression
		Recurrent laryngeal nerve compression (cardiovocal syndrome)
		Anterior mediastinal masses
		Lymphoma
		Thymoma
		Teratoma
		Middle mediastinum
		Lymphoma
		Lymphadenopathy
		Tuberculosis
		Mycoses
		Histoplasmosis
		Blastomycosis
		Coccidiomycosis
		Sarcoidosis
		Posterior mediastinum
		Neurogenic tumors
		Esophageal duplication cyst
		Bronchogenic cyst
Intramural lesions	Uncommon	Tracheomalacia
		Primary (congenital)
		Cartilaginous defect: Campbell–Williams syndrome
		Muscular defect: Mounier–Kuhn syndrome
		s/p Tracheoesophageal fistula repair
		External compression
		Secondary (acquired)
		Chronic inflammation
		Recurrent infections
		Gastroesophageal reflux
		Recurrent aspiration
		Prolonged positive pressure ventilation
		External compression
		Complete tracheal cartilaginous rings
Intraluminal lesions	Foreign bodies	Tracheal granulomas
	Irregularly shaped	Artificial airway and "deep suctioning"
	Elongated	Hemangioma
	Bacterial tracheitis	Papillomatosis
	Chronic tracheostomy	Tracheal web
	tube usage	
	Pseudomonas	
	aeruginosa	
	Serratia marcescens	
Bronchi/bronchioles	Viral bronchiolitis	Asthma
	Respiratory syncytial virus	Bronchopulmonary dysplasia
	Parainfluenza virus	Bronchomalacia
	Influenza virus	Prolonged positive pressure ventilation
	Adenovirus	Chronic inflammation
	Pneumonia	Carcinoid
	Viral	Adenoma
	Mycoplasma	
	Foreign body	
	Small size	
	Tumor	

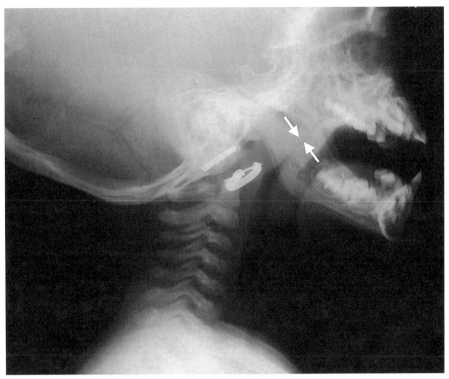

Figure 2-8   Lateral neck radiograph demonstrating adenoidal enlargement with nasopharyngeal narrowing (between arrows) in a 5-year-old child with snoring at night. (Courtesy of Raanan Arens, M.D.)

choanal stenosis and midface hypoplasia, and nasal tumors. Nasal obstruction, however, may not be as clinically evident as infants get older and are no longer obligate nose-breathers. Older infants and children with severe obstruction bypass the nasal obstruction by breathing through their mouths chronically.

Oropharynx

Acute

Peritonsillar and retropharyngeal abscesses, and palatine tonsillitis are important to consider in patients presenting with a "muffled" voice, often described as a "hot-potato" voice. Children with tonsillitis may have fever and can be ill-appearing, but their constitutional illness usually is not as severe as that seen in children with a peritonsillar or retropharyngeal abscess.

Chronic

Persistent sounds of similar character with a muffled or hyponasal voice can be heard in children with severe adenotonsillar hypertrophy. Sonorous or stridulous sounds during inspiration occur when the oral airway is narrowed from macroglossia or micrognathia.

When nasal and oral obstructions are both present, they represent a set of resistances in series. As such, the pressure drop across the nasal obstruction can accentuate the magnitude of the oral obstruction. Conversely, "unloading the nasal airway" by use of decongestants can also markedly improve symptoms resulting from oropharyngeal obstruction.

Nasopharyngeal and oropharyngeal lesions often will present first during sleep, as the tone in the support musculature of the pharynx decreases and the airway collapses during inspiration, producing snoring and perhaps obstructive apnea.

Hypopharynx

Acute

Hypopharyngeal obstruction can occur in patients with an otherwise normal hypopharynx when another obstruction occurs more proximally in the airway, as described above. This process causes a dynamic hypopharyngeal obstruction and produces a rattling stridulous sound or snore. Anything that causes acute nasopharyngeal or oropharyngeal obstruction can also cause noisy breathing from the hypopharynx due to airway collapse during inspiration.

Chronic

Hypopharyngeal obstruction can be prominent in patients with intrinsic airway hypotonia. Hypopharyngeal hypotonia is a common source of obstruction in patients with a variety of central nervous system abnormalities, including both cerebral and cranial nerve abnormalities. This hypotonia causes hypopharyngeal narrowing or collapse under a normal pressure gradient across the hypopharyngeal wall. Hypopharyngeal narrowing is accentuated during periods of decreased airway muscle tone, such as when the child is sedated or asleep. Furthermore, tone falls to its nadir during the stage of rapid eye movement (REM) sleep. As a result, children with hypopharyngeal hypotonia can develop sleep hypoventilation or obstructive apnea requiring therapy with non-invasive positive pressure, a nasopharyngeal airway, or tracheostomy tube. Hypopharyngeal collapse is also made worse with the addition of a second site of extrathoracic obstruction, such as nasal obstruction (Figure 2-6).

The obstruction caused by glossoptosis, or prolapse of the tongue into the posterior pharynx, is often hard to distinguish from the obstruction from hypopharyngeal hypotonia. Turning the head to the side to move the tongue out of the posterior pharynx can relieve the glossal obstruction present in glossoptosis. A jaw thrust can decrease the sound from hypopharyngeal hypotonia by putting tension on the pharynx and can also elevate the tongue. Extrinsic compression of the hypopharynx from the increased soft tissue mass in obesity or neoplasia can cause a fixed obstruction that will produce biphasic sounds.

Larynx
Acute

Epiglottitis (Figure 2-9) occurs most commonly from an infection with *Haemophilus influenzae* type B, and less commonly due to other *Haemophilus* species,

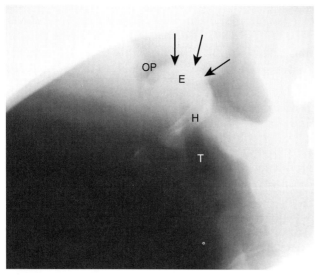

Figure 2-9 Lateral neck radiograph showing epiglottitis (E) with a positive "thumb sign" (below arrows) in a 2-year-old child. OP, oropharynx; H, hyoid bone; T, trachea. (Courtesy of Ian Jacobs, M.D.)

Staphylococcus aureus and group A *Streptococcus*. With modern immunization practice for *Haemophilus influenzae* type B, epiglottitis is now very rare. The typical presentation includes a "muffled" voice, significant respiratory distress or respiratory failure, and generalized toxicity. Epiglottitis is a true medical emergency and airway stabilization is of utmost importance. Maintaining the child in a calm state can minimize his or her work of breathing and prevent or delay the onset of respiratory failure. Epiglottitis may be confused with other disorders such as retropharyngeal abscess or laryngotracheobronchitis (croup), but patients with epiglottitis are more toxic-appearing, they have dysphagia and drool, and they often sit in a tripod posture to help maintain an open airway.

Croup is caused by a viral infection (parainfluenza types 1 and 3, respiratory syncytial virus (RSV), or influenza) that leads to laryngeal and subglottic edema and marked subglottic narrowing. It usually responds promptly to adrenergic agonists and steroids, which help to reduce the airway swelling. Croup may be discriminated from epiglottitis by the presence of a viral prodrome.

Where foreign bodies lodge in the airway depends on their size and contour. Large and round or asymmetric foreign bodies typically lodge in the larynx or posterior pharynx (Figure 2-10) because they have difficulty passing into the esophagus or between the vocal cords and into the trachea. As with any fixed obstruction, the patient with a laryngeal foreign body will produce biphasic sounds with a more prominent inspiratory component. Smaller foreign bodies may pass between the vocal cords and lodge in the distal trachea at the carina (Figure 2-11) or in the bronchi (Figure 2-12). Broad and flat foreign bodies often lodge in the esophagus (Figure 2-13) and can cause biphasic sounds if they are large enough to cause compression or displacement of the adjacent airway.

Acute obstruction with stridor can occur from laryngospasm during anaphylaxis. In such situations, life-threatening respiratory distress requiring immediate airway stabilization can also occur.

Chronic

Laryngomalacia is the most common cause of stridor in infants[2]. It presents as a rattling, vibratory or high-pitched inspiratory sound that is made louder with exertion and crying but is usually absent during restful breathing and sleep. The noise results from prolapse of laryngeal tissues into the airway during inspiration. Laryngomalacia is proposed to occur because of delayed maturation of the laryngeal cartilage and muscle[3], which results in inadequate support of the laryngeal tissue. It can also occur in children with gastroesophageal reflux (GER), perhaps due to upper airway hypotonia[2] similar to the lower esophageal sphincter hypotonia that often occurs in GER.

Laryngoscopic findings include arytenoid cartilage prolapse during inspiration and curling of the epiglottis

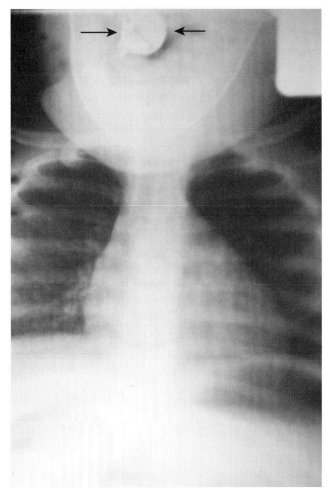

Figure 2-10 Anteroposterior neck radiograph which shows aspiration of a small bell (between arrows) that lodged in the posterior pharynx. (Courtesy of Ian Jacobs, M.D.)

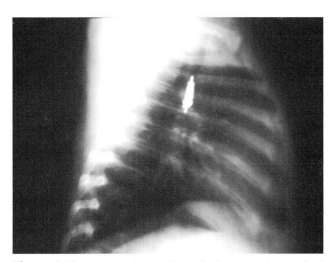

Figure 2-11 Lateral chest radiograph demonstrating tracheal aspiration of a small whistle, with positioning just above the carina. (Courtesy of Ian Jacobs, M.D.)

into an omega shape. Primary (congenital) laryngomalacia usually presents shortly after birth and can worsen during the first year of life as a result of the infant's increased activity and respiratory effort. It often completely resolves by the end of the first or second year of life. In rare cases when obstruction is severe enough to cause respiratory embarrassment or growth failure, surgery ("epiglottoplasty") is performed to remove redundant tissue that prolapses into the airway. Even less commonly, a tracheostomy may be required to bypass the laryngeal obstruction. Secondary laryngomalacia can occur after any chronic inflammatory process that causes weakening of the laryngeal tissue, such as recurrent aspiration or prolonged endotracheal intubation.

Papillomas from human papillomavirus infection can cause biphasic sounds when the masses grow on the vocal cords and narrow the glottic opening. If the papillomas grow large enough the airway narrowing can cause respiratory difficulty. Although papillomas can occur throughout the respiratory tract, they are most common in the upper airway due to exposure during the birthing process.

Airway hemangiomas can displace the laryngeal structures causing inspiratory and expiratory sounds, depending on the size of the lesion. They should be considered in any child who also has a cutaneous hemangioma and stridor or wheezing.

Patients receiving aggressive oropharyngeal "deep" suctioning may develop granulomas where the suction catheter contacts the airway, such as at the epiglottis or glottis. These lesions would cause biphasic sounds of variable severity, depending on the size of the lesion.

Other less common causes of laryngeal obstruction include congenital lesions such as laryngeal cyst, laryngeal web and laryngocele. Each would likely cause a biphasic noise because of its fixed nature and position in the airway.

Glottis
Acute

The vocal cords can cause airway obstruction and a variety of different abnormal sounds. Changes in voice will be most clear in children who are beyond infancy and have clear vocal characteristics. Infants with dysfunctional vocal cords can present with a weak or absent cry. Paralyzed vocal cords can be fully abducted, in which case no abnormal sounds will be present during quiet inspiration, or in a paramedian or median (fully adducted) position. The closer to the median position the vocal cords are fixed, the more audible the sounds will be during relaxed breathing, due to the narrowing of the airway opening. During forced inspiration (e.g., crying), even fully abducted paralyzed cords can cause stridor as the structures are passively drawn together when transmural pressure across the glottis becomes negative. Vocal cord paresis can occur after traumatic or prolonged endotracheal intubation due to direct injury to or inflammation of the vocal cords.

Vocal cord inflammation from overuse during repetitive periods of loud speaking, often referred to as "laryngitis," can occur in vocalizing children of any age. Multiple episodes can cause polyps to develop on the vocal cords. Therapy involves vocal cord rest.

Chronic

Vocal cord dysfunction (paradoxical vocal cord motion) is disordered movement of the vocal cords that causes vocal cord adduction, as opposed to abduction, during inspiration. The chief complaint is often mistaken as "wheezing." Patients often are unsuccessfully treated with bronchodilator and anti-inflammatory therapy and diagnosed as having "refractory" asthma. With a good history, however, the findings can usually be isolated to inspiration and to the suprasternal region (glottis). The symptoms can sometimes be reproduced during a physical examination or lung function testing with hyperventilation or exertion. Spirometry when symptoms are present discloses limitation of inspiratory peak flow, but expiratory flows are normal, indicating a variable extrathoracic obstruction. The noise is usually accompanied by acute respiratory distress during periods of physical or emotional stress and reverses with calming techniques and speech therapy.

Brainstem compression from an intracranial mass or structural abnormality or injury at the locus of the vagus

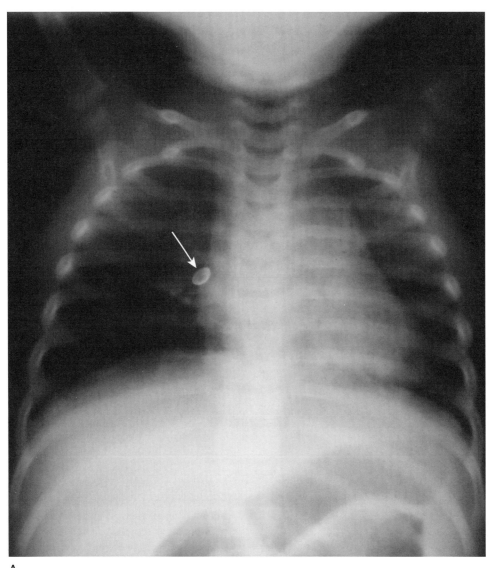

A

Figure 2-12 Anteroposterior (**A**) and lateral (**B**) chest radiographs demonstrating right main bronchus aspiration of a button. (Courtesy of Ian Jacobs, M.D.)   (*Continued*)

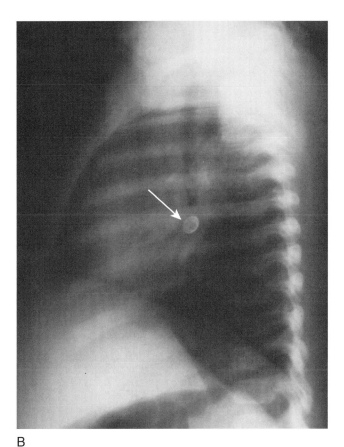

B

Figure 2-12 Cont'd

and glossopharyngeal nerves can cause vocal cord paresis or paralysis with stridor and/or a hoarse voice. Excessive neck traction during delivery or previous cardiac or mediastinal surgery can cause recurrent laryngeal nerve injury and ipsilateral vocal cord paresis or paralysis. Compression of the left recurrent laryngeal nerve from enlarged pulmonary arteries will cause left vocal cord paralysis (cardiovocal syndrome, see below).

Since the infection from human papillomavirus can occur at any point along the airway, glottic involvement is certainly possible.

Subglottis/Extrathoracic Trachea
Acute
Endotracheal intubation in and of itself can cause mucosal inflammation. If the inflammation is moderate to severe, acute respiratory distress and stridor can be quite prominent after extubation. This occurs most significantly at the level of the cricoid cartilage because the mucosal inflammation and edema can only extend into the center of the tracheal lumen. Direct trauma to the glottis itself and to the mucosa above and below the cricoid cartilage can further contribute to the acute airway obstruction post-extubation. Resolution can occur

spontaneously over time if the patient's ventilatory status remains adequate. Steroids or adrenergic agents can be used to reduce the mucosal swelling, accelerate resolution, and avoid the need for reintubation. Placing a patient on a helium and oxygen mixture can stabilize or improve respiratory status until the inflammation in the airway resolves.

Croup and bacterial tracheitis cause narrowing in the immediate subglottic area, and may additionally involve the distal trachea and bronchi. Patients with either condition can present with stridor and/or a "barking" cough. Because of the airway narrowing patients often present with markedly increased work of breathing to overcome the increased airways resistance. Infectious croup, or laryngotracheobronchitis, is caused by a viral infection (parainfluenza types 1 and 3, RSV, or influenza) leading to glottic and subglottic edema and marked laryngeal and subglottic narrowing, with further inflammation possible throughout much of the respiratory tract. It usually responds to adrenergic agonists and steroids, which reduce the swelling. Some patients have positive, calming responses when exposed to cool and/or humidified air; however, there is no conclusive evidence of the efficacy of either intervention.

Patients with bacterial tracheitis (usually resulting from infection with *Staphylococcus aureus*) begin their illness with similar respiratory complaints to those who present with croup. Several days into the illness, however, they develop new onset of fever and respiratory distress returns. These children are usually more ill-appearing with high fever and do not respond to standard croup therapy since the infection is of bacterial origin, and is one with a large purulent component. Treatment requires aggressive airway clearance, antibiotic therapy and airway stabilization, preferably in a controlled intensive care or operating room environment.

Any lesion that causes glottic narrowing produces increased airways resistance and alteration in the flow patterns in the affected airways. Airflow is laminar in peripheral airways, with the flow vectors all directed in the same direction. In this setting, airways resistance is directly proportional to the flow rate. However, in the trachea, where flow is turbulent, with vectors in multiple directions, the resistance is related to the *square* of the flow rate. Therefore, when a child with croup or bacterial tracheitis tries to inhale rapidly because of anxiety or air hunger, resistance across the narrowed airway segment will rise dramatically and make it more difficult to inspire effectively. Thus, anxiety worsens the child's dyspnea and leads to further clinical deterioration. For this reason, patient calming is an important intervention that can often cause substantial relief of symptoms.

Since the infection from human papillomavirus can occur at any point along the airway, tracheal involvement is certainly possible.

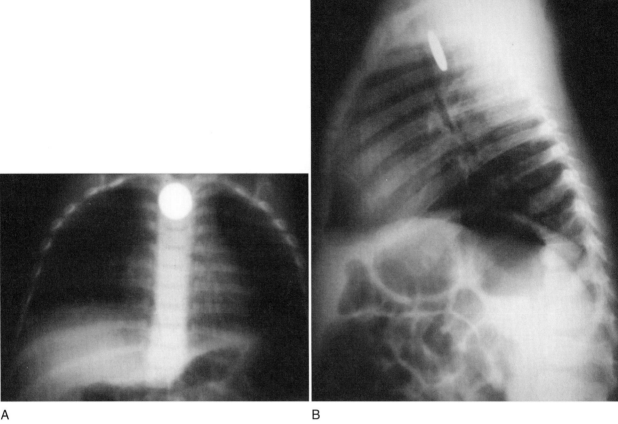

A   B

Figure 2-13   Anteroposterior (**A**) and lateral (**B**) chest radiographs of a patient who swallowed a coin and the typical positioning in the esophagus. Note that on the anteroposterior radiograph, the face of a coin lodged in the esophagus will be seen, whereas a coin lodged in the airway will appear "on edge" as it lines up between the vocal cords. (Courtesy of Ian Jacobs, M.D.)

Chronic

As a fixed airway obstruction, subglottic stenosis (Figure 2-14) causes both inspiratory and expiratory sounds. It can present as a congenital lesion with abnormal tracheal formation such as with complete tracheal rings in the extrathoracic trachea. Though it is often associated with other congenital midline lesions and vascular abnormalities, it can occur as an isolated lesion. It can also occur after endotracheal tube placement of any duration with the sequence of mucosal irritation, inflammation, fibrosis, scarring, and narrowing. Tracheostomy placement is a temporizing solution to bypass the obstruction and to allow the patient to breathe with less effort. With growth subglottic stenosis can resolve spontaneously or become easier to repair. When subglottic stenosis does not improve spontaneously, several surgical approaches are available to increase airway diameter. An anterior cricoid split, in which the anterior subglottic trachea is incised down to the mucosa, can enlarge the airway enough in cases of mild subglottic stenosis to

avoid tracheostomy placement. When the stenosis is more severe, a staged laryngotracheoplasty may be needed to increase tracheal diameter to a caliber that allows adequate ventilation. During laryngotracheoplasty, the stenotic section of trachea is incised longitudinally and cartilage grafts, the number depending on the severity, are inserted to increase the tracheal diameter.

Intrathoracic Airway

The intrathoracic airway starts as the trachea passes through the thoracic inlet and includes a portion of the trachea, the main bronchi, smaller bronchi, and bronchioles (Table 2-2). Dynamic and fixed obstruction of intrathoracic airways produces expiratory sounds; however, fixed obstruction can also produce inspiratory sounds. The amplitude of the sound can increase through exhalation due to the progressive narrowing of the intrathoracic airway through exhalation (Figure 2-5). The opposite circumstance occurs during inspiration (Figure 2-4).

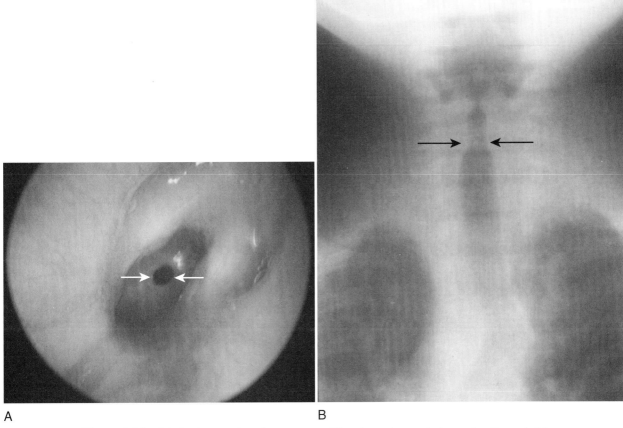

A   B

Figure 2-14 Subglottic stenosis on laryngoscopy (**A**) and on anteroposterior neck radiograph (**B**) with the functional airway outlined by arrows. (Courtesy of Howard Panitch, M.D. (**A**) and Ian Jacobs, M.D. (**B**).)

Obstruction can result from extrinsic compression, an intrinsic defect of the airway wall, or an intraluminal process.

Trachea: Extrinsic Compression

Acute

The common lesions causing tracheal compression are chronic processes. Extrinsic compression may be completely asymptomatic when the patient is well but becomes clinically apparent during acute respiratory difficulty, as in a respiratory tract infection. Clues to an extrinsic compression include atypical physical findings on examination of a patient with "acute" wheezing, such as homophonous biphasic wheezing, that would be associated more with a fixed central airway obstruction than with an acute respiratory infection.

Chronic

The numerous etiologies of tracheal compression can be divided into two broad groups: cardiovascular and non-pulsatile fixed compression. Because these lesions are fixed obstructions, they cause biphasic sounds with more prominent expiratory sounds. Computed tomography (CT) and magnetic resonance imaging (MRI) are useful in differentiating the different mediastinal masses.

Vascular rings (Table 2-3) cause a fixed but pulsatile compression of the trachea in a variety of ways depending on the specific defect. Children with these abnormalities present with chronic coughing and can have prominent inspiratory sounds and homophonous wheezing.

Table 2-3 Common Types of Vascular Abnormalities[4]	
Lesion	**Relative Prevalence**
Double aortic arch	43%
Anomalous innominate artery	15%
Right aortic arch with aberrant subclavian artery	11%
Right aortic arch with left ligamentum arteriosum	11%
Pulmonary artery sling	7%
Other	13%

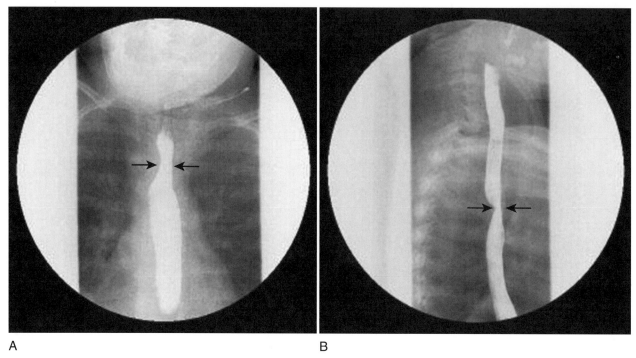

A   B

Figure 2-15   A barium esophagram demonstrating a double aortic arch, represented as bilateral compression in anteroposterior (**A**) and posterior compression in lateral (**B**) images of the esophagus.

In many series, the most common vascular anomaly is the double aortic arch, followed by anomalous innominate artery, right aortic arch with an aberrant left subclavian artery or with mirror image branching and a left ligamentum arteriosum, and pulmonary artery sling[4]. Although tracheal and bronchial compression may not be visible on the chest radiograph, vascular anomalies often are associated with a right descending aorta, which should be visible directly along the spine or indirectly as a medially displaced trachea. A barium esophagram is helpful in confirming compression (Figure 2-15), but a CT scan or MRI study (Figure 2-16) is often necessary to identify the course of the vessels with more certainty. Some institutions are able to perform three-dimensional reconstruction of the trachea and vascular structures allowing for even easier understanding of the anatomy (Figure 2-17).

Because complete vascular rings with vessels or remnants of vessels encircle both the trachea and esophagus, the biphasic sounds are made worse with swallowing as the bolus in the esophagus compresses the trachea within the ring. Dysphagia will also be a prominent symptom if the ring is tight, as solids and even liquids may not pass easily beyond the esophageal obstruction. A double aortic arch encircles the trachea and esophagus proximal to the carina (Figures 2-15, 2-16) and may cause marked bilateral tracheal compression (Figure 2-18), compromising airway clearance from the

distal airways. In such situations recurrent pneumonia or atelectasis can occur. Between 70% and 90% of double aortic arches have a right descending aorta[4].

The anomalous innominate artery leaves the aortic arch more distally than normal and courses across the anterior portion of the proximal trachea slightly to the right of midline (Figure 2-19). It can present with a homophonous wheeze or stridor, especially in infants. About 95% of patients with congenital heart disease have

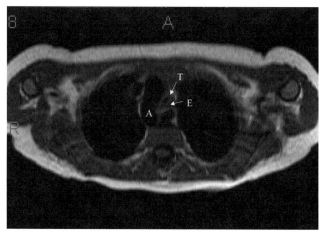

Figure 2-16   Right aortic arch (A) passing posterior to and compressing the esophagus (E) and trachea (T) on a CT scan of the chest.

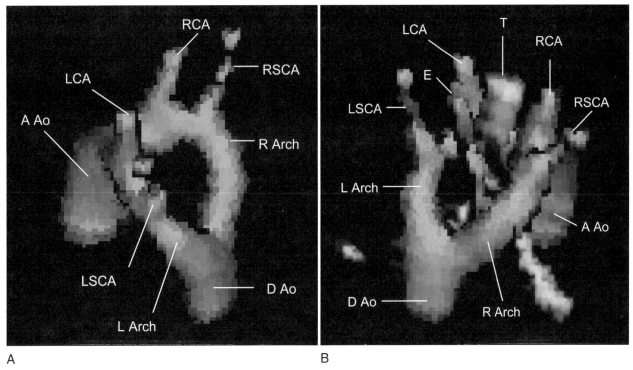

A   B

Figure 2-17   3-Dimensional MRI reconstruction of the double aortic arch (**A**) and with the trachea and esophagus (**B**). D Ao, double aortic arch; A Ao, ascending aorta; R Arch, right aortic arch; L Arch, left aortic arch; LSCA, left subclavian artery; RSCA, right subclavian artery; RCA, right carotid artery; LCA, left carotid artery; T, trachea; E, esophagus. (Courtesy of Paul Weinberg, M.D., reprinted with permission from: Aortic arch abnormalities, in Moss and Adams' Heart disease in infants, children and adolescents, 6th edition, p 724, 2001.)

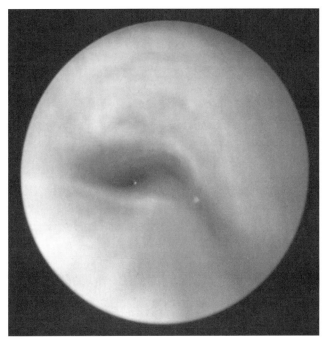

Figure 2-18   Bronchoscopic view of double aortic arch with anterior tracheal compression. The compression causes widening and invagination of the posterior muscular wall of the trachea.

an anomalous innominate artery[4]. Although it is involved in 20% of cases of infant stridor and apnea[4], it usually is not severe enough to require surgical correction. Additionally, an anomalous innominate artery can be asymptomatic and discovered incidentally on bronchoscopy when the airway compression is mild. One can diagnose an anomalous innominate artery by using the bronchoscope to press on the right anterolateral pulsatile compression while palpating the right brachial or radial pulse[5]. The pulse will diminish or be absent if the compression is from an anomalous innominate artery[5].

The right aortic arch with mirror image branching causes left anterolateral compression, opposite to that of anomalous innominate artery. A left descending aorta with a ligamentum arteriosum forms a complete vascular ring and may present similarly to a double aortic arch. In approximately 90% of cases this type of ring is associated with congenital heart disease[4].

In patients with a right aortic arch with an aberrant left subclavian artery, the left common carotid artery arises from the ascending aorta and also causes left anterolateral compression just above the carina. As with the right aortic arch with mirror image branching, a complete vascular ring is formed if there is a left descending

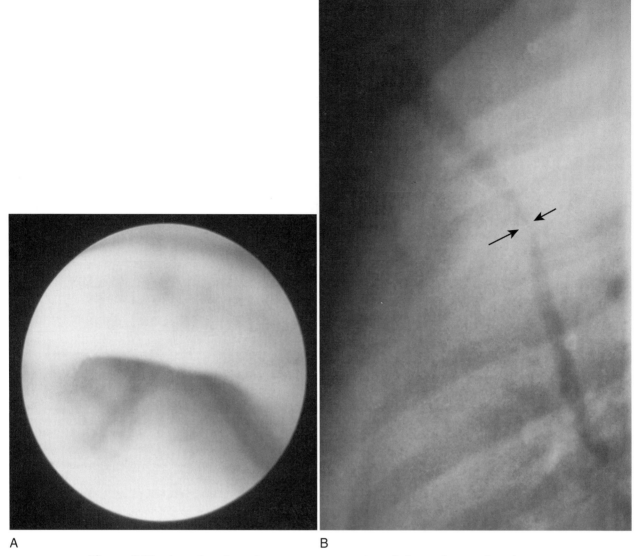

A   B

Figure 2-19 Anomalous innominate artery compression of the trachea on bronchoscopy (**A**) and on airway fluoroscopy (**B**). (Courtesy of Howard Panitch, M.D. (**A**) and Ian Jacobs, M.D. (**B**).)

aorta and a ligamentum arteriosum. Because the compression caused is not as severe as that of a double aortic arch, the right aortic arch with an aberrant left subclavian or with mirror image branching causes less severe respiratory symptoms.

A pulmonary sling results when the left pulmonary artery arises not from the main pulmonary artery but from the right pulmonary artery instead. The left pulmonary artery then courses between the trachea and esophagus just above the carina and can cause right bronchial compression and a focal homophonous wheeze. This lesion is associated with complete tracheal rings (Figure 2-20), congenital heart disease, as well as other congenital anomalies, and an overall poor prognosis. It is unique in that it causes an *anterior* compression

of the esophagus and a posterior compression of the trachea. This can clearly be seen on the lateral view of a barium esophagram.

Large vessel dilation can cause compression of the distal trachea or central bronchi and a fixed obstruction. The right and left main pulmonary arteries may be dilated in situations of increased flow, owing to a left to right shunt from atrioseptal or ventriculoseptal defects, a patent ductus arteriosus, or partially corrected congenital heart disease, such as a Stage 2 Norwood repair of left ventricular hypoplasia. Main pulmonary artery dilation can also occur with peripheral branch pulmonic stenosis and conditions causing pulmonary hypertension.

The left main bronchus can be compressed by the left pulmonary artery, and the bronchus intermedius can be

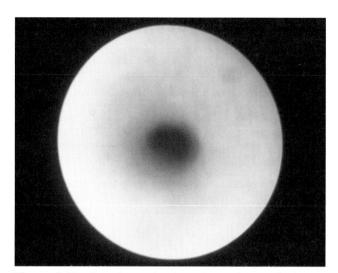

Figure 2-20 Bronchoscopic view of complete tracheal rings demonstrating the absence of the posterior membrane and the typical "U"-shaped tracheal cartilage.

compressed by the right pulmonary artery. The right upper lobe bronchus is free from potential compression, because it is positioned superior to the corresponding pulmonary artery branch. Vascular compression can cause a focal, homophonous wheeze, but if the obstruction is large enough there may also be a history of recurrent lobar pneumonia or chronic atelectasis depending on the location and extent of the compression. Pressure on the recurrent laryngeal nerve from an enlarged pulmonary artery medially displacing the aorta can result in left vocal cord paralysis with stridor (the cardiovocal syndrome).

Left ventricular dysfunction and left atrial enlargement can also cause left main bronchus compression from below and clinical findings similar to those seen with left pulmonary artery compression.

Anterior mediastinal masses, such as lymphoma, teratoma, and thymic masses, cause a fixed compression on the proximal trachea and are difficult to differentiate from vascular abnormalities without CT or MRI scans or direct visualization during bronchoscopy.

In the middle mediastinum, the high concentration of peritracheal and perihilar lymph nodes can be the focus of lymphoma or lymphadenopathy from any of a number of sources and may cause a central wheeze and an inspiratory sound. Other non-infectious etiologies of lymphadenopathy, such as sarcoidosis, can cause clinically significant wheeze or stridor if the lymph node is large enough to displace the trachea or compress the main bronchus.

Although lymphadenopathy secondary to infection more commonly presents without remarkable auscultatory findings, airway compression can occur. Tuberculosis should be at the top of an infectious disease differential

of lymphadenopathy, but other chronic respiratory infections need to be considered as well. Chief among these in North America are regional endemic mycotic disease from histoplasmosis in the Midwestern states, blastomycosis in the South Central and Midwestern states, and coccidiomycosis in the Southwestern states.

Posterior mediastinal masses such as neurogenic tumors and esophageal duplication or bronchogenic cysts are rarely symptomatic unless they are large. Symptomatic lesions usually lie adjacent to the main carina and cause main bronchus compression.

Masses that cause extrinsic compression tend to present as chronic processes. They may remain subclinical with slow growth, but can present as acute processes with a lower respiratory tract infection. One should strongly consider chest radiography in any child with a homophonous wheeze of unclear etiology, since the physical finding points to a problem involving the central airways.

Trachea: Intramural Airway Lesions
Acute
Intramural lesions tend to be chronic, but acute respiratory changes with infection or other abnormality may cause acute worsening of tracheal intramural lesions.
Chronic
Tracheomalacia is the most common intrinsic airway lesion and causes a dynamic airway obstruction. It worsens with the increased transmural pressure gradients created during forceful exhalation, such as with crying, agitation, or increased exertion. The patient with intrathoracic tracheomalacia produces a homophonous wheeze that is made louder with vigorous exhalation. It can be made worse after bronchodilator therapy due to tracheal smooth muscle relaxation, which makes the trachea more compliant or collapsible.

In contrast, increasing tracheal smooth muscle tone reduces compliance, making the trachea more rigid and less collapsible. Tracheal smooth muscle stimulation causes the posterior tracheal muscle to shorten and pulls the posterior edges of the tracheal cartilage together. Both of these make the trachea less compliant and therefore less susceptible to collapse when exposed to high transmural pressure gradients[6].

The rigidity of the trachea is primarily due to the presence of the C-shaped tracheal cartilage "rings." The posterior tracheal muscle then spans the two posterior ends of the tracheal cartilage (Figure 2-21). Tracheomalacia can result from a muscular or cartilaginous defect, or in association with tracheoesophageal fistula or tracheal compression from vessels or other lesions. It can also arise from a defect in the tracheal smooth muscle or its mechanics.

Secondary or acquired tracheomalacia can also occur after chronic inflammation, from infections or chemical damage as occurs in gastroesophageal reflux with chronic aspiration, or after exposure to positive pressure

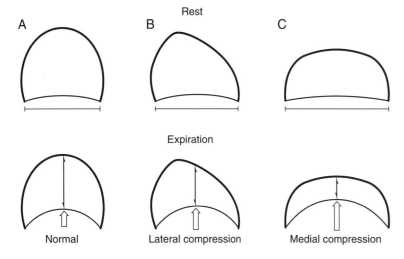

Rest

A B C

Expiration

Normal   Lateral compression   Medial compression

Figure 2-21 The effect of distortion and tracheal collapsibility. In the normal trachea (**A**) during expiration, there is a small amount of invagination of the posterior membrane (trachealis muscle) and narrowing of the tracheal lumen. Both lateral (**B**) and medial (**C**) compression of the trachea cause distortion of the trachea and broadening of the posterior membrane at rest and more narrowing of the tracheal lumen during expiration.

in a premature infant. All of these can weaken the cartilage and disrupt the interaction between cartilage and airway smooth muscle.

In some instances, the collapsibility of the trachea can be related to an increased muscle-to-cartilage ratio within the tracheal wall[5]. An altered ratio can result from abnormal formation (i.e., in tracheoesophageal fistula), or from external distortion. For example, anterior pressure on the cartilage can cause the posterior tips to separate and the posterior tracheal membrane to broaden (Figure 2-18). The smooth muscle would then comprise a greater percentage of the tracheal circumference. Tracheal compliance would increase and the tracheal membrane would be prone to invaginate with changes in transmural pressure (Figure 2-21).

Following removal of a mass compressing the trachea, tracheomalacia can persist and the distortion of the trachea (increased muscle-to-cartilage ratio) or abnormal cartilage mechanics may not resolve completely. Prior repair to the tracheal wall, such as after a tracheoesophageal fistula repair or tracheostomy decannulation, may leave a residual distortion or defect in the continuity of the tracheal wall. Furthermore, a tracheoesophageal fistula in and of itself can be associated with an increased muscle-to-cartilage ratio and increased tracheal compliance (Figure 2-21) even after repair. Both situations can adversely affect tracheal mechanics and cause tracheomalacia.

Complete tracheal rings, where the posterior membrane is absent (Figure 2-20), cause airway narrowing and a fixed obstruction with sounds that are most prominent during exhalation. Although uncommon, they are often associated with pulmonary arterial sling, tracheal bronchus, and pulmonary hypoplasia.

The intramural airway lesions also are primarily chronic processes; however, as with any airway obstruction, they are made worse during respiratory tract infections. As is often the case with tracheomalacia, the homophonous wheeze may only be evident with increased effort of breathing associated with agitation or with more distal small airway obstruction. In these situations, the increased positive intrathoracic pressure generated during exhalation will favor compression of a malacic trachea.

Intraluminal Airway Lesions
Acute
Intraluminal lesions typically cause biphasic sounds or just expiratory sounds if less severe.

Tracheal foreign bodies (Figure 2-11) are uncommon, for anything that is able to pass between the vocal cords is substantially smaller than the tracheal caliber and therefore should lodge in a bronchus. Irregularly shaped or elongated foreign bodies, however, can rotate and become trapped in the trachea with the long axis in the anteroposterior plane (Figure 2-22). As with the rest of the intrathoracic airway, tracheal foreign bodies usually present with biphasic noisy breath sounds, more prominent during expiration because of dynamic narrowing of the intrathoracic airway.

Tracheitis or tracheal aspiration of upper airway secretions is associated with a low-pitched wheeze with a rattling character. Bacterial colonization of the trachea is common in patients with an artificial airway, and on occasion the colonizing bacteria can increase in number and cause a tracheitis. The tracheitis that occurs in patients with an artificial airway is typically caused by Gram-negative organisms (e.g., *Pseudomonas aeruginosa*, *Serratia marcescens*) and is not associated with the same generalized toxicity as that caused by *Staphylococcus aureus* in otherwise healthy children without an artificial airway. This tracheitis is associated with an increase in tracheal secretions and clinically

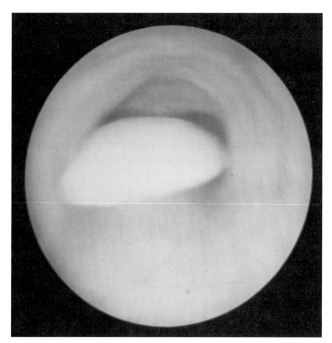

Figure 2-22   Pumpkin seed lodged in the distal trachea at the carina.

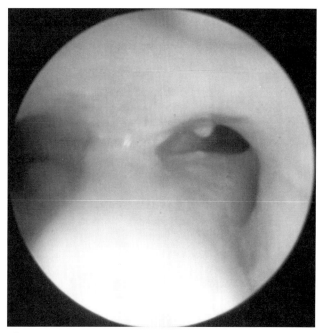

Figure 2-23   Granuloma formation in the right main bronchus of a child with a tracheostomy tube and a history of "deep" tracheal suctioning past the end of the tracheostomy tube.

significant respiratory difficulty, often with coarse wheezing and crackles and oxyhemoglobin desaturation.

Chronic

Tracheal granulomas are a common cause of intraluminal obstruction, especially in patients who are subjected to "deep" tracheal suctioning. The American Thoracic Society recommends endotracheal or tracheal tube suctioning only to within 0.5 cm of the distal tip of the airway[7]. The points of trauma from deep suctioning usually occur at the carina or in the right main bronchus (Figure 2-23), and can cause unilateral crackles, biphasic wheezes, and decreased breath sounds if large enough. Segmental and/or lobar atelectasis can also occur due to complete obstruction or to compromised airway clearance distal to the obstruction.

Patients with an artificial airway for any duration may develop granulation tissue at the tip of the tube from the artificial airway rubbing against and/or injuring the native airway wall. These lesions lie within the midtrachea at the typical positioning of the distal tip of the artificial airway. Auscultatory findings are typically symmetric, homophonous and biphasic.

Patients with cutaneous hemangiomas and wheezing or stridor should be evaluated closely for airway hemangiomas using direct visualization by flexible or rigid bronchoscopy. These lesions typically present in infancy and many lesions regress spontaneously within the first decade; however, symptomatic lesions may require therapy with local steroid injection, laser cautery, Interferon-α, or other sclerosing agents to bring about regression.

Other less common intraluminal tracheal lesions include tracheal papillomas from infection with human papillomavirus, and tracheal web, which is most likely to present in the newborn period.

Bronchi/Bronchioles

Acute

Viral bronchiolitis can present similarly to an asthma exacerbation with coarse heterophonous wheezing, but typically there is a viral prodrome, prominent airway secretions and occasionally crackles. Viral culture or direct fluorescent antigen testing for common respiratory viruses, will help distinguish viral bronchiolitis from asthma. Therapy for bronchiolitis is supportive with supplemental oxygen, fluid therapy and bronchodilator and anti-inflammatory drug administration, based on patient response. There are antiviral medications that can be used to limit the course of the disease caused by many viral pathogens. Their efficacy is limited unless they are initiated early in the course of disease, and they are not widely used. There is a use for antiviral agents in subjects who have not had leukocyte engraftment after bone marrow transplant, since untreated viral bronchiolitis is almost universally fatal in such patients.

Bacterial pneumonia usually presents as focal crackles that can be localized to a particular lobe or lung region. Viral or *Mycoplasma* pneumonia, however, often presents with diffuse crackles. The inflammatory reaction that accompanies pneumonia can also cause airway wall edema and wheezing. This occurs most commonly in patients with viral pneumonia. It is also important to assess for lung regions in which there is decreased aeration or tubular breath sounds, representing enhanced transmission of larger airway sounds through a consolidated region of lung.

Small foreign bodies that enter the trachea commonly become wedged in one of the main bronchi as opposed to the trachea due to the typically small caliber of foreign bodies that are able to pass between the vocal cords. In adults, foreign bodies more commonly wedge in the right main bronchus because of the less acute angle it takes from the trachea compared with the left main bronchus. This predilection does not exist in children, however, and foreign bodies are found in either main bronchus with near equal frequency.

Chronic

Asthma is a disease of small airway obstruction, and though by definition it is a chronic disease it frequently presents with acute exacerbations and is a common cause of acute onset of wheezing. The hallmark of asthma is recurrent heterophonous wheezing, airway obstruction that is reversible with bronchodilator therapy, and airway smooth muscle reactivity to an exposure. Airway obstruction in asthma results from bronchoconstriction, inflammation, mucosal edema and increased mucus secretion. Usually, the wheeze in asthmatic children responds to bronchodilator therapy. With a more severe exacerbation, mucosal edema and mucus in the airways can cause wheezing that is less sensitive to bronchodilator therapy. Mucus in the airway can cause a deeper-sounding wheeze as well as crackles due to opening and closing of airways throughout the respiratory cycle. Both wheezing and crackles can occur during an asthma exacerbation.

Bronchopulmonary dysplasia (BPD) is associated with obstructive lung disease primarily in small airways. BPD is seen most commonly in prematurely born infants who required mechanical ventilation in the newborn period, a prolonged (>1 month) use of supplemental oxygen, and who have persistent clinical findings at 1 month of age. BPD has clinical similarities to asthma, including increased airway smooth muscle tone, frequently demonstrable bronchodilator responsiveness, and heterophonous wheezes during acute illnesses.

If there is a diffuse process, such as bronchomalacia or airway wall edema from inflammation or cardiac failure, homophonous wheezing will be present, reflecting central airway disease.

Prolonged positive pressure ventilation in premature infants can lead to bronchomalacia, and produce a homophonous wheeze. Secondary bronchomalacia from chronic regional inflammation or infection will be asymmetrically distributed and cause a localized homophonous wheeze. As with tracheomalacia, the wheezing may worsen after a bronchodilator treatment since the airway will be more compliant due to smooth muscle relaxation.

EVALUATION

Diagnosing a respiratory abnormality can often be accomplished with a comprehensive history and physical examination; however, additional studies can be helpful in confirming or further elucidating the diagnosis. Chest radiography should be performed in any patient with asymmetric wheezing or air entry, especially if it is new in onset. Children with a symmetric respiratory examination, especially those with a history of asthma, do not necessarily need a chest radiograph. Because the chest radiograph only shows one plane at a time, it may miss more complicated, inhomogeneous or early disease with small areas of airway damage, such as bronchiectasis, or parenchymal damage, such as areas of subsegmental atelectasis or necrosis. With chest radiography one can evaluate the aortic arch and descending aorta, cardiothymic silhouette, mass lesions, pulmonary parenchyma and vessels, and large airway position.

Chest CT gives a clearer view of the pulmonary parenchyma and delineates healthy from diseased lung, as well as mediastinal structures and other relationships to more central and larger airways. When airway compression is a concern, a CT scan can often document airway narrowing and clearly show the compressing mass. Three-dimensional reconstruction from a CT scan or MR image can more clearly show the mediastinal structures and their interrelationships, especially with vascular abnormalities.

Using a barium esophagram one can evaluate for vascular compression, gastroesophageal reflux, and for abdominal anatomic abnormalities. A barium esophagram will demonstrate compression of the esophagus resulting from a fixed intrathoracic lesion such as a vascular abnormality or a mediastinal lesion.

A video feeding study can be used to evaluate swallowing function for a variety of textures and consistencies of food and liquids. This is helpful in assessing for aspiration, which can cause recurrent lower airway infection and inflammation. Non-contrast fluoroscopy can also give a dynamic view of the central airway to evaluate for dynamic tracheal narrowing non-invasively. When direct endoscopic airway visualization is not available, airway fluoroscopy is a reasonable alternative evaluation. It must be remembered, however, that even normal infants can narrow their airways by up to 50% during crying, so that fluoroscopic presence of luminal narrowing may not be abnormal.

Direct visualization of the central airway using flexible bronchoscopy under conscious sedation is the best method to show how the airways behave under dynamic conditions. Bronchoalveolar lavage using flexible bronchoscopy provides a sample for culture of pathogens, especially in subjects with persistent lower respiratory symptoms. In addition, a lavage specimen can be sent for cytologic analysis to evaluate for lipid-laden macrophages, an indication of recurrent aspiration, or for a preponderance of neutrophils or lymphocytes that also would indicate chronic inflammation.

Rigid bronchoscopy is performed under general anesthesia and is less helpful for evaluating dynamic conditions. For foreign body removal, however, rigid bronchoscopy is preferable since the working channel is larger to allow for better instrumentation. Furthermore, rigid bronchoscopy is the safer technique for foreign body removal, since it is performed under general anesthesia and with a controlled airway in place through which assisted ventilation can be delivered.

Pulmonary function testing is helpful in evaluating respiratory system mechanics, determining the severity of a particular disorder, and assessing its change with interventions, such as after bronchodilator, anti-inflammatory or antibiotic administration. Spirometry is a useful initial test in which patients perform a maximal expiratory flow volume maneuver (MEFVM). It provides an accurate measure of airway mechanics and obstructive airway disease. Obstructive lung disease is usually present when the ratio of forced expiratory volume in the first second of exhalation (FEV_1) to forced vital capacity (FVC) is below 0.8. Post-bronchodilator increase in FEV_1 of greater than 12%[7] is a statistically significant change and defines reversible airway obstruction, one of the central components of asthma.

Examination of the flow–volume curve can also help to diagnose airway obstruction (Figure 2-24). Normal spirometry (Figure 2-24a) involves a rapid increase in expiratory flow at the onset of expiration with a gradual deceleration of flow through lower lung volumes, and a more gradual increase in flow during inspiration with peak inspiratory flow occurring midway through inspiration. A rapid decrease in expiratory flow after reaching peak flow (i.e., a "concave" expiratory flow–volume curve) is diagnostic of peripheral intrathoracic airway obstruction (Figure 2-24b). A truncated inspiratory flow?volume curve, where peak flow is low and the loop is flattened, together with a normal expiratory flow-volume curve (Figure 2-24c), is diagnostic for a variable *extrathoracic* obstruction such as a supraglottic tumor or vocal cord paralysis. Conversely, expiratory peak flow limitation, with a normal inspiratory flow–volume loop (Figure 2-24e), represents a variable *intrathoracic* obstruction seen in large intrathoracic airway obstruction. Truncation of both inspiratory and expiratory peak flows (Figure 2-24d) is diagnostic of a fixed obstruction.

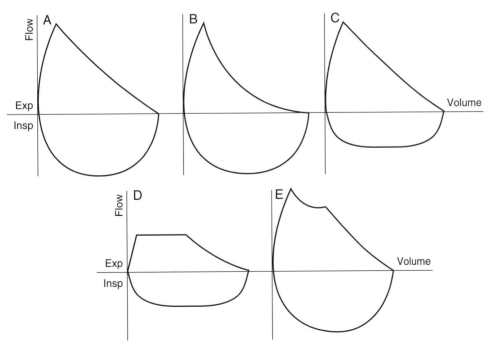

Figure 2-24   Representative flow–volume curves: (**A**) normal; (**B**) intrathoracic peripheral airway obstruction; (**C**) variable extrathoracic airway obstruction; (**D**) fixed airway obstruction; and (**E**) variable intrathoracic central airway obstruction. By convention, flow is represented on the y-axis, volume on the x-axis, expiration as an upward deflection, and inspiration as a downward deflection.

These measurements require that the subject willfully be able to take a deep breath and exhale with maximal effort for at least 6 seconds[8], a task which is challenging for children 6 years and under and impossible for toddlers and infants to perform. Some have suggested adapting the American Thoracic Society end-of-test criterion for spirometry to the capabilities of younger children, but no criteria have been widely accepted yet. Similar measurements can be performed in sedated infants and toddlers using equipment that applies positive pressure to the mouth to inflate the lungs and external compression to the chest and abdomen to forcefully deflate the lungs.

There are a variety of laboratory studies that can be helpful in evaluating for an infectious cause of noisy breathing. In the fall, winter and early spring months, viral antigen testing from the nasal secretions for common viral pathogens (RSV, parainfluenza types 1 and 3, influenza, and adenovirus) is diagnostic in the acute setting. Bacterial serologic antigen testing for *Mycoplasma* and pertussis is widely offered. PPD (purified protein derivative) intradermal testing for tuberculosis exposure and or infection is an important part of the evaluation for any chronic pneumonia, parenchymal lesion, or lymphadenopathy. A positive test must be reported to local public health authorities for infection control and to insure that definitive therapy is initiated.

If recurrent wheezing is associated with chronic or recurrent sinusitis and otitis, a deficiency of the immune system may be present. Quantitation of the amount of circulating immunoglobulins (IgG, IgA, IgM and IgE) will detect deficiencies or excess of antibodies. IgM and IgG deficiencies can cause clinically significant disease. Although IgA deficiency is the most common immunodeficiency, it rarely causes clinically significant disease. An elevated IgE level is associated with many chronic inflammatory conditions such as asthma and atopy.

Sweat chloride testing is a definitive test for cystic fibrosis and is an important part of any evaluation of chronic respiratory disease that is not responsive to standard asthma therapy or is associated with failure to thrive, chronic diarrhea, or nasal polyps. Testing should be performed in a recognized Cystic Fibrosis Center, which is experienced in the proper collection and analytic techniques in order to maximize the accuracy of the results.

CONCLUSION

Evaluating the child with noisy breathing can be daunting because of the wide range of presentations and etiologies. With a focused history and physical examination, however, one should be able to diagnose most of the causes of noisy breathing and reserve testing for confirmation or refinement of the diagnosis.

MAJOR POINTS

1. Although there is a wide range of etiologies of noisy breathing, with a focused history and physical examination one should be able to come very close to a diagnosis before any evaluations are performed.
2. By history, be able to discriminate between acute, recurrent and chronic processes and whether the noisy breathing is occurring during inspiration, expiration or both.
3. On the physical examination determine whether the noisy breathing is focused in the intrathoracic or extrathoracic airway and describe the quality of the sound (wheeze, stridor, or crackle).
4. Use evaluations judiciously to augment, but not to replace, a thorough history and physical examination.
5. Reassess the diagnosis after initial therapy to evaluate the response.

REFERENCES

1. Pasterkamp H. The history and physical examination. In Chernick V, Boat T, editors: Kendig's disorders of the respiratory tract in children, 6th edition, pp 85-106. Philadelphia: WB Saunders, 1998.
2. Mancuso R. Stridor in neonates. In Isaacson G, editor: Pediatric otolaryngology. Pediatr Clin North Am 43:1339-1356, 1996.
3. Clements B. Congenital malformations of the lungs and upper airway. In Taussig L, editor: Pediatric respiratory medicine, pp 1106-1136. Philadelphia: Mosby, 1999.
4. Valletta E, Pregarz M, Bergamo-Andreis I, et al. Tracheoesophageal compression due to congenital vascular anomalies (vascular rings). Pediatr Pulmonol 24:93-105, 1996.
5. Holinger L, Green C, Benjamin B, et al. Tracheobronchial tree. In Holinger L, Lusk R, Green C, editors: Pediatric laryngology and bronchoesophagology, pp 187-213. Philadelphia: Lippincott-Raven, 1997.
6. Panitch H, Keklikian E, Motley R, et al. Effect of altering smooth muscle tone on maximal expiratory flows in patients with tracheomalacia. Pediatr Pulmonol 9:170-176, 1990.
7. American Thoracic Society. Care of the child with a chronic tracheostomy. Am J Respir Crit Care Med 161:297-308, 2000.
8. American Thoracic Society. Standardization of spirometry. Am J Respir Crit Care Med 152:1107-1136, 1994.

OTHER RESOURCES

Chernick V, Boat TF, editors. Kendig's disorders of the respiratory tract in children, 6th edition. Philadelphia: W. Saunders, 1998.

Taussig LM, LI Landau, editors. Pediatric respiratory medicine. Philadelphia: Mosby, 1999.

West JB. Respiratory physiology: the essentials, 6th edition. Philadelphia: Lippincott, Williams and Wilkins, 2000.

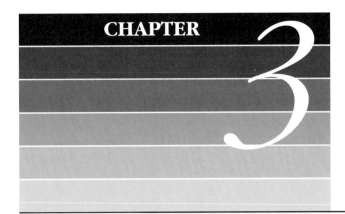

CHAPTER 3

Congenital Malformations of the Lung and the Airway

ANITA BHANDARI, M.D.

Congenital malformations of the lung are a part of the differential diagnosis of lung masses on the chest radiograph in infants and children. Though usually easy to spot, differentiation is a challenge, and may require further diagnostic testing.

EMBRYOLOGY OF THE LUNG

Lung development is divided into five stages (Table 3-1). The lung develops as a ventral outpouching of the primitive gut during the embryonic period (stage 1, day 26 to day 52). Over this period, the trachea appears first as a respiratory diverticulum. Its distal end then divides into the two main bronchi. These elongate into the mesenchyme and form lobar and segmental bronchi. In the pseudoglandular stage (stage 2, day 52 to 16 weeks) the branching continues such that by the end of this stage all the airway branching is complete and conducting airways and the terminal bronchioles are now completely formed. During this phase of development the arteries can be seen running alongside the conducting airways. Within the canalicular stage (stage 3, 16 weeks to 28 weeks) the respiratory bronchioles are formed. These end in primitive alveoli called saccules and the lung develops a vascular bed that is closely associated with respiratory bronchioles. During the saccular stage (stage 4, 28 weeks to 36 weeks), as the pulmonary capillaries proliferate, close contact between the airspaces and the blood supply develops. As the epithelium thins, a rich vascular supply is established and gas exchange is now possible. During this stage elastic fibers that are responsible for further alveolar growth are also laid down. In the alveolar stage (stage 5, 36 weeks to 2–8 years), secondary septation of the alveoli occurs thereby increasing the surface area for gas exchange. A knowledge of the stages of airway and pulmonary parenchymal development is crucial to an understanding why various congenital malformations occur, and how they may affect lung physiology.

LARYNGEAL AND TRACHEAL MALFORMATIONS

Laryngeal Atresia and Web

Laryngeal atresia occurs as a result of failure of recanalization of the larynx around 10 weeks of gestation and is usually associated with a normally developed lung, although lung hyperplasia has been reported (Figure 3-1). Cases of partial recanalization may result in the formation of a laryngeal web.

The typical clinical presentation of laryngeal atresia is development of respiratory distress immediately after birth. The baby has a voiceless cry and no air movement despite respiratory effort. If pulmonary hyperplasia is present, hydrops fetalis can occur, presumably from compression of the vena cava by the massively enlarged

Table 3-1 The Stages of Lung Development

	Stages of Lung Development	Gestational Age
Stage 1	Embryonic stage	Day 26 to day 52
Stage 2	Pseudoglandular stage	Day 52 to 16 weeks
Stage 3	Canalicular stage	16 weeks to 28 weeks
Stage 4	Saccular stage	28 weeks to 36 weeks
Stage 5	Alveolar stage	36 weeks to postnatal

lungs (see the section on CHAOS, below). The infant with a laryngeal web will present with stridor and a weak cry at birth. If the web causes severe airway narrowing, respiratory distress can develop soon after birth.

Diagnosis

Diagnosis is confirmed by direct visualization in both cases. In the case of laryngeal atresia, a fibrous membrane occluding the lumen of the larynx can be visualized on laryngoscopy. Laryngeal webs are most commonly located in the glottic area and are anteriorly placed, revealing a concave posterior glottic opening on laryngoscopy.

Treatment

Treatment of laryngeal atresia involves tracheostomy placement to bypass the obstruction. Once the child is large enough (usually 10 kg or more), laryngeal reconstruction can be undertaken. Treatment involves excision of the web in cases of partial occlusion, and should be curative.

Prognosis

The outcome of patients with laryngeal atresia will depend in part on the presence of other associated anomalies. Patients with partial recanalization do better than those with complete occlusion of the laryngeal lumen. The rapidity with which the airway is established at birth will also impact long-term prognosis. Reconstructive surgery in some cases may allow development of speech.

Congenital High Airway Obstruction Syndrome

Congenital high airway obstruction syndrome (CHAOS) is a syndrome of prenatally diagnosed complete or near-complete upper airway obstruction. Airway obstruction is usually caused by laryngeal atresia, a laryngeal web, or severe subglottic stenosis. Prenatal sonographic findings include bilateral enlarged lungs, dilated airways and flattened diaphragms with associated non-immune hydrops or fetal ascites. Ex utero intrapartum therapy (EXIT), which involves tracheostomy placement during delivery while the infant is still supported by the placenta, and positive pressure ventilation, has been tried with some success in these cases[1].

Tracheal Agenesis

Tracheal agenesis is a rare congenital abnormality of the airway that is incompatible with life. It is thought to occur because of a malformation of the laryngotracheal groove. Thus, this lesion occurs early in the embryonic stage of lung development. There is usually an incomplete presence or complete absence of a trachea below the cricoid cartilage or the larynx with or without main-stem bronchi. There is also an associated tracheoesophageal fistula in 80% of these cases. Clinically, patients have respiratory distress at birth, and usually die soon after birth.

Treatment

Reconstructive surgery has been attempted with poor results.

Prognosis

Tracheal agenesis carries a poor prognosis and is uniformly fatal.

Tracheal Stenosis

Congenital stenosis of trachea most commonly occurs as a result of the presence of tracheal webs causing narrowing of the airway. These webs are typically fibrous in nature and occur most commonly in the subglottic region.

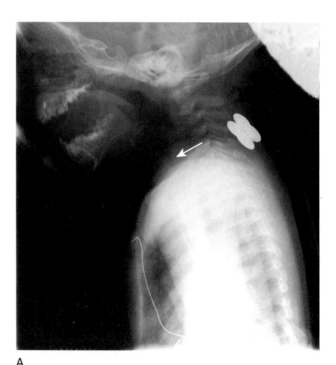

A

Figure 3-1 (**A**) Lateral neck radiograph of an infant with laryngeal atresia. Note the abrupt cessation of the air column at the level of the larynx (arrow). (**B**) Serial CT images of the same patient, progressing caudally from just above the lesion. Note the disappearance of the air column in images 6 through 10, with its reappearance and placement of a tracheostomy tube in the last two panels. (Images courtesy of Avrum Pollock, M.D., FRCPC.)

(Continued)

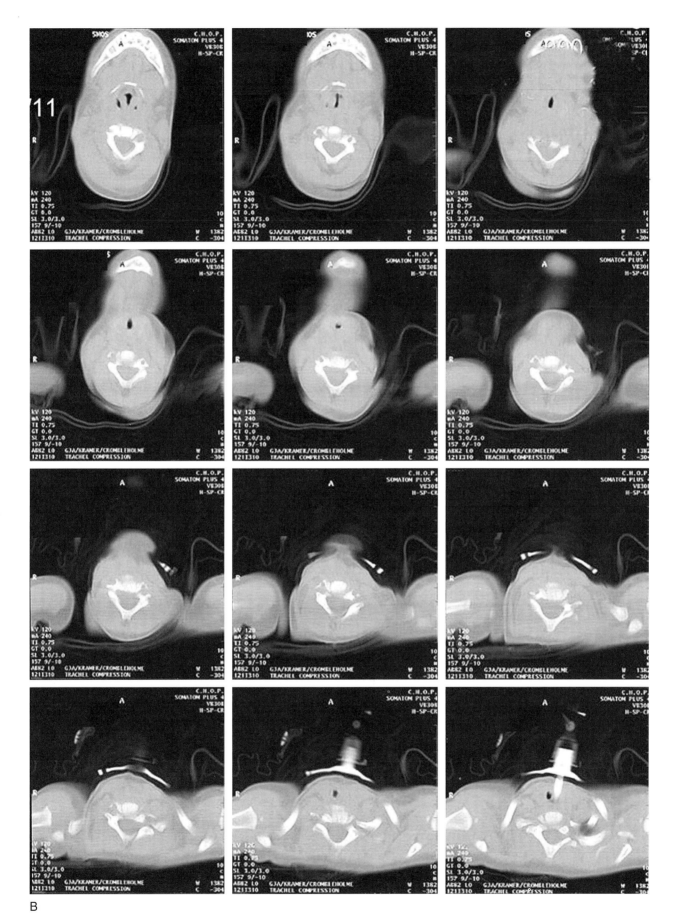

B

Figure 3-1 Cont'd

Clinically, patients present shortly after birth with respiratory difficulty and stridor suggesting an upper airway lesion.

Diagnosis

A plain chest and neck radiograph can suggest airway narrowing. Bronchoscopy is definitive and reveals narrowing of the airway on direct visualization. In situations where the stenosis is too small to permit the entry of a bronchoscope, a tracheogram with water-soluble contrast can be used to confirm diagnosis and define the extent of the narrowing (Figure 3-2).

Treatment

Conservative management is preferred, since the tracheal lumen may widen enough with time to alleviate respiratory distress. Intraluminal stenting and high doses of intralesional steroids as well as inhaled steroids have been tried. Tracheostomy may be necessary if the patient presents in acute respiratory distress.

Tracheomalacia

Tracheomalacia is the commonest tracheal abnormality. It may be congenital or acquired. Acquired tracheomalacia can occur secondary to extrinsic compression by, for example, a vascular ring. The intrathoracic tracheal lumen dilates during normal inspiration and narrows during normal expiration. In patients with intrathoracic tracheomalacia, this normal expiratory process will be exaggerated because of lack of tracheal support, resulting in pronounced narrowing during

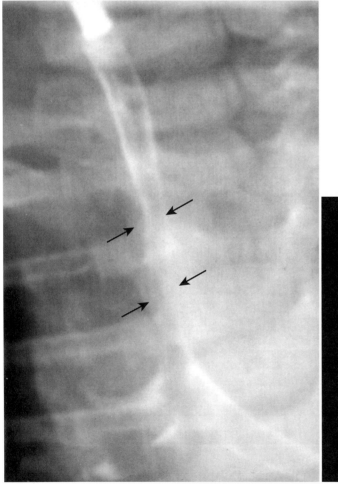

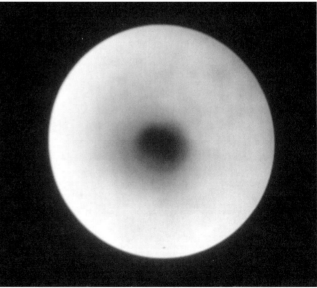

A   B

Figure 3-2   (**A**) Tracheobronchogram with water-soluble contrast medium (Omnipaque) in a 3-month-old infant with distal tracheal stenosis. Note that the caliber of the distal trachea is smaller than that of the left main bronchus. The bronchoscope, which has a diameter of 3.6 mm, can be seen at the top of the airway for a size reference. (**B**) Bronchoscopic view of the trachea. The tracheal lumen was too small to allow the bronchoscope to be advanced through it. In this patient, the stenosis was associated with a series of complete tracheal rings. The posterior tracheal membrane (pars trachealis) that normally spans the ends of the C-shaped cartilages, is absent. (Images courtesy of Howard B. Panitch, M.D.)

exhalation. For similar reasons, patients with extrathoracic tracheomalacia will experience airway narrowing during inspiration. This condition can present with symptoms of persistent wheeze, cough, stridor, dyspnea or tachypnea. Symptoms typically worsen with high-airflow activities, e.g., during feeding or crying. In contrast, symptoms will improve during sleep. They may also worsen with intercurrent upper respiratory infections.

Diagnosis

The diagnosis is generally made based on clinical history and presence of stridor (extrathoracic tracheomalacia) or a homophonous wheeze (intrathoracic tracheomalacia) on clinical examination. The presence of an easily collapsible tracheal wall can be confirmed by flexible bronchoscopy. Airway fluoroscopy, demonstrating a narrowing of the tracheal air column, has also been used as a diagnostic test (Figure 3-3). Symptoms usually improve with age and resolve spontaneously by 12 months of life.

Differential Diagnosis

1. Vascular rings, especially double aortic arch and right aberrant subclavian artery, may cause symptoms of tracheal compression and should be ruled out. A normal upper gastrointestinal series rules out most significant vascular rings but will miss an anterior tracheal compression by an anomalous innominate artery. Presence of a pulsatile mass on bronchoscopic examination suggests the presence of a vascular ring.

2. Tracheal webs and congenital tracheal stenosis also cause narrowing of the tracheal lumen. On clinical examination, the noise will often be bi-phasic. These lesions can be ruled out by direct visualization during bronchoscopy.

Treatment

If symptoms are mild, anticipatory guidance is adequate. In cases of severe tracheomalacia, infants and children may have life-threatening episodes of airway collapse. In such situations, prolonged treatment with continuous positive airway pressure (CPAP) via tracheostomy may be required. The application of CPAP can improve forced expiratory flows by acting as an intraluminal stent or by increasing lung volume (or both). When measured, there has been no increase in the forced vital capacity (FVC) detected with institution of CPAP, but there is a decrease in inspiratory capacity (IC) suggesting an increase in functional residual capacity (FRC). Together, these mechanisms help prevent airway collapse especially during forced expiratory maneuvers such as crying[2-4].

Bronchoconstrictors, such as bethanechol and methacholine, cause an increase in airway smooth muscle tone

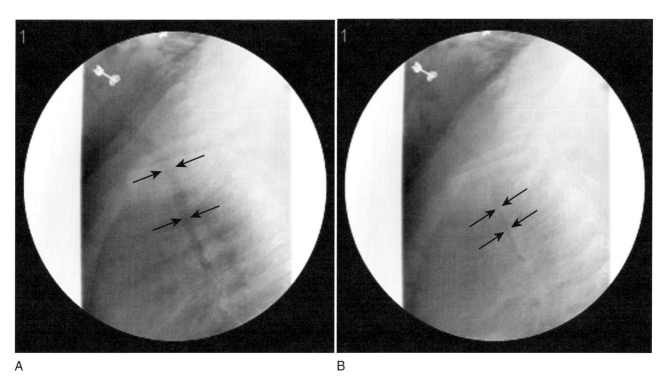

A   B

Figure 3-3 (**A**) Chest fluoroscopy in the lateral position during inspiration, demonstrating a tracheal air column of normal caliber (arrows). (**B**) Expiratory view of same patient, showing marked narrowing of the intrathoracic airway (arrows), consistent with intrathoracic tracheomalacia. Care should be taken to avoid the patient crying during the examination, since the airway caliber can narrow by as much as 50% in normal babies under such conditions. (Images courtesy of Avrum Pollock, M.D., FRCPC.)

which in turn stiffens the trachea. This intervention has been shown to improve expiratory flow in patients with tracheomalacia when the narrowed trachea is the major site of obstruction[5].

The surgical approach to treatment of tracheomalacia includes placement of a tracheostomy tube, which if long enough, can preserve the airway lumen by stenting the trachea. Aortopexy has also been used successfully in patients with distal tracheomalacia. Suspension of the aorta to the anterior chest wall can relieve vascular compression as well as preventing anterior tracheal wall collapse. A marked improvement in clinical symptoms as well as evidence of relief of tracheal obstruction has been documented on infant pulmonary functions, controlled ventilation CT scans and MRI postoperatively.

Since tracheomalacia may result in poor airway clearance, intercurrent infections need to be treated with aggressive airway clearance maneuvers. Occasionally, antibiotics may be required, especially if the patient has a history of recurrent pneumonia and bronchitis.

Prognosis

The prognosis is excellent for infants with isolated tracheomalacia. In most cases, symptoms resolve spontaneously by 12 months of age. Tracheomalacia associated with vascular compression or tracheoesophageal fistula, however, may persist for years. In patients with severe tracheomalacia requiring tracheostomy and mechanical ventilation, the course is usually prolonged and resolution of tracheomalacia takes months to years.

Tracheoesophageal Fistula

Tracheoesophageal fistula (TEF) results from the failure of the digestive and the respiratory tracts to separate from each other during the embryonic stage of development. Four different types of TEF have been recognized. The commonest type involves the esophagus ending in a blind proximal pouch while the distal esophageal remnant communicates with the trachea. This type accounts for 85% of all TEFs (Figure 3-4). The distal and the proximal esophageal pouches may be attached by a fibrous band and the distance between the distal pouch and the proximal pouch is variable. The fistula runs from the distal esophageal segment to the posterior wall of the trachea and enters the airway typically just above the carina or the proximal part of either one of the main-stem bronchi.

Esophageal atresia with the TEF originating from the proximal esophageal pouch is uncommon (Figure 3-4E). Here, the fistula opens either in the mid-portion of the trachea or close to the carina depending upon the length of the proximal esophageal pouch.

Three to six percent of all TEFs occur as an H-type fistula, where both the esophagus and the trachea maintain patent lumens throughout their lengths, but there exists

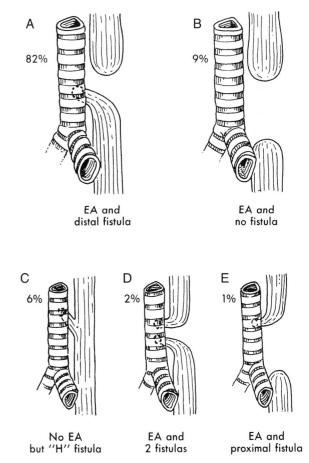

Figure 3-4 The common (**A**, **B**) and less common (**C**, **D**, **E**) combinations of esophageal atresia (EA) and tracheoesophageal fistula (TEF). (From Blickman H, editor: The requisites: pediatric radiology, 2nd edition, p 93. Philadelphia: Mosby, 1998.)

a fistula between the trachea and the esophagus (Figure 3-4C). The fistula usually runs upwards from the esophagus towards the middle of the trachea and appears as an opening in the posterior tracheal wall. The epithelium lining the fistula is usually esophageal. The tracheal epithelium in patients with TEF reveals multiple areas of squamous metaplasia with loss of ciliated epithelium. There is also often a greater proportion of muscle to cartilage in the tracheal wall at the site of the fistula, resulting in an area of tracheomalacia. Together, these factors result in poor airway clearance, thus contributing to recurrent bronchitis and pneumonia.

Esophageal atresia with both the proximal and the distal esophageal pouch communicating with the trachea occurs rarely (Figure 3-4D). Approximately 10% of esophageal atresia is not associated with any TEF.

Clinical Features

About 30% of the cases of TEF with esophageal atresia are complicated by hydramnios and 50% of the patients may have associated cardiovascular, renal, gastrointestinal, and central nervous system abnormalities[6,7]. Infants with esophageal atresia usually present with copious oral secretions and, when attempted, there is a failure to pass an orogastric tube. There may be recurrent vomiting and/or respiratory distress. Recurrent aspiration of oral secretions occurs because of pooling of secretions in the proximal blind pouch. Patients may present with a history of recurrent bronchitis and pneumonia. There may be history of intermittent choking with food and symptoms are usually worse with ingestion of fluids rather than solids.

Clinical presentation of an H-type fistula is usually more subtle, consisting of cough in association with ingestion of formula or food. Affected patients are usually full-term infants and patients may not be diagnosed until adulthood.

Diagnosis

The plain chest radiograph can disclose aspiration pneumonia or chronic scarring from recurrent episodes of aspiration pneumonia. There will be an associated gasless abdomen in cases of TEF with proximal esophageal atresia whereas esophageal atresia with a distal TEF is associated with presence of gas in the abdomen (Figure 3-5).

A fistulous opening between the trachea and the esophagus can often be demonstrated by bronchoscopic examination. Esophagoscopy can also reveal an orifice.

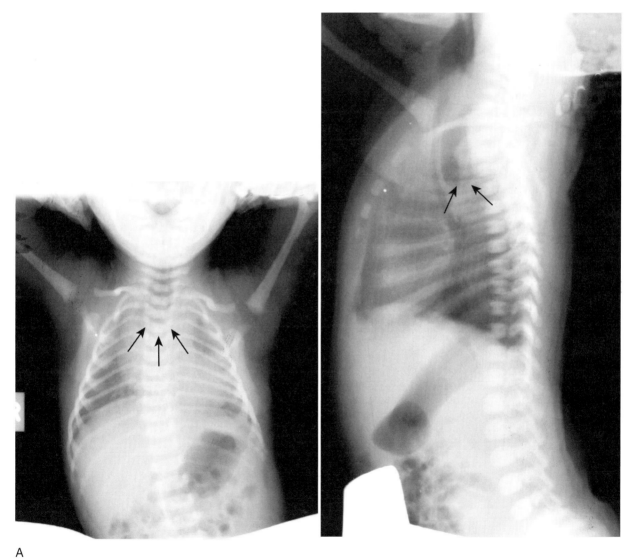

A

Figure 3-5 (**A**) Anteroposterior and lateral chest radiographs of a newborn with esophageal atresia and distal TEF. The proximal pouch can be seen as a lucency that abruptly ends on both views (arrows). Presence of gas in the abdomen suggests that the distal esophageal segment must be in connection with the airway. (**B**) Anteroposterior and lateral chest radiographs of the same infant after an attempt to pass an orogastric tube. The tube loops back upon itself in the proximal fistula, demonstrating the pouch. (Images courtesy of Avrum Pollock, M.D., FRCPC.)   *(Continued)*

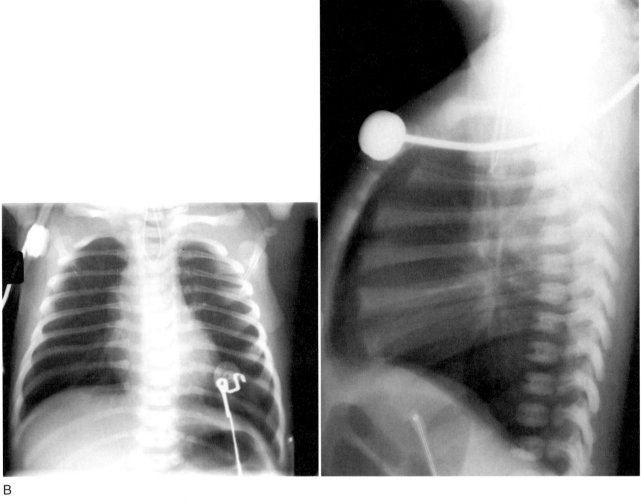

B

Figure 3-5 Cont'd

If methylene blue dye instillation through one orifice is recovered from another, especially when the distal esophagus is occluded with a Foley catheter, the diagnosis is confirmed.

Continuous imaging and videotaping with a contrast medium swallow helps differentiate between filling of the trachea via a fistulous opening and tracheal filling seen in overflow aspiration. Instillation of contrast medium under pressure via a feeding tube (Figure 3-6) can demonstrate a fistula too small to be identified endoscopically. The combination of this technique with bronchoscopy will detect >90% of cases of TEF.

Differential Diagnosis

1. A vascular ring that includes both the airway and esophagus, such as a double aortic arch or right aberrant subclavian artery, may cause tracheomalacia and gastroesophageal reflux

disease (GERD) symptoms because of compression of the esophagus and the trachea. An upper gastrointestinal series with contrast helps rule out a vascular ring or sling.
2. Cystic fibrosis should be considered when patients present with recurrent pneumonia and failure to thrive. A negative sweat test will rule out cystic fibrosis in most cases.
3. Immunodeficiency should be considered in patients presenting with recurrent pneumonia.

Management

Surgical repair is the treatment of choice and operative mortality is low. Surgical repair may be carried out as a primary repair or as a staged procedure in premature infants or infants with other associated anomalies. Prompt diagnosis and operative management are crucial to minimize development of chronic pulmonary disease.

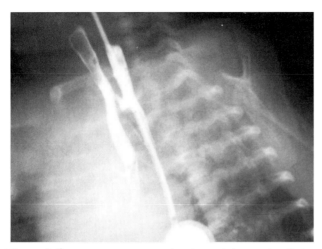

Figure 3-6 Upper gastrointestinal series with barium instillation via a tube demonstrates an H-type TEF with filling of both the esophagus and the airway. Placement of the tube beyond the fistula, with retrograde filling, allows for differentiation between the fistula and possible aspiration of contrast material into the airway during swallowing. (Image courtesy of Avrum Pollock, M.D., FRCPC.)

Prognosis

Recurrence of TEF after surgical repair occurs in 4–10% of cases. Postoperative strictures at the site of the anastomosis are common[6,8,9]. Persistent tracheomalacia at the fistula site occurs frequently as well. It has been reported that 60% of affected children, after successful surgical repair, have persistent GERD symptoms until late adulthood[10]. Recurrent bouts of pneumonia and bronchitis are seen in about half of these patients postoperatively[11]. The rate of postoperative complications is lower in patients with H-type fistula compared with patients with associated esophageal atresia.

Without surgery, TEF with esophageal atresia is fatal; however, patients with H-type fistula may survive many years without surgery. When promptly diagnosed 95% of term infants with TEF survive. Survival rates in premature babies with moderate pneumonia or congenital abnormalities are lower.

ABNORMALITIES OF THE LUNG

Pulmonary Agenesis

Pulmonary agenesis is characterized by underdevelopment of lung. In cases of pulmonary agenesis there is no development of the bronchial tree or pulmonary tissue[12], whereas in pulmonary aplasia there may be a rudimentary pouch with no pulmonary tissue. Both these entities may be associated with other congenital abnormalities. Pulmonary agenesis and aplasia both occur during the embryonic stage of lung development[12-14]. Agenesis can affect either a single lobe, an entire lung or

both lungs. The unaffected lobes or lung usually demonstrate compensatory hypertrophy. Agenesis of the right lung is more likely to be associated with other congenital abnormalities than is agenesis of the left lung.

Patients are usually symptomatic and present with tachypnea, respiratory difficulty or recurrent pulmonary infections. As the patient gets older, the chest examination can reveal an abnormal chest contour because of lack of lung growth on the affected side. The hemithorax that lacks the lung may be filled with the hypertrophied contralateral lung that herniates over to the affected side. The mediastinal structures may also shift to fill the empty hemithorax. There are decreased breath sounds on the affected side, though often there may not be complete absence of breath sounds because of air movement in the herniated lung that is filling the empty hemithorax.

Diagnosis

The chest radiograph shows approximation of the ribs, elevation of the diaphragm and presence of a uniform dense opacity on the affected side (Figure 3-7). There is deviation of the mediastinal structures towards the affected side[12,15].

On bronchoscopic examination, there is absence of bronchi (agenesis) or presence of a rudimentary pouch on the affected side (aplasia). Bronchography can outline the tracheobronchial tree and confirm findings seen on bronchoscopy. Angiography has been used to demonstrate absence of pulmonary vasculature[14]. Chest CT is useful in showing absence of lung parenchyma and the tracheobronchial tree.

Differential Diagnosis

1. Pneumonia presents as a large opacity on a plain chest radiograph. However, close approximation of ribs and an elevated hemidiaphragm, or deviation of trachea and the mediastinal structures, all reflect loss of volume on the side of the opacification and therefore are suggestive of lung agenesis. In contrast, acute pneumonia is not associated with ipsilateral volume loss.
2. Atelectasis may be difficult to distinguish from pulmonary agenesis radiographically. Bronchoscopy will demonstrate both main bronchi, and probably also reveal a central airway obstruction leading to the atelectasis.

Treatment

Intervention is aimed at supportive care. If respiratory insufficiency is present, tracheostomy tube placement will facilitate chronic mechanical ventilation. Aggressive airway clearance is recommended for adequate pulmonary toilet. If there is an isolated lobar agenesis, resection of the abnormal lobe may be helpful[16].

Prognosis

Outcome depends on the extent of agenesis and the presence of associated congenital malformations.

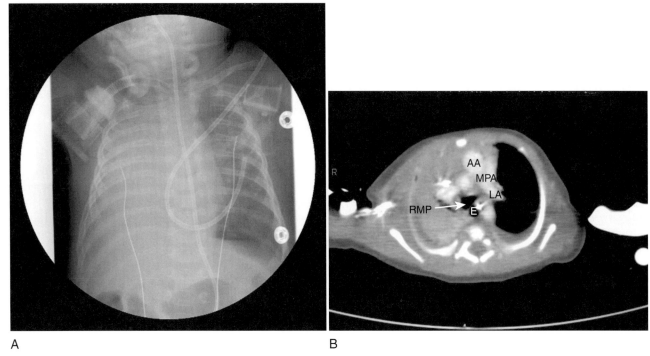

A   B

Figure 3-7 (**A**) Anteroposterior chest radiograph of a newborn infant with right-sided pulmonary aplasia. The right hemithorax is uniformly opacified. Endoscopic evaluation demonstrated a rudimentary bronchial bud on the right, with a normal left main bronchus. (**B**) Chest CT scan of the same patient. The rudimentary right main bronchus can be seen as well as a normal-sized left main pulmonary artery. The right main pulmonary artery is absent. AA, aortic arch; E, esophagus; MPA, main pulmonary artery; LPA, left pulmonary artery; RMB, right main bronchial bud. (Images courtesy of Avrum Pollock, MD, FRCPC.)

Right-sided agenesis causes a greater degree of mediastinal shift. Because of the shift, the risk for spillage of the contents of the right bronchial pouch into the left lung will be increased and can lead to recurrent lung infections[13,17].

Pulmonary Hypoplasia

Hypoplastic lungs are small, have a decreased alveolar number, lower DNA content, and a decreased number of airway generations. Reduction in airway number, when present, suggests an injury before 16 weeks gestation. Isolated lung hypoplasia is unusual but is more likely to occur as a secondary event. A number of clinical conditions result in pulmonary hypoplasia. For example, congenital neuromuscular diseases that result in decreased fetal movements and decreased expansion of the chest and the lungs in utero will lead to pulmonary hypoplasia. Renal and congenital genitourinary diseases can lead to oligohydramnios, which is also associated with a decreased alveolar number. A space-occupying lesion in the chest cavity, such as diaphragmatic hernia or pleural effusion (as in hydrops), can also impair lung growth and result in lung hypoplasia. Abnormal pulmonary artery

formation or congenital heart disease can lead to impaired pulmonary perfusion and decreased lung growth. An abnormal bronchus can also interfere with lung development and lead to pulmonary hypoplasia.

Since there are many causes of pulmonary hypoplasia, clinical features will depend on the underlying cause of the hypoplasia. The spectrum of clinical presentation is wide and depends on the severity of associated lesions and the degree of hypoplasia. Thus patients may be completely asymptomatic or may present with significant respiratory distress.

Diagnosis

The chest radiograph or CT scan shows poorly aerated lungs or findings of the associated abnormality responsible for the hypoplasia, such as pleural effusion or diaphragmatic hernia. The main pulmonary arteries may also appear small.

Treatment

The mainstay of care is supportive; therapy depends upon the degree of hypoplasia and associated anomalies, if any. Some children with pulmonary hypoplasia may require supplemental oxygen only initially whereas others require chronic mechanical ventilation to maintain adequate gas exchange.

Prognosis

Outcome depends upon the cause of hypoplasia and presence of other associated anomalies.

Congenital Lobar Emphysema

Congenital lobar emphysema (CLE) makes up 14% of all bronchopulmonary malformations. The emphysematous lobes are commonly left-sided and usually occur in the upper lobes. This malformation is most often characterized by overdistension of the affected lobe and the alveoli are otherwise normal anatomically. Occasionally, there may be a reduced number of alveoli within the lobe. The pathogenesis of CLE is thought to be secondary to an obstruction of the bronchus leading to secondary hyperinflation. This obstruction of the airway may be the result of an intrinsic lesion or extrinsic compression (Table 3-2). Intrinsic lesions result either from abnormal characteristics of the bronchial wall or intraluminal causes. Extrinsic lesions cause compression of the airway by vascular or mass structures. Vascular compression can result from abnormal structures (e.g., rings, slings) or from enlarged vessels associated with left-to-right shunts.

Clinical presentation depends on the degree of lobar overdistension and resultant compression and impairment of ventilation of normal areas of lung. Symptoms can range from mild tachypnea in the neonatal period to significant respiratory distress, wheezing and cough. Early presentation with significant respiratory distress in the neonatal period can occur because of progressive air trapping and shift of mediastinal structures, often requiring emergency surgical intervention. About 50% of patients are diagnosed by 1 month of age[13]. Rarely, CLE may escape early diagnosis and present with recurrent respiratory infections in an older child. Physical examination reveals asymmetric chest wall prominence on the side of the lesion, and mediastinal shift away from the affected side. On auscultation, breath sounds are decreased on the affected side and the ipsilateral hemithorax may be hyper-resonant on percussion. Associated congenital cardiovascular abnormalities can further complicate the clinical picture.

Diagnosis

An area of hyperlucent lung with lung markings throughout the lesion is characteristic on the chest radiograph (Figure 3-8). Shortly after birth, the lesion may be opacified because of abnormal drainage of fetal lung fluid. CT scan of the chest with contrast can reveal an area of bronchial narrowing and air trapping. MRI can exclude abnormal vasculature or the presence of a vascular ring causing bronchial compression.

Differential Diagnosis

1. Polyalveolar lobe is considered to be a distinct entity where there is a true increase in the number of alveoli instead of increased distension of the terminal alveolar spaces. The pathogenesis of polyalveolar lobe is poorly understood.
2. Swyer-James-Mcleod syndrome. This syndrome occurs as a result of obliterative bronchiolitis, where both terminal airways and their attendant blood vessels become irreversibly scarred and obliterated. As a result, there is decreased pulmonary blood flow to the affected areas. The decreased pulmonary blood flow in turn causes hyperlucency of the affected region. Here, the affected lung is hyperlucent but smaller compared with the normal lung (Figure 3-9). In contrast, in CLE the affected lung is hyperlucent and larger than the unaffected lung.

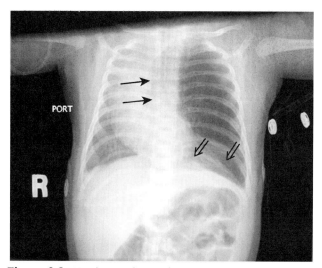

Figure 3-8 Newborn infant with congenital lobar emphysema involving the left upper lobe. Although the area is hyperlucent, lung markings can still be identified within the lesion. The overdistended left upper lobe crosses the midline (thin arrows), compresses the left lower lobe and lingula (thick arrows), and causes a right-ward shift of the mediastinal structures. (Image courtesy of Avrum Pollock, M.D., FRCPC, and Howard Panitch, M.D.)

Table 3-2	**Causes of Bronchial Obstruction**
Intrinsic	**Extrinsic**
Hypoplastic/dysplastic bronchial cartilage	Patent ductus arteriosus
Inspissated mucus plugs	Pulmonary artery sling
Bronchial stenosis/ atresia	Pulmonary stenosis
Bronchial granulations	Tetralogy of Fallot with absent pulmonary valve
	Bronchogenic cyst
	Mediastinal teratoma
	Neuroblastoma
	Mediastinal lymphadenopathy
	Esophageal duplication cyst
	Accessory diaphragm

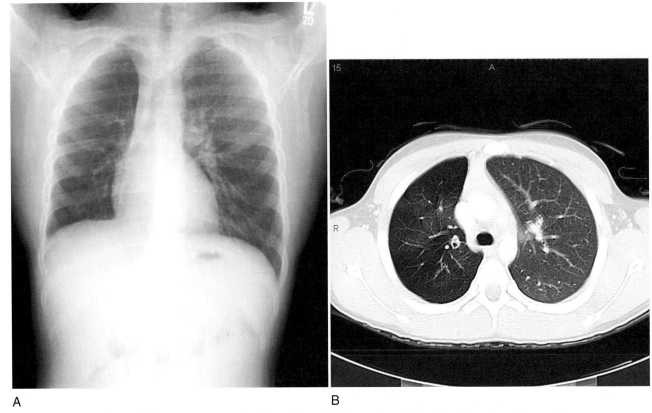

Figure 3-9 (**A**) Posteroanterior chest radiograph of Swyer-James-Mcleod syndrome in a 13-year-old. Note that the right lung is both hyperlucent and smaller, compared with the left lung. (**B**) CT scan of the same patient, again demonstrating the smaller hyperlucent right lung. The vascular markings are diminished in the right lung, giving it its hyperlucent appearance. (Images courtesy of Avrum Pollock, M.D., FRCPC.)

Management

Surgical excision of the affected lobe is recommended. Elective resection before respiratory distress occurs is safe and associated with low mortality. Surgical intervention may be needed urgently if the patient presents with significant respiratory distress.

Prognosis

Untreated, patients may do well. However, in such situations acute respiratory infection can worsen the obstruction, resulting in enlargement of the emphysematous lobe and creation of life-threatening respiratory distress. For those patients who undergo excision of the emphysematous lobe, the prognosis is good. Long-term follow-up after lobectomy reveals compensatory lung growth[18-20]. Although some other investigators report evidence of obstructive lung disease on pulmonary function tests on follow-up[21,22] most patients are asymptomatic postoperatively.

Bronchogenic Cysts

Bronchogenic cysts occur as a result of abnormal budding of the bronchial tissue. This abnormal budding may occur either in early or late gestation. If the abnormal bud separates from the embryonic bronchial tissue early, it results in formation of central (mediastinal) bronchogenic cysts whereas tissue separation later in gestation results in formation of peripheral (pulmonary) cysts. Bronchogenic cysts can be multilocular or unilocular. Histologically, they are thin-walled cysts lined with cuboidal epithelium or secretory ciliated epithelium. The cyst can contain mucus glands, smooth muscle, elastic tissue and cartilage. Gastric or respiratory epithelium may also be found in the cyst depending upon the time of development. The cyst fluid is usually thin, clear or mucoid; recurrent hemorrhage results in thick, dark-brown cyst contents. There is typically no communication between the cyst and the tracheobronchial tree, but on occasion one may occur.

Bronchogenic cysts usually are found in the mediastinum, and are typically located subcarinally in paraesophageal, paratracheal, and hilar regions (Figure 3-10). Intrapulmonary cysts are uncommon and are usually found in the lower lobes. A case of intraluminal tracheal cyst, which presented with tachypnea and stridor in a 7-month-old otherwise healthy baby has recently been reported[23].

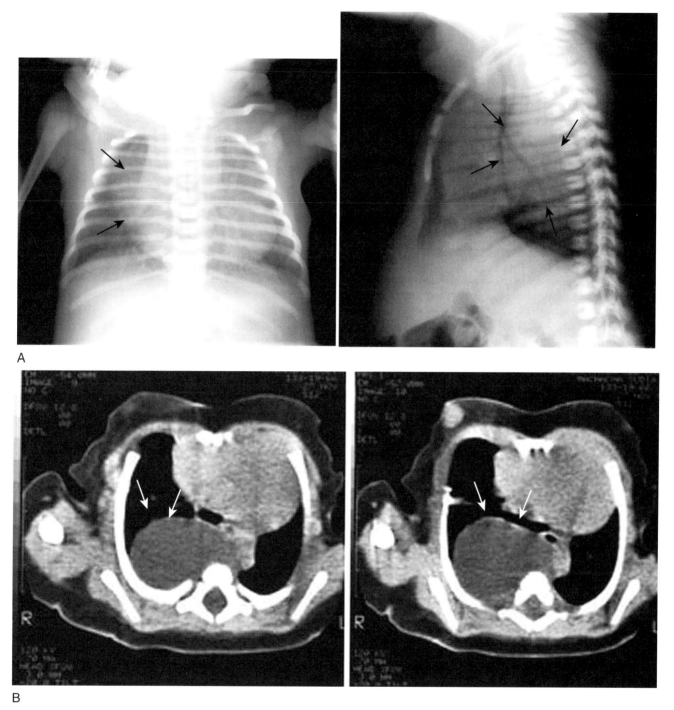

A

B

Figure 3-10   (**A**) Anteroposterior and lateral chest radiographs of an infant with a bronchogenic cyst (arrows). (**B**) The lesion's position in the mediastinum is confirmed by CT scan (arrows). It is of uniform density and is without loculations. (Images courtesy of Avrum Pollock, M.D., FRCPC, and Richard Markowitz, M.D.)

Clinically, small cysts are mostly asymptomatic and present as an incidental radiographic finding in adulthood. If the cyst is large enough or positioned in such a way as to cause compression and distortion of the tracheobronchial tree, however, the infant will present with severe respiratory distress. This compression results in a check-valve type mechanism, causing enlargement of the cyst and further impairment of gas exchange as the offending mass lesion increases in size. Such acute enlargement of the cyst is commonly seen in infancy; as children get older, enlargement of the cyst is less common. In older children, a bronchogenic cyst can present with signs of infection, cough, fever, hemoptysis or recurrent attacks of pneumonia[24].

Diagnosis

Chest radiography is the most useful modality for diagnosing a cyst[25]. The radiographic appearance of a bronchogenic cyst usually is of a round or oval structure of uniform density located peripherally. Mediastinal cysts are located more centrally and may be difficult to visualize on a plain chest radiograph. An air–fluid level may be visualized in an infected bronchogenic cyst. CT scan with contrast allows identification of the cyst and its differentiation from mediastinal structures. MRI can also be helpful, although it does not add much more to the information provided by a CT scan. Occasionally esophagoscopy and bronchoscopy have been used to delineate cysts that may be poorly visualized by other modalities[26,27].

Differential Diagnosis

1. Encapsulated empyema can be confused with an infected bronchogenic cyst, since the radiological appearance is similar on a plain chest radiograph. Anatomic location of the lesion will help distinguish between the two if the cyst is subcarinal. A thoracic CT scan with contrast can also help differentiate between the two entities.
2. Post-infectious pneumatoceles after staphylococcal pneumonia may be mistaken for an air-filled cyst. These commonly resolve spontaneously whereas an air-filled bronchogenic cyst is unlikely to resolve spontaneously.
3. Loculated pneumothorax is also important to differentiate from an air-filled bronchogenic cyst; the important distinguishing point for a pneumothorax is the presence of a compressed lung, which may be seen as a hilar shadow on a plain chest radiograph.

Treatment

Excision of the cyst, whether mediastinal or pulmonary, is recommended. Intrapulmonary lesions may require segmental or lobar excision. Excision is preferentially performed electively, before compression of normal structures results in significant respiratory distress and the need for emergency excision.

Prognosis

In general, outcome is good following surgery. Patients who present with significant air trapping show gradual improvement following surgical excision. Residual bronchomalacia and tracheomalacia can lead to persistent symptoms. Without surgery, mortality rate in symptomatic patients is 100%.

Congenital Cystic Adenomatoid Malformation

Congenital cystic adenomatoid malformation (CCAM) occurs secondary to the cystic adenomatous overgrowth of terminal bronchioles, which results in the secondary inhibition of alveolar growth[28,29]. These cysts communicate with each other and also with the tracheobronchial tree. Grossly, a CCAM appears as a firm mass without normal lobar configuration. It mostly affects one lobe, although no lobar predilection is known (Figure 3-11). Occasionally, it can affect an entire lung. Histologically, there is an interspersion of adenomatous areas and cysts. Two types of cysts have been described, the first of which is characterized by cuboidal respiratory epithelium lining the cyst with no elastic tissue or smooth muscle in the cyst wall[28,30-33]. In the second type of cyst, the lining contains primarily pseudostratified columnar epithelium with papillary projections into the cyst lumen and large amounts of elastic tissue as well as some smooth muscle present in the cyst wall. However, there is complete lack of cartilage. The adenomatous areas consist of tubular structures similar to terminal bronchioles but with complete absence of mature alveoli, suggesting developmental arrest in the second (pseudoglandular) stage of lung development.

There is no known race or gender predilection for CCAM but there is a known association with maternal polyhydramnios. Polyhydramnios is thought to occur as a result of compression of the esophagus by the mass lesion, causing impairment in fetal swallowing and fluid accumulation in the amniotic sac. Compression of the heart by the lesion can also result in hydrops. Normal lung surrounding the CCAM is commonly compressed, atelectatic, and hypoplastic. Polyhydramnios is also thought to occur because of impaired fluid absorption from this atelectatic normal lung surrounding the CCAM.

There are three types of CCAM as described by Stocker et al.[28]:

Type I: Characterized by presence of large cystic spaces interspersed with large alveolar spaces with few or no adenomatous components. This accounts for 50% of all cases of CCAM.

Type II: Characterized by mixed cystic and adenomatoid components. It is the subtype most commonly associated with other congenital abnormalities.

Type III: Characterized by entirely adenomatous structures with no cystic lesions.

Clinical Presentation

Patients with CCAM typically present with tachypnea or respiratory distress soon after birth or in infancy. There may be a history of maternal hydramnios complicating

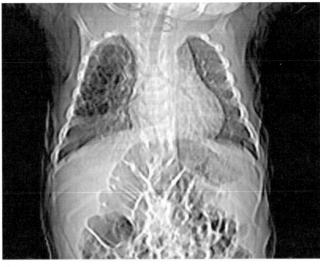

A

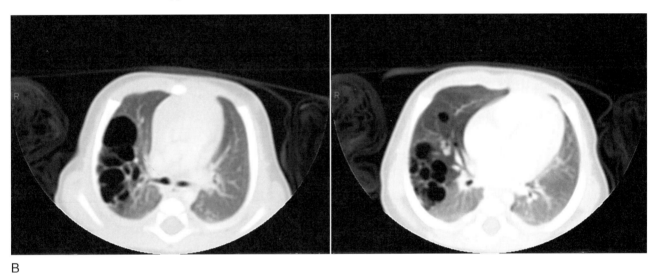

B

Figure 3-11 CT scout film (**A**) and axial images (**B**) of a congenital cystic adenomatoid malformation (CCAM) in a 6-week-old infant. A large multicystic structure involves much of the right upper lobe. The right lower lobe is spared, and there was no evidence of a feeding systemic vessel. The largest cyst was estimated to measure 1.5–1.8 cm. (Images courtesy of Avrum Pollock, M.D., FRCPC.)

the pregnancy. Stillbirth and premature birth are commonly associated with CCAM. The presence of microcystic lesions as identified on prenatal ultrasonography has been reported to be associated with hydrops and stillbirth, whereas the presence of macrocystic lesions prenatally is associated with a more stable clinical condition after birth[34-36].

Since the cysts in CCAM communicate with the tracheobronchial tree, the lesions can rapidly enlarge after birth and cause significant respiratory distress. Most cases present by early infancy, but others with smaller areas of involvement can present with recurrent pneumonia in the same lobe during adolescence or adulthood. CCAM is associated with other congenital pulmonary defects such as pulmonary hypoplasia and also cardiovascular and genitourinary anomalies. Rarely, it is diagnosed as an incidental finding on a chest radiograph in adulthood.

Diagnosis

Radiographic findings vary depending upon the size of the cyst. Typically the chest radiograph shows a multicystic lesion. Lesions may also be solid-appearing or present as a single cystic lesion. The surrounding normal lung may be compressed and atelectatic with evidence of mediastinal shift. A barium swallow with contrast will help differentiate between a congenital diaphragmatic hernia and a CCAM. Ultrasonography can distinguish cystic versus solid lesions in the thorax. Prenatal ultrasonography can reveal the presence of microcystic or macrocystic lesions, thus aiding in predicting outcome in the perinatal period.

Chest CT scan with contrast can differentiate between the different types of CCAM based on the different sizes of the cysts visible on the examination, especially type III lesions[37,38].

Differential Diagnosis

1. Diaphragmatic hernia: Loops of bowel migrate through the diaphragmatic defect into the chest cavity and can be confused with a multicystic CCAM (Figure 3-12). An upper gastrointestinal series with contrast or a barium enema can help differentiate between the two entities.

2. Post-infectious pneumatoceles: Pneumatoceles that form after acute infection are frequently seen following staphylococcal pneumonia. These can present as numerous small air-filled cysts on a chest radiograph.

3. Bronchogenic cyst: In some cases an air-filled cyst may be difficult to differentiate from a CCAM though, typically, bronchogenic cysts appear as opaque dense shadows.

4. Mesenchymal hamartomas are lesions characterized by nodules and cysts. The cysts are lined by respiratory epithelium with an underlying layer of mesenchymal cells, while the nodules are made of primitive mesenchymal cells. These lesions usually enlarge with time and may be bilateral, unlike CCAMs which are rarely bilateral or progressive. The radiographic appearance may be very similar to that of a CCAM.

Treatment

Surgical resection is the treatment of choice. Since most patients present in the neonatal period with respiratory distress, excision is done urgently in most cases. Observation and stabilization of the patient is not advised since expansion of the lesion can occur, further worsening the respiratory status of the patient. Elective excision is recommended even in asymptomatic cases because of the reported potential for malignant transformation[39]. Once the diagnosis is suspected, early intervention is recommended since excision allows decompression of the compressed normal lung surrounding the CCAM, thus maximizing the potential growth of normal lung tissue.

Prognosis

As noted above, the presence of microcystic lesions on prenatal ultrasonography has been reported to result in a poorer prognosis and is usually associated with

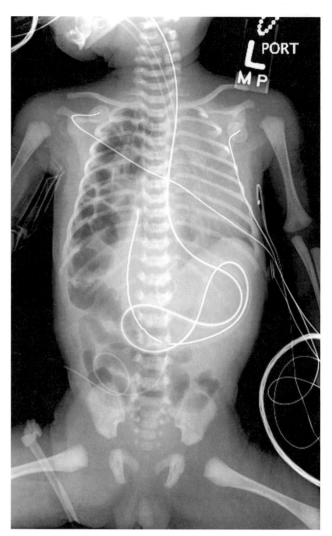

Figure 3-12   Anteroposterior view of the chest and abdomen of a newborn with right-sided congenital diaphragmatic hernia. The bowel has entered the right hemithorax and appears like a multicystic mass. The mediastinum is displaced to the left. (Image courtesy of Avrum Pollock, M.D., FRCPC, and Howard Panitch, M.D.)

hydrops and stillbirth. In contrast, the presence of macrocystic lesions prenatally portends a better prognosis with a more stable clinical condition after birth[34-36].

CCAM type I carries the best prognosis. Patients with CCAM type II have the worst prognosis since the lesion is most likely to undergo a malignant change and to be associated with other congenital abnormalities.

Long-term prognosis following resection of the CCAM is good, with evidence of compensatory lung growth on follow-up pulmonary lung function testing[40,41].

Pulmonary Sequestration

Pulmonary sequestration is defined as a mass of nonfunctioning lung tissue that has a systemic vascular supply but usually no connection with the tracheobronchial tree. Sequestrations are classified as either intralobar or extralobar (Table 3-3). Intralobar sequestrations occur within the borders of the pleural membrane surrounding the normal lung, while extralobar sequestrations exist outside of the lung tissue surrounded by the pleura. Extralobar sequestrations are usually invested with their own pleural membrane. Extralobar sequestration is thought to occur later in gestation compared with an intralobar sequestration[31]. Intralobar sequestrations are far more common than the extralobar type, although both types of sequestrations are uncommon. Both types occur twice as frequently on the left side compared with the right. Ninety-eight percent of all intralobar sequestrations occur in the lower lobes. Extralobar sequestrations are also thought to occur more commonly in the lower lobes, although they may occasionally occur in the upper lobes. Intra-abdominal extralobar lung sequestrations have also been reported.

Intralobar sequestrations are clearly distinguishable from the surrounding normal lung on gross pathologic examination; their texture is variable depending on whether or not there is any air in the sequestration. Grossly, extralobar sequestrations are gray or dark brown and firm to the touch. Histologically, the extralobar sequestration has embryonic lung tissue with evidence of a single or multiple cysts, while intralobar sequestrations characteristically demonstrate areas of bronchiectasis and cysts, the walls of which may contain cartilage, muscle, bronchial glands, and alveolar structures.

Clinical Presentation

Patients with intralobar sequestration rarely present in infancy. About one third present before 10 years of age and 15% of sequestrations are found incidentally on a chest radiograph taken for another reason. The most common clinical presentation is one of recurrent pneumonia. Patients typically present with fever, cough, and chest pain. In occasional patients, hemoptysis may be present. Congestive cardiac failure, cyanosis, and digital clubbing may be present in patients who have a significant systemic arterial-to-pulmonary arterial shunt.

Extralobar sequestrations are usually diagnosed in the neonatal period in infants with other congenital abnormalities. Much less commonly, these lesions can present with respiratory distress in an otherwise normal newborn. Infection of the sequestered lobe can occur, especially if there is a communication with the gastrointestinal tract.

Diagnosis

Sequestrations are usually first detected on a plain chest radiograph. They appear as a solid mass or cystic structure on the plain film. It is difficult to differentiate extralobar from an intralobar sequestration on a plain chest radiograph, but an extralobar sequestration is more often seen as a solid lesion whereas an intralobar sequestration more often appears as a cystic lesion.

Definitive diagnosis of a sequestration is made by demonstration of a systemic vessel leading to the mass. A chest CT scan with contrast can reveal the presence of the systemic feeding vessel to the sequestration (Figure 3-13). Although a CT scan is less invasive, it is also a less reliable procedure than an angiogram in identifying the vessel[37].

Since a pulmonary angiogram or an aortogram can delineate both small and large vessels feeding the sequestration, it has the best success rate in making the definitive diagnosis of a sequestration[25,31,37,42-44].

MRI is much less invasive than an angiogram or aortogram and has a good success rate, especially when the feeding vessels are large and arise directly from the aorta[45]. However, 15% of smaller vessels may be missed during imaging with CT or MRI.

Differential Diagnosis

1. Post-infectious pneumatoceles: Air-filled pulmonary sequestrations may be confused with post-infectious pneumatoceles. Sequestration is more likely to persist on serial imaging studies, while post-infectious

Table 3-3 Characteristics of Pulmonary Sequestration

Characteristics	Extralobar	Intralobar
Incidence	Rare	Uncommon
Gender	Male > female	Male = female
Pleural covering	Separate from the lung	Same as the lung
Arterial supply	Systemic	Pulmonary artery/systemic
Venous drainage	Systemic	Pulmonary vein/systemic
Communication with tracheobronchial tree	A small patent opening may be present	Does not communicate with the airway
Associated anomalies	50% (30% associated with diaphragmatic hernia)	Isolated
Age at presentation	Usually neonatal	Adolescent/young adult
Clinical features	Respiratory difficulty	Recurrent lung infections

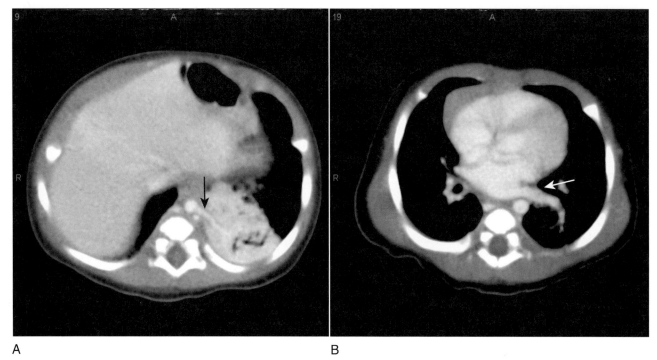

A   B

Figure 3-13 Contrast-enhanced CT scans of a pulmonary sequestration in the left lower lobe of a 5-week-old infant. (**A**) The lesion has arterial feeders from the aorta (arrow) and peripheral cystic components are present. (**B**) There is a large draining vein emptying into the left inferior pulmonary vein (arrow). (Images courtesy of Avrum Pollock, M.D., FRCPC.)

pneumatoceles regress over time. The presence of a feeding vessel originating from the systemic blood supply to the lesion confirms a sequestration.

2. Diaphragmatic hernia: The loops of bowel in the chest cavity may be confused with an air-filled sequestration. An upper gastrointestinal series with contrast or a barium enema can help differentiate between the two entities. Extralobar sequestrations, however, are often associated with diaphragmatic hernias.

3. CCAM should be ruled out in cases of air-filled sequestration, although CCAM is usually multicystic and only rarely appears as a unilocular cyst.

4. Bronchogenic cyst: A bronchogenic cyst may be difficult to distinguish from a sequestration; again, presence of systemic blood supply confirms a sequestration. A thoracic CT scan may also reveal a stalk connecting a bronchogenic cyst with the tracheobronchial tree.

5. Pulmonary arteriovenous malformation (AVM): A pulmonary AVM also appears as a solid structure with systemic arterialization; however, the clinical manifestations of AVM are distinct from that of a pulmonary sequestration. Patients with pulmonary AVM typically present with dyspnea, exercise intolerance, cyanosis, clubbing, and an

unremarkable cardiac examination. Polycythemia, with a hematocrit of 60–80%, and low arterial oxygen saturation occur because of an intrapulmonary right-to-left shunt. A bruit may be present over the lesion. Since it is a vascular abnormality, a pulmonary AVM may appear as a pulsatile lesion on fluoroscopy and it can decrease in size during a Valsalva maneuver.

Treatment

Excision of the sequestration is recommended in all cases. In cases of extralobar sequestration, the lesion may be removed completely since the pleural covering is separate from the rest of the lung. A lobectomy may be required for removal of an intralobar sequestration, since the sequestered lobe shares the same pleural covering as the rest of the normal lung[43].

Prognosis

The prognosis is excellent if there are no associated abnormalities. Risk of bleeding from accidental severing of the systemic artery is the commonest cause of intraoperative mortality[7]. If pulmonary sequestration is left untreated, there is a risk of recurrent serious infection.

Vascular Rings

Vascular rings usually occur as anomalies of the aortic arch. Although many variations from normal develop-

	Table 3-4	Vascular Rings producing Tracheal and Esophageal Compression	

Type of Vascular Ring	Tracheal Compression	Esophageal Compression
Double aortic arch	+	+
Right aortic arch with ductus arteriosus	+	+
Left aortic arch with ductus arteriosus	+	+
Anomalous innominate artery	+	−
Aberrant subclavian artery	−	+

ment of the arch have been reported, only a few distinct patterns produce tracheal and esophageal compression (Table 3-4). The double aortic arch is the most common vascular ring. In this condition, both the fourth branchial arch and dorsal aortic root persist on both sides, so that a tight ring of vascular structures is formed around the trachea and esophagus (Figures 3-14).

A right-sided aortic arch with persistent left ductus arteriosus or ligamentum arteriosum from the descending aorta also results in the formation of a complete vascular ring. In this situation, persistence of the right fourth branchial vessel results in compression of the trachea anteriorly. The persistent left ductus or ligamentum, which now runs behind the esophagus, results in the formation of a circular ring around the trachea and esophagus producing symptoms of both tracheal and esophageal compression.

An anomalous innominate artery does not represent a vascular ring, but it produces direct anterior pressure on the tracheal wall. In this situation, the origin of the innominate artery arises to the left of its normal position. It must traverse the anterior trachea to reach its

destination, and in so doing can produce tracheal compression. The aberrant right subclavian artery does not cross over the trachea and so does not produce any respiratory symptoms. It does, however, cause constriction of the posterior esophageal wall as it courses behind the esophagus and can produce dysphagia. A pulmonary artery sling is the least common of all vascular rings. Here the left pulmonary artery arises from the right pulmonary artery. In order to reach the left lung, it must cross over the right main bronchus, the left main bronchus, and the esophagus. In so doing, it can cause compression of one or more of these structures. It usually does not cause any esophageal compression.

Clinically, patients with a double aortic arch anomaly and right aortic arch with ligamentum arteriosum present early, from 2 to 9 months of age. Earlier presentation correlates with a greater degree of compression of the trachea or esophagus. Thus, presenting symptoms include respiratory distress, tachypnea, stridor or cyanosis. Because the esophagus is included in the ring, feeding intolerance or dysphagia is often present. Symptoms worsen with an intercurrent infection, during feeds, and with crying. Flexion of the neck can also worsen respiratory symptoms.

The presence of the vascular ring typically causes compression of the tracheoesophageal complex resulting in obstruction to airflow especially during exhalation. Esophageal distension from feeding and swallowing can further compress the trachea and exacerbate its narrowing[17]. Thus, double aortic arch, right-sided aortic arch with persistent left ductus arteriosus from the descending aorta, and left aortic arch with right persistent ductus arteriosus from the descending aorta present early. In contrast, children with anomalous innominate artery present later, and patients with right aberrant subclavian artery may be completely asymptomatic, or have only dysphagia. A syndrome of reflex apnea has been

Figure 3-14 Various anomalies of the aortic arch and pulmonary artery. (**A**) Normal left arch. (**B**) Double aortic arch. (**C**) Right aortic arch with aberrant subclavian artery. (**D**) Right aortic arch with mirror-image branching and left ductus arteriosus. (**E**) Left aortic arch with aberrant right subclavian artery with left ductus arteriosus. (**F**) Left pulmonary artery arising from right pulmonary artery (pulmonary artery sling). A, aorta; LC, left common carotid artery; L Ductus, left ductus arteriosus; LPA, left pulmonary artery; LS, left subclavian artery; L Arch, left aortic arch; PT, pulmonary arterial trunk; RC, right common carotid artery; RPA, right pulmonary artery; RS, right subclavian artery; R Arch, right aortic arch. (From Valletta EA, et al. Tracheoesophageal compression due to congenital vascular anomalies [vascular rings]. Pediatr Pulmonol 1997;24:93-105. ©1997 John Wiley & Sons, Inc. Reprinted with permission of Wiley-Liss, Inc., a subsidiary of John Wiley & Sons, Inc.)

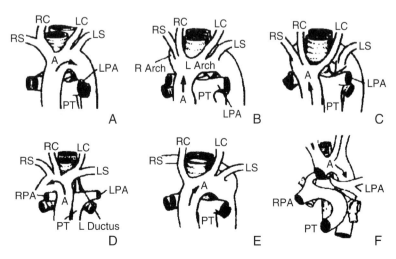

described especially in patients with double aortic arch and anomalous innominate artery[46]. This is thought to be a reflex respiratory arrest initiated by irritation of the area of tracheal compression by a bolus of food or pooling of secretions[47].

Diagnosis

Plain chest films may show well-aerated or even hyperinflated lungs, pneumonia or scattered atelectasis. If present, a right-sided aortic arch can be detected on a plain chest radiograph. Other clues on an anteroposterior film include a midline trachea and disappearance of the air shadow of the distal trachea and main carina because of the overlying vascular ring. The lateral chest radiograph shows narrowing or anterior buckling of the trachea just above the carina (Figure 3-15).

The contrast esophagogram (barium swallow) is traditionally the most helpful study to detect a vascular ring. A normal esophagogram effectively rules out a vascular ring of a magnitude significant enough to cause respiratory compromise. An anterior indentation of the esophagus is pathognomonic for a pulmonary artery sling, and a double lateral indentation of the esophagus and trachea at the same level is typical of a double aortic arch (Figure 3-16). The aberrant subclavian appears as a fixed posterior esophageal indentation. The anomalous innominate artery cannot be detected by the contrast esophagogram.

Bronchoscopy demonstrates a posterolateral pulsatile mass in cases of double aortic arch (Figure 3-17). A right anterolateral pulsatile compression approximately 2 cm proximal to the main carina is typical for an anomalous innominate artery. Here, the diagnosis is confirmed by compressing the vessel with the bronchoscope and noting the disappearance of the right radial artery pulse. Angiography helps define vascular anatomy, especially small vessels that may not be readily seen on an aortogram. Thoracic CT with contrast and MRI, however, have become the diagnostic imaging modalities of choice for vascular rings (Figure 3-18). They are less invasive than an angiogram and allow

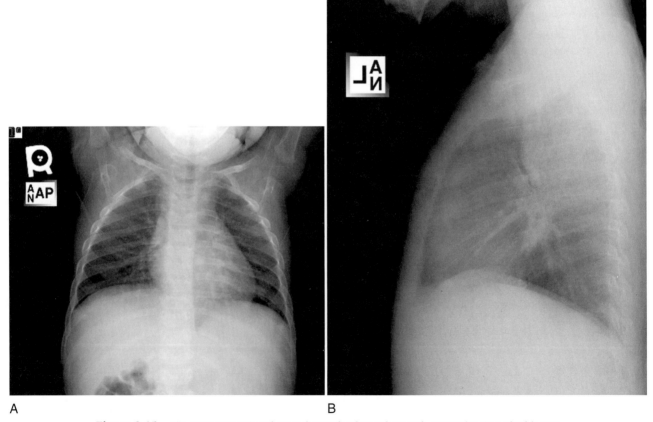

A   B

Figure 3-15 (**A**) Anteroposterior chest radiograph of an infant with a vascular ring (double aortic arch). The trachea is deviated to the right by the right-sided aortic arch, so that it is positioned in the midline. There is loss of definition of the distal tracheal air column and main carina because of the overlying vascular ring. (**B**) Lateral chest radiograph demonstrates anterior buckling of the tracheal air column resulting from the vascular ring. (Images courtesy of Avrum Pollock, M.D., FRCPC.)

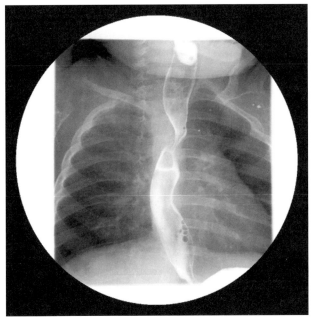

Figure 3-16 Anteroposterior view of a barium esophagogram, demonstrating bilateral lateral indentations of the esophagus at the same level, typical of a double aortic arch. (Image courtesy of Avrum Pollock, M.D., FRCPC.)

good visualization of the airways and the esophagus. A ligamentum arteriosum and the atretic part of the aortic arch will not be well visualized, but can be inferred. Both modalities can be used to provide three-dimensional reconstruction of the airway.

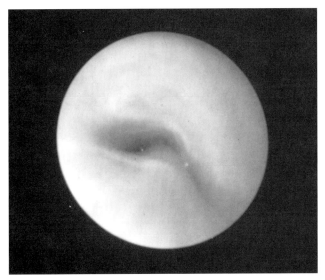

Figure 3-17 Endoscopic image of a double aortic arch. The main carina cannot be visualized clearly because of the pulsatile compressions of the anterior tracheal walls. There is also invagination of the posterior membrane, further narrowing the airway lumen. (Image courtesy of Howard Panitch, M.D.)

Differential Diagnosis

Lesions that produce wheezing along with dysphagia include:

1. Mediastinal tumors, if they compress the tracheoesophageal complex. These can be ruled out by a plain chest radiograph or CT scan.
2. Retained foreign bodies produce symptoms of tracheal obstruction. The plain chest radiograph may demonstrate an area of atelectasis or unilateral hyperlucent lung that fails to empty on a lateral decubitus film. Bronchoscopy confirms the diagnosis in the absence of a significant choking history and when the chest radiograph is normal.
3. TEF without esophageal atresia may also produce similar clinical symptoms. A barium swallow can show a fistulous tract or presence of barium in the airway in case of a TEF. In contrast, fixed indentations on the barium esophagogram point towards a vascular ring.
4. Tracheal stenosis should also be considered as a cause of bi-phasic central airway noise. Thoracic CT scan with three-dimensional reconstruction can define the stenosis. Direct visualization with a flexible bronchoscope confirms the diagnosis of stenosis. Non-invasive studies to confirm this diagnosis include radiographs of the chest and lateral neck.
5. Tracheomalacia without vascular compression can present in a similar manner. Direct visualization of the airway is often necessary to distinguish this dynamic cause of airway obstruction from other fixed lesions.

Management

Surgical ligation and takedown of the ring is standard. In cases of a double aortic arch the division of the smaller arch, which is usually the anterior one, is performed and provides relief of symptoms. In cases involving a right aortic arch with ligamentum arteriosum, the ligamentum is divided and that provides relief of symptoms. In patients with anomalous innominate artery, surgery may be necessary in 10% of cases.

Prognosis

The mortality and morbidity with surgical intervention is low. Relief of symptoms following surgery is usually immediate. The most commonly seen postoperative problem results from residual tracheomalacia, especially following surgery for double aortic arch. Tracheomalacia frequently persists for months to years after surgery.

In untreated cases death may occur suddenly because of airway compression or sepsis.

Pulmonary Lymphangiectasis

Pulmonary lymphangiectasis is a rare condition involving congenital dilatation of pulmonary lymphatics.

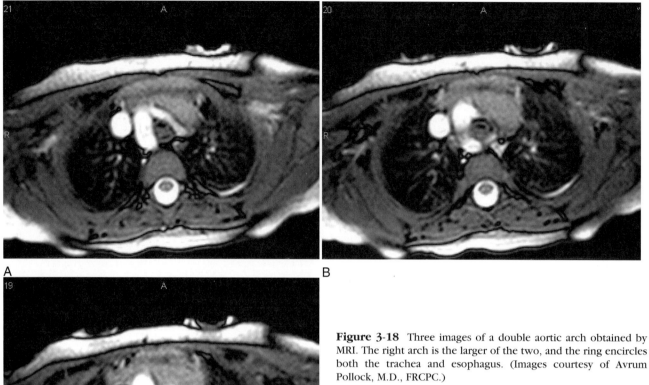

Figure 3-18 Three images of a double aortic arch obtained by MRI. The right arch is the larger of the two, and the ring encircles both the trachea and esophagus. (Images courtesy of Avrum Pollock, M.D., FRCPC.)

It is seen more commonly in males than females, and it is usually lethal. Familial occurrence has been reported. Three different types of pulmonary lymphangiectasis have been recognized:

1. Generalized lymphangiectasia. This is the rarest type of lymphangiectasis. Both pulmonary and intestinal involvement as well as hemihypertrophy have been reported with this form. Involvement of lungs may also be seen as part of a syndrome of generalized angiomatosis predominantly involving the bones.

2. Lymphangiectasia in association with congenital heart disease occurs when pulmonary venous obstruction causes obstruction of lymph flow. The most commonly associated congenital heart disease is total anomalous pulmonary venous return (TAPVR). An association with hypoplastic left heart

syndrome, atrioventricular canal, and other septal defects has also been reported.

3. Lymphangiectasia can occur as an isolated pulmonary abnormality where there is no associated heart abnormality.

The lungs in this case are bulky and the subpleural surface has a dense network of lymphatic vessels. On histologic examination, the lung parenchyma is riddled with dilated lymphatic vessels and increased connective tissue in the perivascular, interlobular, and sub-pleural areas. Other congenital defects such as urogenital malformations, facial anomalies, and asplenia have also been reported to occur in association with pulmonary lymphangiectasis.

Most patients with isolated pulmonary lymphangiectasis present soon after birth with severe respiratory distress and usually do not survive for more than 2 weeks. Those with associated congenital heart disease present

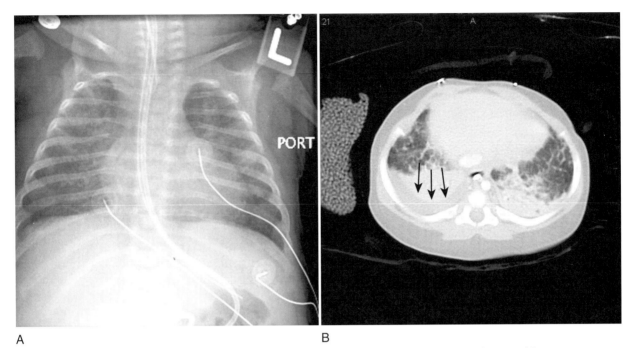

Figure 3-19   (A) Anteroposterior chest radiograph of an infant with Noonan syndrome and lymphangiectasis. There is a fine reticular pattern present in both lungs. (B) Chest CT image of the same patient. In addition to intraparenchymal linear densities related to abnormal lymphatics, bilateral dependent atelectasis is present. There is a pleural effusion in the right hemithorax (arrows). Analysis of the fluid was consistent with a chylous effusion. (Images courtesy of Avrum Pollock, M.D., FRCPC, and Howard Panitch, M.D.)

somewhat later. Here, respiratory difficulty is thought to be secondary to decreased compliance of the lung, and blood gas analysis reveals low oxygen content and carbon dioxide retention supporting hypoventilation.

Pulmonary involvement is usually less severe in patients with systemic lymphangiectasis and angiomatosis, and long-term survival has been reported in these patients.

Diagnosis

The chest radiograph demonstrates a non-specific reticular pattern with small areas of atelectasis or areas of patchy infiltration (Figure 3-19). Lung biopsy is diagnostic.

Differential Diagnosis

Disorders that present early in life and cause prominence of the interstitium on the chest radiograph must be considered.

1. Meconium aspiration syndrome is usually seen in term or post-term infants who have undergone extreme perinatal stress. Infants have a history of fetal hypoxia, and pulmonary hypertension with persistence of the fetal circulation is common. Meconium is passed before delivery, staining the amniotic fluid. Often, thick meconium is also aspirated, adding to respiratory compromise.

2. Hyaline membrane disease or neonatal respiratory distress syndrome is usually seen in premature infants and is the result of surfactant deficiency. The infant demonstrates respiratory distress and the chest radiograph has a typical "ground-glass" appearance with low lung volumes, reflecting the low compliance of the lungs. Respiratory distress typically resolves or improves over the first week of life.

3. Neonatal pneumonia: The clinical picture is very similar and the chest radiograph findings are non-specific.

4. Veno-occlusive disease can also cause prominence of the pulmonary interstitium and respiratory compromise. Obstructed veins can occasionally be detected by echocardiogram, but a cardiac catheterization is diagnostic.

Diagnosis

Lung biopsy is diagnostic.

Management

Severe cases are uniformly fatal. Atrial septostomy has been tried in cases with pulmonary venous obstruction. No specific treatment is known.

MAJOR POINTS

1. Congenital abnormalities form an important group of disorders that cause respiratory problems in infants and children.
2. Though easy to spot on a radiograph, they are hard to differentiate without further testing.
3. Abnormalities that affect airway number result from defects that occur within the first 16 weeks of gestation.
4. Lung sequestration and CCAM occur most commonly in the lower lobes.
5. Congenital lobar emphysema occurs most commonly in the upper lobes.
6. Congenital abnormalities of the lung are frequently associated with other extra-pulmonary congenital abnormalities.

REFERENCES

1. Lim FY, Crombleholme TM, Hedrick HL, Flake AW, Johnson MP, Howell LJ, Adzick NS. Congenital high airway obstruction syndrome: natural history and management. J Pediatr Surg 38:940-945, 2003.
2. Davis S, Jones M, Kisling J, Angelicchio C, Tepper RS. Effect of continuous positive airway pressure on forced expiratory flows in infants with tracheomalacia. Am J Respir Crit Care Med 158:148-152, 1998.
3. Panitch HB, Allen JL, Alpert BE, Schidlow DV. Effects of CPAP on lung mechanics in infants with acquired tracheobronchomalacia. Am J Respir Crit Care Med 150:1341-1346, 1994.
4. Zinman R. Tracheal stenting improves airway mechanics in infants with tracheobronchomalacia. Pediatr Pulmonol 19:275-281,1995.
5. Panitch HB, Keklikian EN, Motley RA, Wolfson MR, Schidlow DV. Effect of altering smooth muscle tone on maximal expiratory flows in patients with tracheomalacia. Pediatr Pulmonol 9:170-176, 1990.
6. Ein SH, Freidberg J. Esophageal atresia and tracheoesophageal fistula. Review and update. Otolaryngol Clin North Am 14:219-249, 1981.
7. Lierl M. Congenital abnormalities. In: Pediatric respiratory disease, diagnosis and treatment, 1st edition, pp 457-498. Philadelphia: WB Saunders, 1993.
8. Daum R. Postoperative complications following operation for oesophageal atresia and tracheo-oesophageal fistula. Prog Pediatr Surg 1:209-237, 1970.
9. Hicks LM, Mansfield PB. Esophageal atresia and tracheoesophageal fistula. Review of thirteen years' experience. J Thorac Cardiovasc Surg 81:358-363, 1981.
10. Orringer MB, Kirsh MM, Sloan H. Long-term esophageal function following repair of esophageal atresia. Ann Surg 186:436-443, 1977.
11. Holder TM, Ashcraft KW. Developments in the care of patients with esophageal atresia and tracheoesophageal fistula. Surg Clin North Am 61:1051-1061, 1981
12. Booth JB, Berry CL. Unilateral pulmonary agenesis. Arch Dis Child 42:361-374, 1967.
13. Keslar P, Newman B, Oh KS. Radiographic manifestations of anomalies of the lung. Radiol Clin North Am 29:255-270, 1991.
14. Markowitz RI, Frederick W, Rosenfield NS, Seashore JH, Duray PH. Single, mediastinal, unilobar lung: a rare form of subtotal pulmonary agenesis. Pediatr Radiol 17:269-272, 1987.
15. Maltz DL, Nadas AS. Agenesis of the lung. Presentation of eight new cases and review of the literature. Pediatrics 42:175-188, 1968.
16. Eraklis AJ, Griscom NT, McGovern JB. Bronchogenic cysts of the mediastinum in infancy. N Engl J Med 281:1150-1155, 1969.
17. Krummel TM. Congenital malformations of the lung. In: Disorders of the respiratory tract in children, 6th edition, pp 287-316. Philadelphia: WB Saunders, 1998.
18. Frenckner B, Freyschuss U. Pulmonary function after lobectomy for congenital lobar emphysema and congenital cystic adenomatoid malformation. A follow-up study. Scand J Thorac Cardiovasc Surg 16:293-298, 1982.
19. McBride JT, Wohl ME, Strieder DJ, Jackson AC, Morton JR, Zwerdling RG, Griscom NT, Treves S, Williams AJ, Schuster S. Lung growth and airway function after lobectomy in infancy for congenital lobar emphysema. J Clin Invest 66:962-970, 1980.
20. Tapper D, Schuster S, McBride J, Eraklis A, Wohl ME, Williams A, Reid L. Polyalveolar lobe: anatomic and physiologic parameters and their relationship to congenital lobar emphysema. J Pediatr Surg 15:931-937, 1980.
21. De Muth GR, Sloan H. Congenital lobar emphysema: long term effects and sequelae in treated cases. Surgery 59:601-607, 1966.
22. Eigen H, Lemen RJ, Waring WW. Congenital lobar emphysema: long-term evaluation of surgically and conservatively treated children. Am Rev Respir Dis 113:823-831, 1976.
23. Stewart B, Cochran A, Iglesia K, Speights VO, Ruff T. Unusual case of stridor and wheeze in an infant: tracheal bronchogenic cyst. Pediatr Pulmonol 34:320-323, 2002.
24. Ribet ME, Copin MC, Gosselin BH. Bronchogenic cysts of the lung. Ann Thorac Surg 61:1636-1640, 1996.
25. Bailey PV, Tracy T Jr, Connors RH, deMello D, Lewis JE, Weber TR. Congenital bronchopulmonary malformations. Diagnostic and therapeutic considerations. J Thorac Cardiovasc Surg 99:597-602, 1990.
26. Di Lorenzo M, Collin PP, Vaillancourt R, Duranceau A. Bronchogenic cysts. J Pediatr Surg 24:988-991, 1989.
27. Koval JC, Joseph SG, Schaefer PS, Tenholder MF. Fiberoptic bronchoscopy combined with selective bronchography. A simplified technique. Chest 91:776-778, 1987.

28. Stocker JT, Madewell JE, Drake RM. Congenital cystic adenomatoid malformation of the lung. Classification and morphologic spectrum. Hum Pathol 8:155-171, 1977.

29. Walker J, Cudmore RE. Respiratory problems and cystic adenomatoid malformation of lung. Arch Dis Child 65: 649-650, 1990.

30. Kwittken J, Reiner L. Congenital cystic adenomatoid malformation of the lung. Pediatrics 30:759-768, 1962.

31. Silverman FN. Caffey's pediatric diagnosis, 8th edition, pp 1135-1153. Chicago: Year Book Medical Publishers, 1985.

32. Wesenberg RL. The newborn chest, pp 187-198. Hagerstown: Harper and Row, 1973.

33. Wolf SA, Hertzler JH, Philippart AI. Cystic adenomatoid dysplasia of the lung. J Pediatr Surg 15:925-930, 1980.

34. Adzick NS, Harrison MR, Glick PL, Golbus MS, Anderson RL, Mahony BS, Callen PW, Hirsch JH, Luthy DA, Filly RA, et al. Fetal cystic adenomatoid malformation: prenatal diagnosis and natural history. J Pediatr Surg 20:483-488, 1985.

35. Adzick NS, Harrison MR. Management of the fetus with a cystic adenomatoid malformation. World J Surg 17:342-349, 1993.

36. Duncombe GJ, Dickinson JE, Kikiros CS. Prenatal diagnosis and management of congenital cystic adenomatoid malformation of the lung. Am J Obstet Gynecol 187:950-954, 2002.

37. Haddon MJ, Bowen A. Bronchopulmonary and neurenteric forms of foregut anomalies. Imaging for diagnosis and management. Radiol Clin North Am 29:241-254, 1999.

38. Shamji FM, Sachs HJ, Perkins DG. Cystic disease of the lungs. Surg Clin North Am 68:581-620, 1988.

39. Ueda K, Gruppo R, Unger F, Martin L, Bove K. Rhabdomyosarcoma of lung arising in congenital cystic adenomatoid malformation. Cancer 40:383-388, 1977.

40. Bolande RB, Schneider AF, Boggs JD. Infantile lobar emphysema. AMA Arch Pathol 61:289-294, 1956.

41. Franken EA Jr, Buehl I. Infantile lobar emphysema. Report of two cases with unusual roentgenographic manifestation. Am J Roentgenol Radium Ther Nucl Med 98: 354-357, 1966.

42. Hoeffel JC, Bernard C. Pulmonary sequestration of the upper lobe in children. Radiology 160:513-514, 1986.

43. Piccione W Jr, Burt ME. Pulmonary sequestration in the neonate. Chest 97:244-246, 1990.

44. Savic B, Birtel FJ, Tholen W, Funke HD, Knoche R. Lung sequestration: report of seven cases and review of 540 published cases. Thorax 34:96-101, 1979.

45. Naidich DP, Rumancik WM, Lefleur RS, Estioko MR, Brown SM. Intralobar pulmonary sequestration: MR evaluation. J Comput Assist Tomogr 11:531-533, 1987.

46. Ardito JM, Ossoff RH, Tucker GF Jr, DeLeon SY. Innominate artery compression of the trachea in infants with reflex apnea. Ann Otol Rhinol Laryngol 89:401-405, 1980.

47. Fearon B, Shortreed R. Tracheobronchial compression by congenital cardiovascular anomalies in children: syndrome of apnea. Ann Otol Rhinol Laryngol 72:949-969, 1963.

CHAPTER 4

Bronchopulmonary Dysplasia (Chronic Lung Disease of Infancy)

CARLOS SABOGAL, M.D.

ISAAC TALMACIU, M.D.

The terms bronchopulmonary dysplasia (BPD) and chronic lung disease of infancy (CLDI) are often used synonymously to describe the chronic respiratory disorders primarily associated with premature birth and its therapy. BPD was initially described in 1967 by Northway et al.[1] as a condition seen in premature infants with severe respiratory distress syndrome of the newborn (RDS) treated with mechanical ventilation and supplemental oxygen who subsequently developed clinical, radiologic, and pathologic alterations.

Since the 1960s, there have been many advances in the treatment of neonatal respiratory diseases. These develop-

ments have changed the pattern of BPD presentation and prognosis. Extremely premature infants with severe lung disease now survive more frequently than when BPD was originally described. New definitions and name changes have come up over time, and now the condition is also known as CLDI. In general, the diagnosis of BPD is well defined and is based on clearly distinct criteria. In contrast, CLDI remains a more vague expression that encompasses any long-term pulmonary complication associated with preterm birth and, in some cases, with full-term infants whose course was complicated by perinatal infections, congenital heart disease, aspiration, or other pulmonary insults. This chapter will predominantly focus on BPD.

DEFINITION

The initial definition of BPD used by Northway et al.[1] consisted of a radiologic description in premature infants who had required prolonged mechanical ventilation. Their description included four successive radiographic stages: (1) RDS (1–3 days of life); (2) opacification of both lungs (4–10 days); (3) small rounded bilateral radiolucencies (10–20 days); and (4) enlarged areas of radiolucency together with strands of radiodensity (>30 days).

Bancalari et al.[2] proposed a different definition of BPD which included respiratory failure in the neonatal period requiring assisted ventilation for at least 3 days, followed by persistent respiratory symptoms and oxygen dependence by 28 days of life, in addition to the characteristic radiographic changes described previously.

Over time, with the improved survival of very premature infants, it was noted that many infants who had respiratory symptoms and oxygen dependence at 28 days of life had minimal pulmonary problems and had been weaned to ambient air by the time they were being discharged from the hospital. Shennan et al.[3] generated a new definition that took into account a history of mechanical ventilation in premature infants who remained oxygen-dependent and had radiographic abnormalities at 36 weeks postconceptional age (PCA), rather than at 28 days of life.

More recently, a workshop organized by the National Institute of Child Health and Human Development, the National Heart, Lung and Blood Institute, and the Office of Rare Diseases agreed to retain the name of BPD in order to distinguish this condition clearly from other causes of chronic lung disease of later life[4]. It also proposed a new severity-oriented definition of BPD (Table 4-1). Common criteria for all groups include persistent symptoms of respiratory disease and treatment with supplemental oxygen for at least 28 days. Radiographic abnormalities were felt to be non-contributory to the resolution of this newer definition. Other diagnostic criteria differ for preterm infants less than 32 weeks gestational age (GA) and for those with a GA of 32 weeks and more. For the former group, BPD is defined as: (a) mild, if the infant is breathing room air at 36 weeks PCA, (b) moderate, if the infant is breathing <30% O_2 at 36 weeks PCA, or (c) severe, if the infant requires ≥30% O_2 or positive-pressure ventilation at 36 weeks PCA. For the latter group, BPD severity is based on the oxygen requirement at 56 days of life in a manner similar to that previously explained. Since these newer definitions rely greatly on the persistence of a supplemental oxygen requirement at specific ages, they are limited as they do not provide a precise target for either arterial partial pressure of oxygen (PaO_2) or oxygen saturation (SpO_2). According to the workshop summary, extensive validation is needed to determine whether this BPD definition is superior to prior ones.

INCIDENCE

The incidence of infants who develop BPD is closely related to birthweight and gestational age, as well as the definition of BPD used. There is also variability in the incidence of BPD depending on the reporting institution, since there are no consistent criteria for oxygen supplementation among different neonatal intensive care units. For example, in 1998 the reported incidence of BPD in treated infants with RDS weighing more than 1000 g at Stanford University Medical Center was 18%, and in treated infants weighing less than 1000 g it was 78%[5]. In the Midlands region of England, for infants born at <32 weeks gestation and requiring mechanical ventilation, the rate of BPD remained constant at approximately 40–45% during the 1990s[6].

BPD becomes a more frequent complication as gestational age and birthweight decrease (Table 4-2). The newer definition in which infants are assessed at 36 weeks PCA has undoubtedly decreased the percentage of infants diagnosed with BPD, but the increased number of survivors has counterbalanced this so that the number of patients with BPD has remained relatively constant, with an estimated 3000–7000 new cases each year in the United States.

Table 4-1 Definition of Bronchopulmonary Dysplasia: Diagnostic Criteria

	Gestational Age	
	<32 weeks	**≥32 weeks**
Time point of assessment	36 weeks PMA or discharge to home, whichever comes first	>28 days but <56 days postnatal age or discharge to home, whichever comes first
	Treatment with O_2 >21% for at least 28 days **PLUS**	Treatment with O_2 >21% for at least 28 days **PLUS**
Mild BPD	Breathing room air at 36 weeks PMA or discharge, whichever comes first	Breathing room air by 56 days postnatal age or discharge, whichever comes first
Moderate BPD	Need[a] for <30% O_2 at 36 weeks PMA or discharge, whichever comes first	Need[a] for <30% O_2 at 56 days postnatal age or discharge, whichever comes first
Severe BPD	Need[a] for ≥30% O_2 and/or positive pressure (PPV or NCPAP) at 36 weeks PMA or discharge, whichever comes first	Need[a] for ≥30% O_2 and/or positive pressure (PPV or NCPAP) at 56 days postnatal age or discharge, whichever comes first

(From Jobe AH, Bancalari E. NICHD/NHLBI/ORD workshop summary on bronchopulmonary dysplasia. Am J Respir Crit Care Med, 163:1723, 2001.)
Abbreviations: NCPAP, nasal continuous positive airway pressure; PMA, postmenstrual age; PPV, positive-pressure ventilation.
[a]A physiologic test confirming the oxygen requirement at the assessment time point remains to be defined. This assessment may include a pulse oximetry saturation range.

Table 4-2 Percent of Surviving Infants with BPD in Different Birthweight Groups

Birthweight (g)	O$_2$ Dependence at 28 Days Postnatal Age[35]	O$_2$ Dependence at 36 Weeks PMA for Infant Born <32 weeks[36]
<750	90-100%	54%
750-999	50-70%	33%
1000-1249	30-60%	20%
1250-1499	6-40%	10%

(From Fernandez-Nievas F, Chernick V. Bronchopulmonary dysplasia. Clin Pediatr 41:77, 2002.)

The incidence of BPD appears to be higher in white and male infants[7]. Others have reported a higher incidence of atopic disorders in families of infants with BPD. One study found that a family history of asthma is associated with increased severity of BPD.

PATHOGENESIS

Multiple factors contribute to the pathogenesis of BPD, and most likely act additively or synergistically to cause lung injury. In the pre-surfactant era, "old" or "classic" BPD seemed to be caused primarily by oxidant- and ventilation-mediated damage to the immature lung[4]. Advances in neonatal care have led to changes in the risk factors and pathogenesis of "new" BPD, as well as the extent and type of pulmonary damage encountered.

Oxygen Toxicity

Elevated concentrations of oxygen cause the release of oxygen radical species that can directly injure endothelial and epithelial cells. Endothelial cells are particularly vulnerable to injury, which leads to increased microvascular permeability and development of acute pulmonary edema. Protein leak from edema inhibits the surface-tension-lowering properties of surfactant, thus exacerbating the underlying surfactant deficiency. This acute phase of alveolar damage is followed by a marked proliferative reaction[7]. Long-term exposure to high concentrations of oxygen causes recruitment and activation of lung neutrophils and macrophages, necrosis of type I pneumocytes, hyperplasia of type II cells, and marked proliferation of fibroblasts in the lung interstitium. Since premature infants have lower levels of antioxidant enzymes such as catalase, peroxidase, and superoxide dismutase, they are much more vulnerable to oxygen toxicity.

Positive-Pressure Ventilation

Barotrauma and volutrauma secondary to stretching of the immature lung were strongly associated with the pathogenesis of the "old" BPD. The pathologic lesions of BPD are found even when premature animals are exposed to mechanical ventilation without simultaneous exposure to high levels of supplemental oxygen.

In the presence of low lung compliance, the highly compliant tracheobronchial tree is preferentially distended, leading to distortion of the distal airways. As a result of cyclic bronchiolar stretching, there is terminal airway ischemia and necrosis, followed by pulmonary interstitial emphysema and air leaks that complicate the clinical picture in many patients with BPD[8]. This is associated with maldistribution of ventilation, which results in some areas of the lung being overdistended and others poorly ventilated.

It appears that lung stretch (volutrauma) is the real offender for the damage caused by positive-pressure ventilation. Studies have shown that the newborn lung can tolerate high levels of positive pressure without significant damage if lung stretch is prevented.

With progress in neonatal care that includes antenatal steroids, surfactant treatment, and less aggressive ventilation strategies, the pattern and pathogenesis of BPD has changed. Presently, large premature infants rarely develop BPD, whereas it is a common complication in infants weighing <1 kg who do not appear to have severe lung disease soon after birth. The "new" BPD may be primarily an arrest of lung development[9], resulting in alveolar simplification and "dysmorphic" vascular growth.

Both prenatal and postnatal risk factors probably contribute to the aberration in lung development seen in BPD. Infants dying of BPD have fewer and larger alveoli with less striking fibrosis and inflammation than in the past[10]. The lungs at 24-28 weeks of gestation are in the late canalicular stage or in the early saccular stage. At this time, lung volume and surface area increase considerably secondary to septation and alveolarization. Parallel increases in vascular growth are closely synchronized with alveolarization, but the molecular signals that link distal airspace growth with angiogenesis have not been completely identified.

Research has focused on understanding the regulation of septation and alveolarization. In experimental models, hyperoxia, hypoxia, glucocorticoid treatment, and poor nutrition decrease septation.

Glucocorticoids

The effects of glucocorticoids on the preterm lung are complex because they can interfere with alveolarization while at the same time they induce both the surfactant system and structural maturation by thinning the mesenchyme. Their effects depend on timing during development, dose and other factors. The glucocorticoid-induced inhibition of alveolarization can be blocked in newborn rats with retinoic acid.

Inflammation and Infection

It is known that inflammation is essential to the development of BPD. Multiple proinflammatory and chemotactic factors are found in the lungs of ventilated premature infants, and are present in higher concentrations in infants who go on to develop BPD. Overexpression of cytokines such as tumor necrosis factor-α (TNF-α), pulmonary transforming growth factor-β (TGF-β), interleukins (IL)-6 and 11 results in lungs with fewer and larger alveoli. Infants exposed to prenatal infection or colonization with *Ureaplasma urealyticum* have proinflammatory cytokines in their lungs at the time of delivery and are at a higher risk of developing BPD[11]. Studies in infants exposed to chorioamnionitis have shown that there is a diminished incidence of RDS but increased risk for BPD[12]. Apparently, preterm lungs exposed to inflammatory mediators seem to mature faster but at the same time are more sensitive to exposure to other noxious agents, such as oxygen and mechanical ventilation.

Neutrophils are important in initiating and perpetuating the inflammatory response. The appearance of granulocytes in alveolar washes correlates with pulmonary edema and early lung injury. Proteases, such as elastase, produced by activated neutrophils in the lungs, may contribute to the progression to lung damage.

Nutrition

Animal models have shown that alveolar development is negatively affected by reducing food to the mother and to the progeny. Early nutrition provided to preterm infants may lack important factors that are needed for lung growth, repair and protection against injury.

Vitamin A and E deficiency have been found to lead to hypoplastic alveolar regions. Some studies have shown that administration of parenteral vitamin A may reduce the incidence and severity of BPD[13,14].

Vascular Hypothesis

Recently, a vascular hypothesis for the development of BPD has been proposed. Studies have shown that the lungs of deceased BPD infants have reduced vascular endothelial growth factor (VEGF) mRNA and protein expression, as well as reduced numbers of VEGF receptors[15]. Tracheal VEGF levels are lower in infants with BPD than in premature infants without BPD[16]. VEGF is a potent endothelial-cell-specific mitogen and survival factor that stimulates angiogenesis, and its impaired signaling may contribute to the vascular pathology of BPD. It has been speculated that inhibition of vascular growth itself may directly impair alveolarization, as angiogenesis may be necessary for alveolarization during normal lung development.

In summary, very early preterm birth, together with exposure to positive-pressure ventilation and supplemental oxygen, interferes with normal signaling for lung development, specifically for alveolarization, vascular development, or both. Antenatal and/or early postnatal inflammation appears to aggravate the adverse effects on lung development (Figure 4-1).

CLINICAL MANIFESTATIONS

History

The usual history of BPD is that of a premature infant who develops RDS and associated hyaline membrane disease (HMD). These infants are generally intubated and placed on mechanical ventilation. Before the introduction of surfactant, these infants required long periods of

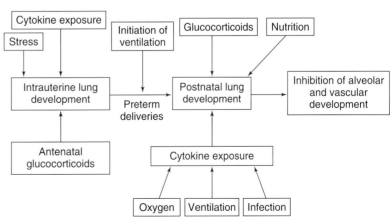

Figure 4-1 Pathogenesis of the new BPD in very low birthweight infants. (From Jobe AJ. The new BPD: an arrest of lung development. Pediatr Res 46:641–643, 1999.)

high positive pressures and oxygen concentrations in order to be adequately ventilated and oxygenated. These factors were the main risk factors for the "old" BPD.

Since the beginning of the 1990s, routine administration of surfactant has meant that infants with RDS improve significantly and can be weaned to minimal ventilatory pressures and low concentrations of oxygen. This period, which may be referred to as a "honeymoon period," usually lasts from several days to a few weeks. Older premature babies usually do not go on to develop chronic pulmonary complications.

Another group of infants, usually younger and smaller premature babies (extremely very low birthweight or EVLBW; birthweight <1000 g) or those with a more convoluted clinical course, are likely to develop complications in the neonatal intensive care unit including apnea, viral or bacterial infections such as pneumonia and/or sepsis, persistence of the ductus arteriosus (PDA) or reopening of a previously closed ductus with secondary heart failure, among other problems. These complications affect the clinical course of preterm infants with secondary deterioration of their respiratory status. Consequently, many of these babies require longer periods of ventilatory support and oxygen supplementation that produce further damage to their immature pulmonary architecture and favor the development of BPD[13,17]. This description applies to the "new" BPD, the type commonly seen nowadays in the post-surfactant era.

Infants with BPD can have multiple problems due to primary and secondary factors. The most common pulmonary complications seen in these infants include atelectasis interspersed with areas of emphysema. Pulmonary interstitial emphysema and other air leaks, including pneumothorax and pneumomediastinum, may develop in relation to increased pulmonary stiffness. Increased airway collapsibility, especially tracheomalacia and bronchomalacia, aggravates airway narrowing and is seen more commonly in these infants compared with those who do not require positive-pressure ventilation in the neonatal period. Pneumonias, which can be viral, bacterial or fungal, may occasionally be associated with secondary sepsis.

In some infants with BPD, right-sided heart failure and pulmonary hypertension become significant problems. All these factors aggravate oxygenation and ventilation, mainly due to ventilation–perfusion mismatch. Very severe cases can also present with aortopulmonary anastomoses due to chronic hypoxemia[14].

Once these babies are discharged from the neonatal intensive care unit they continue to have a higher incidence of pulmonary and non-pulmonary complications. Exacerbations of respiratory symptoms are common in infants with BPD. Potentially the most serious exacerbating factor is viral infection. Viruses such as respiratory syncytial virus (RSV), influenza and adenovirus can be particularly devastating, leading to hospitalization, respiratory failure and further damage to the pulmonary parenchyma. Recurrent wheezing episodes are common. There are reports of a higher incidence of sudden infant death syndrome (SIDS) and apparent life-threatening events (ALTE) among infants with BPD[18].

Non-pulmonary complications found in infants with BPD include gastroesophageal reflux (GER), aspiration, and failure-to-thrive (FTT). GER is common in these infants and may present with obvious vomiting and spitting up, poor feeding, and irritability. It may also cause anemia, hematemesis, esophageal stricture, laryngospasm, stridor, chronic nasal discharge, apnea and ALTE.

FTT may occur as a consequence of behavioral feeding problems, swallowing disorders, GER, chronic or intermittent hypoxemia, heart failure, and elevated metabolic rates. Feeding problems include oral aversion, given that many of these infants remain intubated and receive orogastric or nasogastric feedings for prolonged periods of time due to their underlying prematurity and associated diseases. Resting metabolic expenditure, estimated through measurements of oxygen consumption and indirect calorimetry, appears to be higher in infants with BPD than in age-matched full-term healthy controls. It is important to note that increased work of breathing only partially accounts for this finding and other mechanisms may act to elevate the metabolic expenditure of BPD infants.[19]

Heart failure is common in infants with BPD. Exacerbations caused by cardiac failure may present in a similar way to those caused by infection. Poor feeding, tachypnea, increased oxygen requirements, and inappropriate weight gain may be present. Hepatomegaly is typical of right-sided heart failure. Cyanotic spells are sometimes seen in these babies due to different reasons, such as tracheobronchomalacia, GER, apnea, or cardiovascular problems.

Neurodevelopmental problems are also found among infants with BPD. Developmental delay affects primarily motor, speech, and feeding maturity and appears to be worse in infants treated with dexamethasone, as recently stated by the American Academy of Pediatrics (AAP) Neonatal Committee[20]. Hearing abnormalities have also been found to be more prevalent among infants with BPD. A recent study showed that at 8–12 months of corrected age, 22.1% of infants with BPD had persistent conductive hearing loss compared with 7.7% of non-BPD control infants with a similar gestational age[21]. Other conditions seen in infants with BPD include hernias and retinopathy of prematurity.

Physical Examination

The initial physical examination shows a preterm newborn with RDS: tachypneic with nasal flaring, intercostal retractions, grunting, and irregular respirations with frequent apneas and cyanosis, requiring immediate ventilatory assistance. At this point, the auscultatory findings may include coarse breath sounds with crackles and poor air exchange. The infant's clinical status usually improves after intubation and surfactant administration.

This initial respiratory distress improves with the above-mentioned treatment. After this period, the lung auscultation usually normalizes or some crackles can be heard due to pulmonary edema. Cardiovascular auscultation can reveal a continuous murmur from a PDA. Bounding pulses and wide systolic–diastolic pressure differential are typical findings of a PDA. This PDA can make pulmonary edema worse and at the same time put the baby at higher risk of developing heart failure[13]. The time that the infant stays intubated is variable, usually longer for younger premature babies and those with associated medical complications.

After extubation, many infants persist with tachypnea, intercostal retractions and hypoxemia. On lung auscultation, rhonchi and "Velcro-type" dry crackles are common. Wheezing may be heard during acute respiratory exacerbations, usually triggered by viral infections. Infants with moderate-to-severe BPD usually require oxygen supplementation to keep them normoxemic.

As mentioned previously, pulmonary hypertension and cor pulmonale can be seen in severe cases of BPD. These babies can present with signs of hypoxemia, pulmonary edema, and right ventricular failure. Physical signs include an increased loudness of the second heart sound especially over the pulmonary valve area, hepatomegaly, and fluid retention.

As mentioned before, FTT is seen in some patients with BPD. Weight, length and, in severe cases, head circumference, fall below the 5th percentile for age, even when age is corrected for prematurity. With adequate nutritional support, most infants exhibit catch-up during the first 2 years of life.

Pulmonary Function Testing

BPD produces inflammation and secondary scarring of the lungs affecting its structure and therefore its physiology. Performing pulmonary function testing allows the clinician to characterize these changes and follow their progression over time.

Lung mechanics during tidal breathing have been extensively studied in infants with BPD, usually using sedation with chloral hydrate. Respiratory system compliance is low in the first months of life, a reflection of lung stiffness, whereas resistance is high, an indication of airway obstruction. Both compliance and resistance approach the range of normalcy by 2 years of age[22].

Lung volumes measured by helium dilution or nitrogen washout may underestimate functional residual capacity

(FRC) and are reported to be low in the first 6 months of age, progressing to normal values by 12 months. Lung volumes measured by plethysmography are higher than normal, suggesting air trapping. The ratio of residual volume to total lung capacity (RV/TLC) remains significantly increased at 1 year of age in infants with severe BPD[9], and hyperinflation continues to be a common finding in adolescents with a history of BPD. Partial forced expiratory flow–volume curves obtained by the chest squeeze technique in infants with BPD are clearly abnormal with expiratory flow limitation, as reflected by low values for maximal flow at FRC ($\dot{V}_{max}$FRC) (Figure 4-2)[23]. This expiratory flow limitation does not improve as fast as other parameters, with decreased values still common by 2 years of age[22].

Airway hyperreactivity, as defined by increased responsiveness to a bronchoconstrictor challenge or

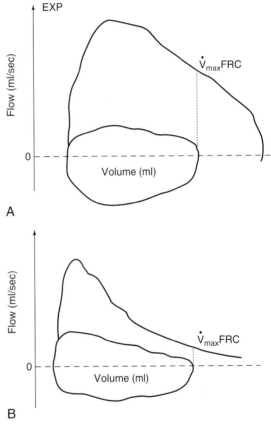

Figure 4-2 Partial expiratory flow–volume curves. The smaller inner curve represents tidal breathing, and the larger curve represents maximal expiratory flow generated by the rapid compression technique. Maximal expiratory flow at functional residual capacity ($\dot{V}_{max}$FRC) is indicated by the dashed line. The difference between tidal breathing and maximal expiratory flow represents expiratory flow reserve. **(A)** Normal control infant has a convex to linear maximal expiratory flow–volume curve, with large expiratory flow reserve. **(B)** Infant with BPD has a concave flow–volume curve, with decreased expiratory flow reserve and $\dot{V}_{max}$FRC, compared with **A**. (From Tepper RS, Morgan WJ, Cota K, et al. Expiratory flow limitation in infants with bronchopulmonary dysplasia. J Pediatr 109:1040–1046, 1986.)

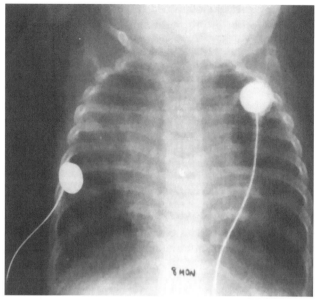

Figure 4-3 Chest radiograph characteristic of stage IV BPD that shows hyperlucency in both bases with strands of radiodensity in the upper lung fields. (From Bancalari E, et al. In Fanaroff AA, Martin RJ, editors: Neonatal-perinatal medicine: diseases of the fetus and infant. St. Louis: Mosby, 1997.)

bronchodilator therapy, is frequently found in BPD infants. Bronchial hyperreactivity may be caused by airway inflammation, altered neurogenic responses, altered maturational responses of airway smooth muscle, and genetic factors. Increased airway reactivity persists in older children and adolescents with a history of BPD.

Radiology

When Northway described the first cases of BPD he clearly showed four different radiological stages that evolved over time[1]. This sequence is no longer seen, mainly due to the use of early surfactant therapy and improvement in ventilatory management.

The first stage is still seen and is characterized by a reticular, granular pattern with ground-glass appearance, associated with air bronchograms and decreased lung volumes. This stage is classically observed in the acute phase of HMD. The second stage was characterized by dense non-specific parenchymal opacification, indistinguishable from pulmonary edema and/or pulmonary hemorrhage. The third stage, rarely seen nowadays, was called the "bubble-like pattern", characterized by cystic-like lesions more noticeable in the upper lobes. Stage four was characterized by hyperlucency in both bases with increased radiopacity in the upper lobes. This last stage is reserved today for infants with severe BPD and, fortunately, is rarely seen[2] (Figure 4-3).

It is more common now to see stage I and, after surfactant administration, clearance of the chest radiograph (Figure 4-4). After some time with mechanical ventilatory support or oxygen supplementation, some radiographic findings start to appear, characteristically as a hazy appearance of both lungs[13] (Figure 4-5).

Several radiographic classifications have been proposed since the introduction of surfactant. The Weinstein score is one of these, which establishes six

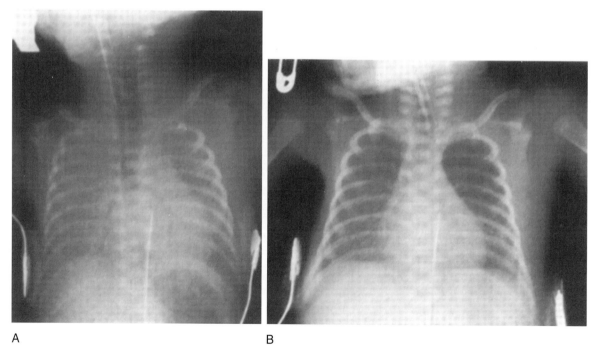

A   B

Figure 4-4 Chest radiographs of an infant with HMD, with ground-glass appearance before (**A**) and marked improvement after (**B**) administration of exogenous surfactant. (From Taussig LM, Landau LI. Pediatric respiratory medicine. St. Louis: Mosby, 1999.)

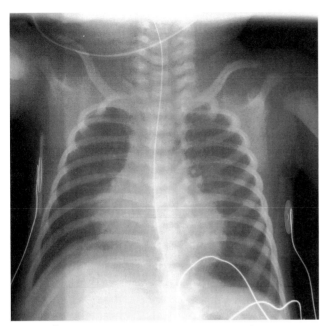

Figure 4-5 Chest radiograph of an infant with "new" BPD. Haziness in both lung fields is noted.

different grades of radiographic abnormalities in BPD[24]. The most benign is grade 1, characterized by faint, not well-defined opacities, which give a hazy appearance to the lung. The most severe is grade 6, characterized by cystic and opaque areas giving the lung a "bubble-like" appearance. In between these grades, gradual appearance of more dense opacities with cystic changes is progressively appreciated.

There are some conditions that can radiographically mimic BPD and should be considered in the differential diagnosis. The most important are: surfactant protein deficiency (more commonly seen in term babies with RDS with a protracted course), Wilson-Mikity syndrome (rarely seen these days), pneumonia, congenital heart disease, pulmonary lymphangiectasis, interstitial lung disease, and aspiration syndromes[14] (Box 4-1).

Studies using high-resolution computed tomography have become a useful auxiliary test. They can provide more detailed information of the actual airway size and

wall thickness, and show hyperinflation caused by gas trapping. At the same time, they reveal the structure of the pulmonary interstitium and provide information on the degree of edema and/or fibrosis affecting the lungs[4].

Other radiology tests frequently ordered in infants with BPD are gastrointestinal studies, especially in babies who have frequent vomiting, FTT, apnea, cyanotic spells, or ALTEs. An upper gastrointestinal series with barium contrast assesses the swallowing mechanism, as well as the anatomy of the esophagus, stomach, and the upper portion of the intestine. It is helpful in the evaluation of swallowing dysfunction, GER, and anatomic abnormalities such as H-type tracheoesophageal fistula and intestinal malrotation. GER nuclear scans can be useful in the diagnosis of GER and aspiration secondary to this condition. More detailed information regarding possible swallowing dysfunction is obtained with video swallowing studies performed fluoroscopically in the presence of a speech therapist.

Laboratory Tests (Box 4-2)

Arterial Blood Gases (ABGs)
Full ABG measurement is most likely to be indicated during the early phase of severe BPD with respiratory failure or during an acute exacerbation. In the early phase, the infant with RDS has respiratory acidosis with

---

Box 4-1 Some Differential Diagnoses of BPD

Pneumonia
Congenital heart disease with pulmonary edema
Surfactant protein deficiency
Wilson-Mikity syndrome
Pulmonary lymphangiectasia
Interstitial lung disease
Aspiration

Box 4-2 Radiology and Laboratory Tests in BPD

Radiology
Acute: Hyaline membrane disease (HMD)
Chronic ("old" BPD): four stages
  HMD
  Dense parenchymal opacification
  Bubble like pattern
  Hyperlucency of bases with radiopacity of the apices
Chronic ("new" BPD): Bilateral haziness of both lungs
Chest CT scan: Evaluates airway and interstitium
Laboratory tests
  Arterial blood gas (ABG) and electrolytes:
    Early: Respiratory acidosis, hypoxemia
    Chronic: Metabolic alkalosis with ↓ Na⁺, ↓ K⁺, ↓ Cl⁻ with use of diuretics
Electrocardiogram (ECG)
  Hypertrophies (i.e., RVH)
  Rhythm disturbances
Echocardiogram
  Congenital heart disease
  PDA
  Pulmonary hypertension
  Other acquired systemic-pulmonary anastomoses

CO_2 retention and hypoxemia, which improve with surfactant administration, oxygen supplementation and ventilatory support. In the infant with established BPD, ABGs may demonstrate CO_2 retention and compensatory metabolic alkalosis with elevated serum bicarbonate (HCO_3^-). In some children, a primary metabolic alkalosis may be present as well, with pH in the normal or slightly alkalotic range. This might result from the use of diuretics, or the presence of heart failure with a low cardiac output state and hyperaldosteronemia. In both cases, the metabolic alkalosis occurs because of volume contraction and depletion of potassium and chloride.

Electrolytes

Electrolyte disturbances are usually caused by the use of diuretics such as furosemide and, to a lesser degree, thiazides. They produce hyponatremia, hypokalemia, and hypochloremia, as well as metabolic alkalosis with elevated serum bicarbonate. Potassium-sparing diuretics and potassium chloride supplements are used to prevent hypokalemia and metabolic alkalosis. Loop diuretics also cause hypercalciuria, which can lead to nephrocalcinosis, increased bone resorption, osteopenia, and rickets.

Electrocardiogram (ECG)

The ECG is a useful tool in the evaluation of associated cardiovascular disease. It provides information about ventricular hypertrophies, rhythm disturbances and, indirectly, pulmonary hypertension (right ventricular hypertrophy and pulmonary "p" wave).

Echocardiogram

This diagnostic test has become very useful and is used almost routinely in premature babies to rule out congenital cardiac disease or a PDA that will require immediate medical care. It is a non-invasive test that supplies information about the heart's and great vessels' anatomy and function, and can provide evidence of pulmonary hypertension.

Pathology

The classical pathologic findings of BPD have changed since the introduction of surfactant for prophylaxis and treatment of RDS. In the pre-surfactant era, the pathologic findings in the lungs were more severe. The lungs had an abnormal appearance with a darker color and an irregular surface showing emphysematous changes alternating with areas of atelectasis (Figure 4-6). Microscopically, the emphysematous areas were seen as distended alveoli, alternating with atelectasis (Figure 4-7). Another finding was a diminished number of alveoli. In the large and small airways, there was evidence of inflammation with metaplasia and hyperplasia of the mucosa, associated with increased numbers of goblet cells and thickening of the basal membrane (Figure 4-8). In the pulmonary interstitium there was pulmonary edema, progressing to fibrosis in the most severe cases.

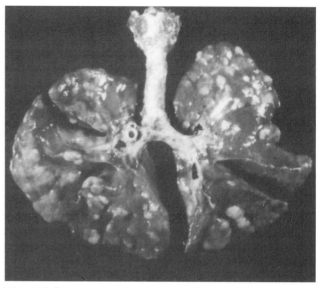

Figure 4-6   Macroscopic appearance of lungs with BPD showing uneven expansion. (From Bancalari E, et al. In Fanaroff AA, Martin RJ, editors: Neonatal-perinatal medicine: diseases of the fetus and infant. St. Louis: Mosby, 1997.)

Pathologic findings also affected the pulmonary vasculature. Pulmonary vessels presented with diminished branching, elastic degeneration, and hypertrophy of the muscular layer. Lymphatic vessels were usually dilated and tortuous. In cases of pulmonary hypertension, there was cardiomegaly with right ventricular hypertrophy (cor pulmonale).

In the post-surfactant era, there is less fibrosis and more uniform inflation of the BPD lungs. The alveoli are enlarged and significantly fewer in number, indicating an interference with septation and alveolarization. The airways, large and small, are usually free of epithelial

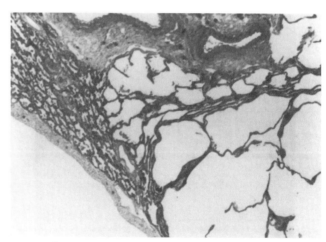

Figure 4-7   Low-magnification view showing areas of emphysema alternating with areas of partial collapse. (From Bancalari E, et al. In Fanaroff AA, Martin RJ, editors: Neonatal-perinatal medicine: diseases of the fetus and infant. St. Louis: Mosby, 1997.)

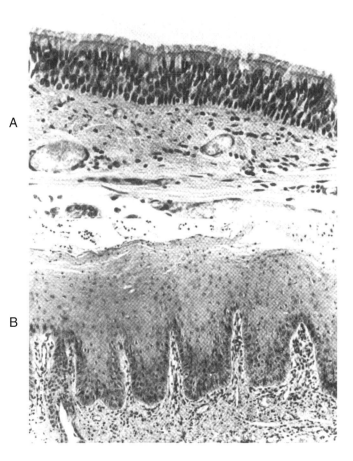

Figure 4-8   Microscopic appearance of airway metaplasia. (**A**) Photomicrograph showing normal ciliated respiratory epithelium. (Hematoxylin–eosin, ×240.) (**B**) Photomicrograph showing mature, keratinizing, stratified squamous epithelium that is markedly thickened from infant with BPD. (Hematoxylin–eosin, ×100.) (From Taussig LM, Landau LI. Pediatric respiratory medicine. St. Louis: Mosby, 1999.)

metaplasia and smooth muscle hypertrophy. In the interstitium, there is an increase in elastic tissue that is proportionate to the severity and duration of the respiratory disease. Finally, a decrease in the pulmonary microvasculature is also noted. More information is needed about the progression of lung injury in survivors of the "new" BPD[4].

TREATMENT

In addition to chronic respiratory disease, infants with BPD may have significant growth, nutritional, neurodevelopmental and cardiovascular problems. The following discussion on clinical management is directed primarily towards the outpatient care of infants and older children with BPD (Box 4-3).

Oxygen Therapy

Patients with BPD have chronic alveolar hypoxia and hypoxemia secondary to ventilation–perfusion ($\dot{V}/\dot{Q}$) mismatch. Over time, chronic hypoxemia leads to altered lung vascular development and an increased response to vasoactive agents that ultimately causes an irreversible increase in pulmonary vascular resistance.

If hypoxemia is left uncorrected, pulmonary hypertension and cor pulmonale develop. Therefore, the risks of uncorrected hypoxemia in patients with BPD are pulmonary hypertension and right ventricular hypertrophy and failure, as well as slow somatic growth and developmental delay.

Box 4-3   The Most Common Therapeutic Modalities for Management of BPD

Oxygen supplementation: if necessary to keep $SpO_2 \geq 92\text{-}95\%$

Diuretics: furosemide, thiazides and/or potassium-sparing diuretics, for patients with recurrent pulmonary edema

Inhaled bronchodilators: β_2-agonists indicated if clinical evidence of reversible airway obstruction

Anti-inflammatory therapy: no definitive benefits of inhaled corticosteroids at this time

Nutrition: maintain caloric intake at 120-140 cal/kg/day

Prevention of intercurrent viral illnesses: RSV prophylaxis, influenza vaccine

Decreased oxygen supply may suppress appetite and increase metabolic demands through neurohumoral stimulation.

Currently, supplemental oxygen is provided to children with BPD by nasal cannula in order to maintain arterial oxyhemoglobin saturation (SpO_2) ≥ 92-95% as measured by pulse oximetry, when the infant is awake, asleep and during feeds. If there is clinical or echocardiographic evidence of pulmonary hypertension, SpO_2 should be kept at a minimum of 95-96% to prevent progression of the condition. These therapeutic ranges are partly based on clinical experience and partly on data from cardiac catheterization studies. Most of the decline in pulmonary vascular resistance with supplemental oxygen occurs with correction of hypoxemia; higher concentrations of inspired oxygen generally do not cause further improvement. Selected patients, however, respond better to higher SpO_2 ($\geq 95\%$), suggesting that higher target oxygen saturations may improve clinical outcome in some infants[25].

Pulse oximetry is used to measure oxygen saturation while the child is quiet and awake. Once oxygen has been weaned to low-flow supplementation ($\frac{1}{8}$-$\frac{1}{16}$ liter per minute or less), this measurement should be done every 2-4 weeks after the patient has been on ambient air for 10 minutes, and if SpO_2 is $\geq 92\%$, oxygen may be discontinued during wakefulness. At first, oxygen therapy is discontinued while the child is awake, since SpO_2 tends to be lower during sleep than wakefulness. SpO_2 needs to be assessed during sleep before complete discontinuation of supplemental oxygen. During the weaning process, it is important to ensure that the infant has normal SpO_2 during feeding and activities; if not, the maintenance dose of oxygen may be too low, the infant may have episodic pulmonary hypertension with transient right-to-left shunting of blood, or other conditions previously mentioned such as GER or airway malacia may exist.

If somatic growth rate slows down or stops in the weeks after discontinuation of oxygen therapy, this may indicate significant intermittent hypoxemia, for which oxygen supplementation should be restarted. If the need for supplemental oxygen rises or fails to decrease during the first few months after discharge from the neonatal intensive care unit, coexisting conditions that may worsen BPD should be excluded, including uncontrolled reactive airways disease, GER and aspiration, congenital heart disease and airway anomalies.

Diuretic Therapy

The role of diuretics in the management of BPD has been extensively reviewed. Although the exact mechanisms by which diuretic therapy improves pulmonary function are incompletely understood, there are data to support the notion that the beneficial effects of diuretics are probably a combination of diuresis and local pulmonary effects[26].

Most infants with established BPD do not have a need for diuretics. Short-term diuretic treatment may be beneficial for infants with established BPD and acute fluid overload. Long-term diuretic therapy is used in infants with more severe BPD, especially those with recurrent pulmonary edema whose pulmonary disease has demonstrated a favorable response to diuretics.

The most frequently used diuretic in the acute phase is furosemide (1 mg/kg/dose IV or IM, or 1-2 mg/kg per dose PO). This drug causes an increase in pulmonary compliance, as well as a fall in resistance and supplemental oxygen requirement. For chronic care, the most frequently used diuretics are furosemide on alternate days or thiazides in combination with spironolactone. Use of a thiazide–spironolactone combination has also been shown to improve pulmonary compliance, with less striking decline in resistance and oxygen requirement when compared with furosemide.

Extended diuretic therapy may produce two serious complications. One includes electrolyte imbalance, volume contraction and metabolic alkalosis, which are treated with supplementation with potassium chloride (KCl) and/or dose adjustments. Although sodium chloride (NaCl) supplements are occasionally used to correct the hyponatremia caused by aggressive diuresis, this therapy seems counterproductive because it leads to fluid retention. The other complication, seen with furosemide, is hypercalciuria with secondary hyperparathyroidism and nephrocalcinosis. The diagnosis of nephrocalcinosis is established by finding echogenic areas during renal ultrasonography. Some clinicians prefer alternate-day therapy with furosemide since it is associated with sustained improvement in lung mechanics without causing alterations in serum electrolytes or high urinary calcium losses. Other practitioners favor thiazide diuretics over furosemide to help reduce urinary calcium losses.

There is no standard weaning process for diuretic therapy. Most clinicians merely allow infants to "outgrow" their therapy and withdraw it when the dose has fallen below the accepted therapeutic range.

Inhaled Bronchodilators

Most infants with CLDI have intermittent wheezing and proof of expiratory airflow limitation on infant pulmonary function testing. Studies have shown that β-agonists produce short-term improvement in pulmonary mechanics in parameters such as respiratory system compliance and airway resistance. It is reasonable to treat infants with BPD who demonstrate clinical evidence of reversible airway obstruction with inhaled β_2-agonists.

The use of β₂-agonists may be associated with potential complications, such as simultaneous induction of pulmonary vasodilation. Prolonged therapy with high doses of β₂-agonists may increase pulmonary blood flow to underventilated lung units, thus aggravating $\dot{V}/\dot{Q}$ mismatch and hypoxemia. Secondly, β₂-agonists may increase airway instability in infants with tracheomalacia. Increased airway smooth muscle tone is necessary in infants with tracheomalacia in order to maintain stability of the large airways. β₂-agonists cause relaxation of the smooth muscle, which may lead to increased collapsibility of the affected airway. This occurrence could explain why inhaled bronchodilators have variable effects on pulmonary mechanics in infants with BPD. Therefore, effectiveness of β-adrenergic therapy for BPD infants needs to be carefully determined on an individual basis. Dysrhythmias and hypokalemia have also been reported with frequent administration of inhaled albuterol.

Atropine and ipratropium bromide have also been studied in infants with BPD. Short-term improvement in pulmonary function has been documented with both medications. There is weak evidence for synergy between β-agonists and anticholinergic agents.

The appropriate dose and means of administration of bronchodilators have not been determined. Deposition of medication into the lower airways depends on inspiratory flow rate, particle size, distance of the nebulizer from the face, and type of spacer and inhaler used. It appears that in infants not mechanically ventilated, all methods of delivery are fairly inefficient.

Anti-inflammatory Therapy

The rationale for the use of anti-inflammatory agents in infants at risk for developing BPD is based on the recognition of the role of lung inflammation in the pathogenesis of BPD. Corticosteroids are the most carefully studied anti-inflammatory agents in the prevention and treatment of BPD.

It has been shown that late administration of high doses of systemic corticosteroids in infants at risk for developing BPD reduces the duration of mechanical ventilation and temporarily improves lung mechanics. However, long-term benefits in terms of duration of oxygen therapy and length of hospitalization have not been demonstrated. When steroids are administered earlier in the course of RDS (as early as day 1 of life), total duration of mechanical ventilation and oxygen may be reduced, as well as the incidence of severe BPD, without a clear influence on mortality[27].

The use of systemic corticosteroids in premature infants is associated with significant side effects such as adrenal suppression, gastrointestinal perforation, hypertrophic cardiomyopathy, somatic growth failure, delayed development of the central nervous system,

higher rate of infections, systemic hypertension, hyperglycemia, and bone demineralization. Long-term consequences of systemic corticosteroid use may include negative effects on neurologic development and function. Systemic glucocorticoids impair alveolar septation in animal models, leading to decreased lung surface area.

Because of the significant side effects associated with systemic steroids, several investigators have looked at the effects of inhaled corticosteroids (ICS) in infants with impending BPD. One of the main problems with this mode of treatment is the variability and difficulty in achieving drug deposition in the distal airways, especially in the presence of airway obstruction. So far, the use of ICS in infants at risk of BPD has produced some enhancement in lung mechanics and gas exchange, as well as improvement in extubation rates, without modifying the incidence or severity of BPD, mortality or long-term outcome in the treated infants[27]. The beneficial effects of ICS are slower and less striking than those of systemic corticosteroids. Likewise, the reported side effects of ICS are substantially milder, but include reversible hypertrophy of the tongue, adrenal suppression, oral candidiasis and growth impairment.

The role of non-steroidal anti-inflammatory medications in the prevention of BPD has been studied as well. Watterberg and Murphy[28] determined that in premature newborns with RDS, cromolyn sodium did not decrease the incidence or severity of BPD, defined as survival to 30 days of life without oxygen dependence. However, a more recent study showed a decline in TNF-α and IL-8 concentrations in lung lavages of infants after 7 days of aerosolized cromolyn sodium therapy in infants ≤1000 g at birth[28].

In established BPD, oral corticosteroids are used during respiratory exacerbations. ICS may be recommended for infants who have recurrent episodes of wheezing and respiratory distress responsive to bronchodilators suggestive of reactive airways disease (RAD), especially if there is a family history of asthma. The role of cromolyn sodium in the treatment of established BPD has not been adequately studied, but could be an alternative for infants with mild RAD in order to avoid the use of ICS.

Nutrition

Altered growth, nutrition, and metabolism may adversely affect the long-term outcome of infants with BPD. Infants with BPD are at risk for malnutrition, failure to thrive and delayed lung repair. Many of these infants have GER, oral aversion, and increased energy expenditure. Oxygen consumption may be increased in proportion to the severity of pulmonary disease.

Since poor nutrition can compromise the development of new alveoli, it is crucial to provide these children with aggressive nutritional support. Nutritional interventions aim to facilitate catch-up growth at a rate of at least 20–30 g/day. Thus, caloric intake should be 120–140 cal/kg/day. Commercial infant formulas with caloric densities higher than 20 cal/oz may be used to avoid excessive fluid intake and the risk of fluid overload. Further increases in caloric density (up to 30 cal/oz) can be achieved by adding medium-chain triglycerides or glucose polymers to the infant's formula. Older children with inadequate caloric intake may be given high calorie formulas such as Pediasure or Nutren Jr. Maintenance elemental iron (2 mg/kg/day) should be given to all infants and iron-deficiency anemia should be treated with 5–6 mg/kg/day. Multivitamins should be given to infants drinking less than 450 ml daily of formula and to breast-fed infants.

Poor caloric intake is often behavioral due to adverse oral stimulation from prolonged endotracheal intubation, gavage feedings and frequent suctioning. Gastrostomy tube placement may be indicated to provide adequate nourishment, while speech therapists work aggressively to resolve oral feeding problems. Fundoplication is often required with gastrostomy for GER that does not resolve with medical management.

When an infant is not gaining weight appropriately despite an adequate caloric intake, coexisting conditions that may interfere with growth and lung healing should be sought. The following should be considered:

- Persistent hypoxemia because of early termination or excessive reduction of supplemental oxygen, or poor adherence to a home oxygen therapy plan.
- Unrecognized intermittent hypoxemia (e.g., obstructive sleep apnea).
- Inadequate oxygen delivery to tissues secondary to anemia.
- Gastroesophageal reflux.
- Unsuspected cardiopulmonary abnormalities, such as congenital heart disease, tracheomalacia, vascular ring, and tracheoesophageal malformations.
- Recurrent aspiration due to swallowing dysfunction.

Prevention of Intercurrent Viral Infections

Infants with BPD have frequent respiratory exacerbations due to recurrent infections of the upper and lower respiratory tract. RSV is a frequent cause of respiratory complications during winter and early spring months in most of the United States, although in some areas such as South Florida RSV is isolated throughout the year. Other viral agents such as influenza A and B, parainfluenza, and adenovirus have also been identified as causes of acute respiratory distress in children with BPD.

In the absence of an effective RSV vaccine, alternative methods of protection have been developed. In the mid-1990s, RSV immunoglobulin (Respigam®) was introduced for infants at risk for severe lower respiratory tract infection by RSV. RSV-IVIG was given as monthly intravenous infusions (750 mg/kg or 15 ml/kg per dose) during the RSV season (November–March in the Northern Hemisphere) and it was able to reduce the number of hospitalizations, number of hospital days, and duration of stay in intensive care units attributed to RSV infections.

Towards the end of the 1990s, palivizumab, a humanized monoclonal antibody against RSV, was developed. The use of palivizumab (Synagis®) as a monthly intramuscular injection (15 mg/kg) during the RSV season resulted in a 35% reduction in RSV admissions and a 42% reduction in hospital days due to RSV disease in the treated group of infants with BPD. At this time, palivizumab has replaced RSV-IVIG for RSV prophylaxis and it is recommended that infants with BPD receive it on a monthly basis during the RSV season in the first 2 years of life.

Infants with BPD 6 months and older should receive the influenza vaccine annually in the early fall months. Many clinicians recommend that parents, siblings and caretakers of these infants also receive the influenza vaccine each year. Routine immunizations should be given to infants with BPD according to their chronological age, regardless of their gestational age. The ultimate effect of prevention of RSV or influenza infections on the long-term prognosis of BPD has not been established, but should be expected to favorably impact final outcome.

In order to decrease the frequency of respiratory infections in children with BPD, advice for their families should include: avoidance of large day-care settings during the winter months, elimination of tobacco smoke exposure, deferral of elective surgical procedures to non-respiratory virus months, and close monitoring for early signs of infection.

LONG-TERM PROGNOSIS

Many of the studies that refer to long-term prognosis in infants with BPD preceded the introduction of surfactant replacement therapy. These reports do not include the EVLBW infants and, at the same time, do not reflect the impact of recent therapeutic approaches that are commonly used these days[30].

Infants who develop BPD are more prone to viral respiratory infections, particularly in the first 2 years of life. These respiratory infections can be severe and can progress to respiratory failure because of poor respiratory reserve.

As mentioned previously, one of the most detrimental respiratory infections seen in these babies is RSV. This virus can not only produce acute disease but can also lead to recurrent inflammation of the airways that can persist for years increasing the likelihood of developing asthma[31].

Reactive airway disease is more common in children with BPD, and presents with recurrent episodes of wheezing and cough, many times in association with respiratory infections.

An interesting study compared pulmonary function at 7 years of age in children with BPD, former premature children who did not have BPD and full-term children. It showed that children with BPD had significantly reduced airflows, particularly forced expiratory volume in 1 second (FEV_1), and forced expiratory flow between 25% and 75% of the vital capacity ($FEF_{25\%-75\%}$). Lung volume measurements showed an elevated residual volume/total lung capacity (RV/TLC) ratio, indicative of air trapping. When bronchodilator responsiveness was evaluated in these groups, children who had BPD had positive responses twice as often as controls. These differences remained significant even after adjustment for birthweight and gestational age[32].

Children with BPD may also have neurodevelopmental sequelae, with problems such as cerebral palsy, impaired vision and hearing, speech delay and learning disabilities. They may also exhibit impaired growth, malnutrition, higher infant mortality rate, and SIDS[8].

Further studies are necessary to determine the long-term outcome of children with the "new BPD", which would include very small premature infants treated with antenatal steroids and surfactant replacement.

PREVENTION

As discussed in the section on the pathogenesis of BPD, there are many factors that play a role in the etiology of BPD. The early recognition of these risk factors should be the main focus of prevention.

The most important risk factor for BPD is prematurity. The younger the infant in terms of gestational age, the more likely he or she is to develop BPD. The main effort should be to prolong the pregnancy as much as possible in cases of preterm labor, cooperating as much as possible with the obstetricians. The use of antenatal steroids effectively reduces the incidence and severity of HMD and reduces the risk of severe BPD. However, this approach has not effectively changed the incidence of the new forms of BPD[13].

We know that proinflammatory cytokines are likely mediators in the pathogenesis of BPD. These cytokines may be induced by many different conditions, one of which is antenatal exposure to infection (chorioamnionitis)[33]. Emphasis should be given to early recognition and treatment of these intrauterine infections, especially in mothers at risk of preterm labor.

Since Northway's original description of BPD, it was recognized that higher ventilatory pressures and oxygen concentrations lead to more severe forms of BPD.

Over time, multiple studies have evaluated different modes of ventilation and types of ventilators. Strategies such as patient-triggered ventilation, permissive hypercapnia and low tidal volume ventilation have not affected the incidence of BPD, even though some patients have been ventilated for shorter periods of time. The efficacy of high-frequency ventilation in preventing BPD still remains controversial. In contrast, use of continuous positive airway pressure (CPAP) immediately after delivery may offer some protection. In one recent study, the group of infants treated in this manner required less surfactant therapy and had a lower incidence of BPD[34]. It must also be remembered that high concentrations and prolonged use of oxygen supplementation inhibit alveolar development.

The use of surfactant replacement therapy in infants with HMD has improved the respiratory course and survival of infants with BPD. It has also changed the course of "classical" BPD, allowing the survival of EVLBW infants. At the same time, the use of surfactant has facilitated less aggressive ventilatory strategies in these infants, making barotrauma infrequent these days[13,17]. Interestingly, surfactant replacement has not decreased the overall incidence of BPD, probably because of the increased survival of EVLBW infants.

Premature infants may require fluid restriction since they are more prone to develop pulmonary edema. Aggressive treatment of a PDA is necessary since its presence can produce pulmonary edema, heart failure and diminished lung compliance. These may translate into longer courses of ventilatory support and oxygen therapy, leading to worse BPD.

Postnatal infections, specifically pneumonias and sepsis, also provoke inflammation in the lungs and worsen the underlying condition. These postnatal infections should be prevented with measures such as general hygiene, isolation, and immunizations. Prophylaxis for certain viral respiratory infections such as RSV and influenza is extremely important as discussed previously.

Adequate nutrition is fundamental in premature infants, essentially for two reasons. It provides enough calories to match the increased metabolic needs of BPD infants, and assures satisfactory somatic and pulmonary growth. It also provides important substrates for the antioxidant mechanisms to protect the lungs against oxidative injury. One of these nutrients is vitamin A, which preserves airway epithelium and promotes alveolar septation, reducing the risk of BPD. Other important antioxidant agents are vitamin E and sulfur-containing amino acids such as glutathione[13].

Postnatal use of systemic steroids, specifically dexamethasone, is no longer recommended as a routine anti-inflammatory therapy due to adverse neurologic outcomes in infants treated with them. Postnatal systemic corticosteroids to aid in weaning an infant from mechanical ventilation should be reserved for the most severe cases that remain oxygen- and ventilator-dependent for prolonged periods of time, and their use should be considered experimental[18].

In summary, BPD describes the chronic respiratory disorders primarily associated with premature birth and its therapy. Its definition, risk factors, radiologic, and pathologic features have evolved over time, mainly related to advances in the care of premature neonates. Its clinical features involve not only the respiratory system but other structures such as the cardiovascular, gastrointestinal and central nervous systems. Its treatment may include oxygen supplementation, diuretics, inhaled bronchodilators and anti-inflammatory medications. As somatic growth is associated with lung development in the first years of life, ensuring adequate nutrition is vital for the resolution of BPD. Prophylaxis against viral infections such as influenza and RSV is very important as well. BPD is unlikely to disappear until preterm delivery of EVLBW infants is prevented. A better understanding of the risk factors for BPD needs to be reached in order for physicians to be able to prevent them or, at least, more successfully treat them.

Acknowledgments

The authors thank Dr. Eduardo Bancalari for his critical review of this chapter, and Dr. Alexander Auais for his assistance with word- and image-processing technology.

MAJOR POINTS

1. Key Aspects in Pathogenesis
   "Old" BPD:
   - Prematurity
   - Oxygen toxicity
   - Positive-pressure ventilation: barotrauma/volutrauma
   "New" BPD:
   - Prematurity
   - Glucocorticoids: antenatal/postnatal
   - Inflammation/infection: chorioamnionitis
   - Nutrition
   - Fluid balance: PDA
2. Key Clinical Findings
   Respiratory:
   - Cough
   - Tachypnea and increased respiratory effort
   - Wheezing
   - Crackles
   - Hypoxemia
   - Recurrent respiratory infections
   - ALTE/SIDS

MAJOR POINTS—Cont'd

   Gastrointestinal: - GER
   - Aspiration
   - Poor feeding
   - FTT
   Cardiovascular: - Heart failure
   - Hepatomegaly
   - Pulmonary hypertension
   - Cor pulmonale
   Neurologic: - Developmental delay
   - Retinopathy of prematurity
3. Key Pathologic Findings
   Pulmonary parenchyma and airways:
   - Decreased alveolarization
   - Alternating areas of emphysema and atelectasis
   - Airway metaplasia
   - Pulmonary edema
   Pulmonary vasculature:
   - Decreased branching
   - Elastic degeneration
   - Hypertrophy of muscular layer
4. Key Treatment
   See Box 4-3
5. Key Preventive Strategies
   Prenatal:
   - Prolongation of gestation
   - Use of antenatal steroids
   - Early recognition and treatment of intrauterine infections
   Postnatal:
   - Surfactant replacement
   - Gentle ventilatory strategies
   - Fluid restriction/aggressive management of PDA
   - Adequate nutrition

REFERENCES

1. Northway WH Jr., Rosan RD, Porter DY. Pulmonary disease following respiratory therapy of hyaline membrane disease: bronchopulmonary dysplasia. N Engl J Med 276:357-368, 1967.

2. Bancalari E, Abdenour GE, Feller R, et al. Bronchopulmonary dysplasia: clinical presentation. J Pediatr 95:819-823, 1979.

3. Shennan AT, Dunn MS, Ohlsson A, et al. Abnormal pulmonary outcomes in premature infants: prediction from oxygen requirement in neonatal period. Pediatrics 82:527-532, 1988.

4. Jobe AH, Bancalari E. NICHD/NHLBI/ORF workshop summary: bronchopulmonary dysplasia. Am J Respir Crit Care Med 163:1723-1729, 2001.

5. Northway WH Jr. Bronchopulmonary dysplasia: thirty-three years later. Pediatr Pulmonol Suppl 23:5-7, 2001.

6. Field T. Trent Neonatal Survey 1999 Annual Report. University of Leicester, 2000.

7. Avery ME, Tooley WH, Keller MPH, et al. Is chronic lung disease in low birthweight infants preventable? A survey of eight centers. Pediatrics 79:26, 1987.

8. Abman SH, Groothuis JR. Pathophysiology and treatment of bronchopulmonary dysplasia: current issues. Pediatr Clin North Am 41:277-315, 1994.

9. Jacob SV, Coates AL, Lands LC, et al. Long-term sequelae of severe bronchopulmonary dysplasia. J Pediatr 133:193-200, 1998.

10. Husain NA, Siddiqui NH, Stocker JR. Pathology of arrested acinar development in postsurfactant bronchopulmonary dysplasia. Hum Pathol 29:710-717, 1998.

11. Yoon BH, Romero R, Jun JK, et al. Microbial invasion of the amniotic cavity with *Ureaplasma urealyticum* is associated with a robust host response in fetal, amniotic and maternal compartments. Am J Obstet Gynecol 179:1254-1260, 1998.

12. Watterberg K, Demers L, Scott S, et al. Chorioamnionitis and early lung inflammation in infants in whom bronchopulmonary dysplasia develops. Pediatrics 97:210-215, 1996.

13. Bancalari E. Changes in pathogenesis and prevention of chronic lung disease of prematurity. Am J Perinatol 18:1-9, 2001.

14. Fanaroff A, Martin R, editors. Neonatal-perinatal medicine, 6th edition. St. Louis: Mosby, 1997.

15. Bhatt AJ, Pryhuber GS, Huyck H, et al. Disrupted pulmonary vasculature and decreased vascular endothelial growth factor, Flt-1, and TIE-2 in human infants dying with bronchopulmonary dysplasia. Am J Respir Crit Care Med 164:1971-1980, 2001.

16. Lassus P, Turanlahti M, Heikkilä P, et al. Pulmonary vascular endothelial growth factor and Flt-1 in fetuses, in acute and chronic lung disease, and in persistent pulmonary hypertension of the newborn. Am J Respir Crit Care Med 164:1981-1987, 2001.

17. Bancalari E, Del Moral T. Bronchopulmonary dysplasia and surfactant. Biol Neonate 80 (Suppl 1):7-13, 2001.

18. Taussig LM, Landau LI, editors. Pediatric respiratory medicine, 1st edition. St. Louis: Mosby, 1999.

19. Kurzner SI, Garg M, Bautista DB, et al. Growth failure in bronchopulmonary dysplasia: elevated metabolic rates and pulmonary mechanics. J Pediatr 112:73-80, 1988.

20. American Academy of Pediatrics, Committee on Fetus and Newborn. Postnatal corticosteroids to treat or prevent chronic lung disease in preterm infants. Pediatrics 109:330-338, 2002.

21. Gray PH, Sarkar S, Young J, et al. Conductive hearing loss in preterm infants with bronchopulmonary dysplasia. J Paediatr Child Health 37:278-282, 2001.

22. Baraldi E, Filippone M, Trevisanuto D, et al. Pulmonary function until two years of life in infants with bronchopulmonary function. Am J Respir Crit Care Med 155:149-155, 1997.

23. Tepper RS, Morgan WJ, Cota, K, et al. Expiratory flow limitation in infants with bronchopulmonary dysplasia. J Pediatr 109:1040-1046, 1986.

24. Weinstein RM, Peters ME, Sadek M, et al. A new radiographic scoring system for bronchopulmonary dysplasia. Pediatr Pulmonol 18:284-289, 1994.

25. Abman SH, Wolfe RR, Accurso FJ, et al. Pulmonary vascular response to oxygen in infants with severe BPD. Pediatrics 75:80-84, 1985.

26. Rush MG, Hazinski TA. Current therapy of bronchopulmonary dysplasia. Clin Perinatol 19:563-590, 1992.

27. Bancalari E. Corticosteroids and neonatal chronic lung disease. Eur J Pediatr 157 (Suppl 1):S31-S37, 1998.

28. Watterberg KL, Murphy S. Failure of cromolyn sodium to reduce the incidence of bronchopulmonary dysplasia: a pilot study. The Neonatal Cromolyn Study Group. Pediatrics 91:803-806, 1993.

29. Viscardi RM, Hasday JD, Gumpper KF, et al. Cromolyn sodium prophylaxis inhibits pulmonary proinflammatory cytokines in infants at high risk for bronchopulmonary dysplasia. Am J Respir Crit Care Med 156:1523-1529, 1997.

30. Fernandez-Nievas F, Chernick V. Bronchopulmonary dysplasia: an update for the pediatrician. Clin Pediatr 41:77-85, 2002.

31. Stein RT, Sherrill D, Morgan WJ, et al. Respiratory syncytial virus in early life and risk of wheeze and allergy by age 13 years. Lancet 354:541-545, 1999.

32. Gross S, Ianuzzi D, Kveselis D, et al. Effect of preterm birth on pulmonary function at school age: a prospective controlled study. J Pediatr 133:188-192, 1998.

33. Jobe A, Ikegami M. Prevention of bronchopulmonary dysplasia. Curr Opin Pediatr 13:124-129, 2001.

34. Van Marter LJ, Allred EN, Pagano M, et al. Do clinical markers of barotrauma and oxygen toxicity explain interhospital variation in rates of chronic lung disease? Pediatrics 105:1194-1201, 2000.

CHAPTER 5

Sleep-Disordered Breathing in Children

RAANAN ARENS, M.D.

Sleep may bring deleterious effects to children with underlying respiratory abnormalities. The term "sleep-disordered" breathing refers to a group of respiratory disorders that are exacerbated during sleep. Important physiologic changes occur during sleep compared to wakefulness including reduced upper airway dilator muscle activity, reduced functional residual capacity (FRC), reduced chemoreceptor sensitivity, and altered arousal threshold during sleep stages. These changes can affect upper airway stability, ventilatory drive, and chest wall mechanics, and lead to immediate significant abnormalities in gas exchange and sleep architecture as well as to long-term consequences on the cardiovascular system and cognitive function.

The most prominent sleep-related breathing disorder in children is obstructive sleep apnea syndrome (OSAS), which affects up to 2% of normal children[1,2]. Other respiratory disorders exacerbated by sleep include: central apnea, hypoventilation, obstructive lung diseases, and restrictive lung diseases. This chapter will discuss the diagnosis and management and the clinical implications of these disorders in children with special emphasis on OSAS.

OBSTRUCTIVE SLEEP APNEA SYNDROME

Obstructive sleep apnea syndrome (OSAS) in children is defined as a breathing disorder characterized by recurrent events of partial or complete upper airway obstruction during sleep that result in disruption of normal ventilation and sleep patterns[3]. OSAS is most frequently diagnosed in normal children between ages 2 and 6 years with adenotonsillar hypertrophy and is sometimes referred to as primary OSAS. "Secondary OSAS" refers to other medical conditions associated with and causing OSAS. Children with secondary OSAS often have craniofacial anomalies and or neurologic disorders affecting upper airway shape, configuration, and collapsibility during sleep. OSAS in this group may present at any time from early infancy throughout childhood.

OSAS has a range of clinical presentations and may be manifested in mild through severe forms. Knowledge and recognition of childhood OSAS has a tremendous impact on child health care since, if untreated, OSAS may have profound neurobehavioral and cardiopulmonary consequences affecting a child's health and lifestyle.

OSAS is not a new disorder. Children with adenotonsillar hypertrophy associated with loud snoring, breathing pauses, and awakenings from sleep were noted in the nineteenth century by W. Hill and W. Osler. However, not until the mid-1960s with the development of polysomnography recording was there an understanding of the relationship between obstructive events during sleep and daytime symptoms in adults. About the same time several reports recognized the association between adenotonsillar hypertrophy and cor pulmonale in children. However, the first detailed description of 8 children (age 5–14 years) with adenotonsillar hypertrophy and OSAS who were diagnosed by means of nocturnal polysomnography was published by Guilleminault et al. only in 1976[4]. Since that report and with the increasing awareness about OSAS among physicians, numerous studies have been published, clearly distinguishing OSAS in children from OSAS in adults with respect to etiology and clinical manifestations (Table 5-1).

Terminology

Obstructive apnea: Absence of oronasal air flow in the presence of continued respiratory effort lasting longer than 2 respiratory cycle times. Obstructive apnea usually but not always is associated with hypoxemia (Figure 5-1).

Hypopnea: A 50% or greater decrease in the amplitude of the oronasal airflow signal often accompanied by hypoxemia or arousal. Some investigators have attempted to subtype hypopnea into obstructive and non-obstructive forms. Obstructive hypopnea is defined as a reduction in airflow without reduction in effort. On the other hand, non-obstructive hypopnea is associated with a reduction in both airflow and respiratory effort by 50% (Figure 5-2).

Central apnea: Cessation of oronasal airflow and respiratory effort lasting for longer than 2 respiratory cycle times. American Thoracic Society consensus suggests central apnea lasting longer than 20 seconds in children is abnormal (Figure 5-3).

Obstructive hypoventilation: Partial airway obstruction leading to a peak end-tidal CO_2 ($P_{ET}CO_2$) >55 mmHg

Table 5-1 Comparison of OSAS in Children and Adults		
	Children	**Adults**
Population characteristics		
Estimated prevalence	2%	1–3%
Common age at presentation	2–6 years	30–60 years
Gender	Male~Female	Male > Female
Weight	Normal, decreased, increased	Overweight
Major cause	Adenotonsillar hypertrophy	Obesity, narrow pharyngeal airway
Associated disorders	Craniofacial anomalies, neurologic disorders	Obesity, hypertension, postmenopause
Polysomnography findings		
Gas exchange abnormalities	Always	Always
Duration of obstructive apneas	Any duration is abnormal	Events >10 seconds are abnormal
Abnormal AI	>1	>5
Abnormal AHI	>5	>20
Sleep architecture	Often normal	Always altered
Movement/arousal	Occasional	Always
Complications		
Neurobehavioral	Excessive daytime sleepiness (EDS), hyperactivity Poor school performance	Severe EDS, cognitive impairment
Cardiopulmonary	Pulmonary hypertension, cor pulmonale	Systemic hypertension, arrythmias
Treatment of choice	Adenotonsillectomy	CPAP, weight reduction

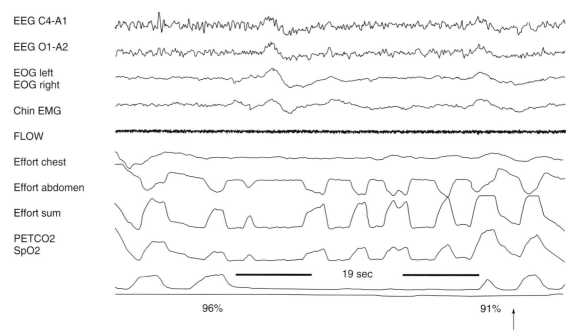

Figure 5-1 A 30 second polysomnography tracing showing an obstructive apnea lasting 19 seconds ending with arterial oxygen desaturation to 91% (arrow). Paradoxical effort continues despite a cessation of flow seen on the oronasal flow and $P_{ET}CO_2$ channels.

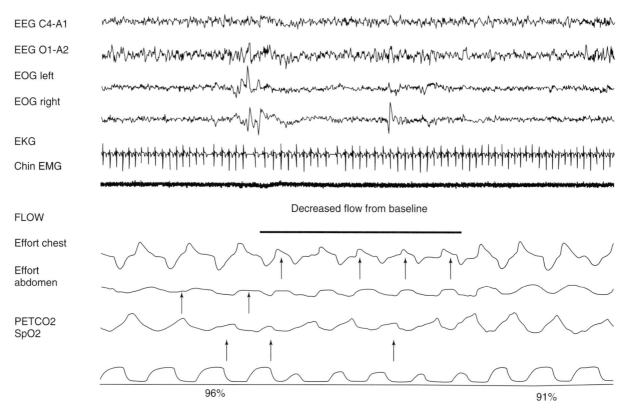

Figure 5-2 A 30 second polysomnography tracing showing an hypopnea followed by arterial oxygen desaturation. Note a 50% reduction in the oronasal flow (arrows) as well as paradoxical breathing and a significant reduction in the chest and abdomen effort channels (arrows).

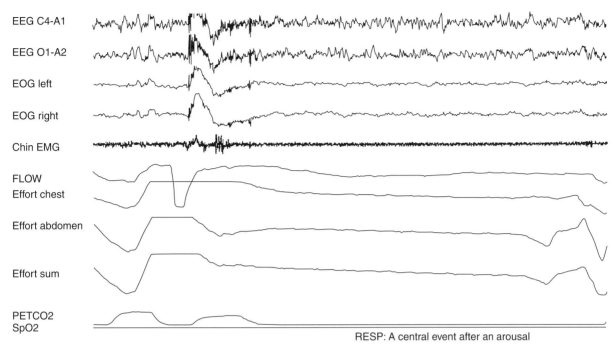

EEG C4-A1

EEG O1-A2

EOG left

EOG right

Chin EMG

FLOW
Effort chest

Effort abdomen

Effort sum

PETCO2
SpO2

RESP: A central event after an arousal

Figure 5-3   A 30 second polysomnography tracing showing a central apnea, following a sigh. Note the absence of oronasal flow and effort.

or $P_{ET}CO_2 > 45$ mmHg for more than 60% of total sleep time (TST), or $P_{ET}CO_2 > 55$ mmHg for more than 10% of TST (in the absence of lung disease).

Non-obstructive hypoventilation: Decreased minute ventilation associated with an increased $P_{ET}CO_2$ due to either a reduction in respiratory drive (central), chemoreceptor function, muscle weakness (neuromuscular), or decreased minute ventilation secondary to a reduction in chest wall movement (restrictive).

Apnea index (AI): Number of obstructive and/or central apneic events per hour of sleep.

Hypopnea index (HI): Number of hypopneas per hour of sleep.

Apnea/hypopnea index (AHI): The summation of apnea index and hypopnea index.

Primary snoring: Also known as habitual snoring, primary snoring is characterized by snoring during sleep without apnea, hypoventilation, hypoxemia, or excessive arousals.

Upper airway resistance syndrome: A respiratory disorder of sleep associated with snoring causing excessive daytime sleepiness due to arousals and sleep fragmentation[5].

Epidemiology

There are no large-scale studies in children assessing the prevalence of OSAS. In pre-school children the incidence of OSAS is estimated to be 2%[1,2], whereas primary snoring is more common and is estimated to occur in 6–9% of school-aged children[6]. OSAS occurs in children of all ages, including neonates. Underlying conditions such as craniofacial anomalies affecting the structure of the upper airway as seen in Pierre–Robin syndrome may manifest symptoms of obstruction early in the neonatal period, while later onset of symptoms may be found in obese children and therefore present in older age. However, the peak incidence of OSAS occurs between 2 and 6 years of age and parallels the prominent growth of the nasopharyngeal lymphoid tissue during these years. Recent data suggest that OSAS may be more common in children with a family history of OSAS, in African-American children, and in children with chronic upper and lower respiratory diseases[2,7]. It is not certain if gender predisposes to OSAS during childhood.

Clinical Features

Although most cases of OSAS in children are secondary to enlarged tonsils and adenoids, many other medical conditions may lead to OSAS. Some of the more common reported conditions associated with OSAS during childhood are listed in Table 5-2. Clinical features of OSAS in children can be divided into nocturnal and daytime signs and symptoms (Table 5-3).

The main physiologic disturbance involves repetitive obstructive apneas and hypopneas (partial obstructions) leading to hypoxemia, hypercapnia, acidosis, and sleep fragmentation. The short- and long-term neurologic,

Table 5-2 Medical Conditions Associated with OSAS in Children

Craniofacial syndromes
Midfacial hypoplasia
    Apert syndrome
    Crouzon syndrome
    Pfeiffer syndrome
    Treacher-Collins syndrome
Macroglossia/glossoptosis
    Down syndrome
    Beckwith-Wiedemann syndrome
    Pierre-Robin sequence
Other
    Achondroplasia
    Hallerman-Streiff syndrome
    Klippel-Feil syndrome
    Goldenhaar syndrome
    Marfan syndrome
Neurologic disorders
Cerebral palsy
Myasthenia gravis
Moebius syndrome
Arnold-Chiari malformation
Miscellaneous disorders
Obesity
Prader-Willi syndrome
Hypothyroidism
Mucopolysaccharidosis
Sickle cell disease
Choanal stenosis
Laryngomalacia
Airway papillomatosis
Subglottic stenosis
Face and neck burns
Postoperatively
Post-adenotonsillectomy in children with secondary OSAS
    and those younger than 2 years
Post-pharyngeal flap
Post-cleft lip repair

Table 5-3 Frequency of Signs and Symptoms in 23 Children with Obstructive Sleep Apnea Syndrome and in 46 Matched Controls

Sign/Symptom	OSAS Group (%)	Control Group (%)	P Value
Difficulty breathing when asleep	96	2	0.001
Snoring	96	9	0.001
Mouth-breathes when awake	87	18	0.001
Frequent upper respiratory tract infections	83	28	0.001
Stops breathing when asleep	78	5	0.001
Restless sleep	78	23	0.001
Chronic rhinorrhea	61	11	0.001
Sweating when sleeping	50	16	0.007
Recurrent middle ear diseases	43	17	0.019
Excessive daytime somnolence	33	9	0.014
Poor appetite	30	9	0.019
Frequent nausea/ vomiting	30	2	0.001
Difficulty swallowing	26	2	0.002
Pathologic shyness/ social withdrawal	22	5	0.027
Hearing problems	13	0	0.014

Modified from Brouillette et al.[9]

cardiovascular, and systemic complications found in children with OSAS are dependent on the severity and duration of these physiologic aberrations.

Nocturnal Symptoms

Breathing During Sleep

Snoring and difficulty breathing during sleep are the most common complaints of parents of children with OSAS, with reports of such symptoms in more than 96% of cases[8,9]. With the exception of young infants, children with OSAS often snore loudly and continuously. In the older child, snoring is often a low-frequency sound produced by the vibration of the soft palate and tonsillar pillars. However, in a young child (<4 years), the snoring sound may have a high-pitched quality if oversized adenoids and tonsils impede movement of the soft palate. Some children do not snore but have other forms of noisy breathing such as grunting, snorting, or gasping.

Furthermore, infants may not produce sufficient flow to produce an easily audible snoring noise. Parents often describe episodes of retractions with increased respiratory effort. At times, absence of respiratory noise despite continued vigorous breathing may be noted. These episodes may be terminated by gasping, movement, or frequent awakenings. The abnormal breathing pattern during sleep may be frightening to parents, resulting in increased vigilance on the part of the family and the perceived need to intervene in order to improve breathing.

When possible, observation of the child during sleep is recommended. Snoring and labored breathing should be noted. This is manifest by visible supraclavicular, suprasternal, and subcostal retractions. Paradoxical rib cage movement has been described as a marker of increased work of breathing. In the presence of a complete or partial upper airway obstruction, inspiratory downward motion of the diaphragm will expand the abdominal wall; however, the sudden increase in negative intrathoracic pressure will cause a paradoxical inward movement of the highly compliant rib cage of the young child.

Children with OSAS are found to have both complete and partial upper airway obstruction causing significant gas exchange abnormalities. Marcus et al.[10] studied 50 healthy children 1 to 17 years of age and found that obstructive apneas were rare and were never longer than 10 seconds, suggesting that obstructive sleep apnea of any length is abnormal in children. Partial obstruction evidenced by snoring appears to dominate the respiratory pattern in children with OSAS[11]. Partial obstruction occurs continuously or it can be interrupted by periods of silence associated with vigorous respiratory effort (obstructive apnea). Variations in esophageal pressures as low as −50 and −70 cm H_2O accompanied by significant abrupt changes in oxygenation have been reported. Although partial obstruction may not result in hypoxemia or hypercarbia in some children, Brouillette et al.[12] showed that prolonged partial airway obstruction is often associated with more severe hypoxemia and hypercarbia than short events of obstructive apnea. Similar findings were noted by Rosen et al.[12], who also reported the more frequent occurrences of partial obstruction compared with complete obstructive events in 36 children with OSAS.

Children with OSAS may have other abnormal breathing patterns in addition to obstructive apnea and evidence of partial obstruction during sleep. Central and mixed apneas (a central apnea followed by an obstructive apnea) can coexist in these children and may account for 17–34% of the total number of apneas, especially in infants and in children with OSAS secondary to craniofacial and neuromuscular syndromes.

In addition, a large number of children may present with increased work of breathing and multiple arousals and sleep fragmentation, unassociated with gas exchange abnormalities. This condition is referred to as the upper airway resistance syndrome (UARS)[5,13]. In UARS, subjects are noted to have multiple short arousals leading to alteration in sleep architecture and impaired neurocognitive function[5,14].

Sleep Patterns

Restless sleep is also commonly reported in children with OSAS. Children appear to be very fidgety during the night, frequently changing sleep positions to those that promote airway patency, such as prone or sideways positions, and hyperextension of the neck[15]. Obese children with significant OSAS may prefer sleeping while sitting upright or at least propped upon pillows.

Nocturnal Sweating

In a study of 50 children with OSAS, nocturnal profuse sweating was noted in 96% of the children[8]. In a controlled study of 23 children with OSAS and 46 controls[16], 50% of those with OSAS had excessive sweating compared with 16% of the controls ($P < 0.007$). Night sweating may be associated with the increased effort required to inspire against resistance over the course of the night. Increased calorie expenditure during sleep has also been demonstrated in children with OSAS[17].

Nocturnal Enuresis

Nocturnal enuresis is a variable finding in children with OSAS. Frank et al.[18] reported that 33% of children older than 4 years with OSAS had bed-wetting and Weider et al.[19] reported a 76% improvement in nocturnal enuresis after tonsillectomy and adenoidectomy. Guilleminault et al.[4] reported that 6 of 8 children with severe OSAS age 5–14 years had enuresis. In a second study on 50 children, 18% presented with secondary enuresis[8]. However, in perhaps the best controlled study, comparing 23 children with OSAS with 46 matched controls, Brouillette et al.[9] could not find a significant difference between the groups with respect to bed-wetting.

Polyuria has been reported in adults with OSAS. Adults with OSAS may make multiple trips to the bathroom during the night. In a recent study, 6 adults with polyuria and severe OSAS were found to have an increased level of atrial natriuretic peptide and catecholamines in the plasma. After initiation of continuous positive airway pressure (CPAP) treatment and resolution of apnea, these levels were significantly reduced and a 50% drop in nocturnal urine volume was noted[20]. It is not known if this mechanism applies to children with OSAS.

Daytime Symptoms

Although respiration in children with OSAS is typically unremarkable during wakefulness, some children with severe OSAS may also experience difficulty breathing when awake, albeit this is less severe than when asleep. These symptoms are most likely related to adenoid and tonsillar hypertrophy. The most common complaints reported by parents of children with OSAS are mouth breathing, frequent upper respiratory tract infections, recurrent ear infections, as well as hearing and speech problems. Enlarged tonsils may cause difficulty swallowing. In addition, nausea and vomiting are commonly reported in children with OSAS and tonsillar hypertrophy.

In contrast to reports in adults, excessive daytime somnolence (EDS) is thought to be uncommon in children with OSAS. However, there has been considerable variability in the reported frequency of this complication in children. In uncontrolled studies, parents and teachers of school-aged children have observed EDS in between 33% and 84% of children with OSAS[8,14]. However, in controlled studies the reported frequency of this complaint is considerably lower compared with that in adults with OSAS[9].

School-aged children may complain of sleepiness, tiredness, and fatigue, but this may be difficult to distinguish from the usual school-week behavior of average adolescents. Abnormal daytime behavior including hyperactivity and aggression has been reported in 31% to 42% of children with OSAS[8,9,12], whereas pathologic shyness and social withdrawal were reported in 22%[9]. Children with underlying genetic disorders, such as those with trisomy 21 or inherited craniofacial malformations, may have an additional impairment in intellectual performance above and beyond that imposed by the underlying syndrome[8]. Morning headaches were reported in 5 of the 8 patients originally described with OSAS by Guilleminault et al.[4]. In a second report on 50 children with OSAS Guilleminault et al.[8] found that 16% of the children had the same complaint. A typical feature of these headaches was that they tended to dissipate completely by late morning. It was hypothesized that the significant swings in intrathoracic pressure during obstructive events could have altered cerebral blood flow and increased intracranial pressures. Moreover, increased intracranial pressure during episodes of obstructive apneas was reported by Pasterkamp et al.[21], who described a 16-year-old girl with OSAS, myelomeningocele, and Arnold–Chiari malformation. After tonsillectomy these elevations in intracranial pressures disappeared. Hypoxemia and hypercarbia during obstructive episodes were considered the mechanisms for pressure changes in this case.

Physical Examination

The physical examination of the child with OSAS is variable. In most cases children have only mildly to moderately enlarged tonsils and adenoids and do not necessarily demonstrate breathing difficulties during the examination. Moreover, at times a significant amount of lymphoid tissue cannot be appreciated directly by the examiner. Therefore, a normal physical examination should not exclude OSAS. Physical examination should include an assessment of the child's growth pattern. Children with OSAS are frequently reported to have delayed growth and weight gain[17]. Obesity, on the other hand, may increase the risk for OSAS in others[22].

The physical examination begins with a general observation of the patient. Mouth breathing and adenoidal facies should be noted. Hyponasal voice is a clue to nasal obstruction and a muffled voice is suggestive of tonsillar enlargement. The lateral facial profile should be inspected for retrognathia, micrognathia, or midfacial hypoplasia. All can affect the nasopharyngeal and oropharyngeal passages and are key findings for diagnosis. The nose is assessed for septal deviation, mucosal thickening, polyps, and patency of either vestibule with the opposite naris occluded. The oral cavity should be observed for tongue and soft palate size and appearance; a large tongue and/or a high-arched or elongated palate may predispose to sleep-disordered breathing. Integrity of the hard palate should be evaluated. A bifid uvula may be associated with submucosal cleft palate.

The size of the tonsils should be assessed. A scale from 0 to a maximum of +4 when the tonsils meet the midline is commonly used[23]. Some simply describe the tonsils' appearance as minimally visible, visible to the pillars, visible beyond the pillars, or visible to the uvula. The nasal passages as well as the oral cavity of children with craniofacial anomalies who have previously undergone repair of these defects should be evaluated carefully in the same manner, since these children may be at risk for recurrent OSAS[24,25].

The chest usually has a normal configuration although pectus excavatum has been reported in some cases. The lungs are usually clear on auscultation. The cardiac examination is usually normal; however, in advanced cases evidence of pulmonary hypertension manifested by a loud second pulmonary heart sound may be present. Systemic hypertension and clubbing have been reported but are uncommon. In children with possible secondary OSAS and in young infants, a neurologic examination is required to exclude any neurologic impairment affecting muscle tone that may contribute to OSAS.

When possible, observation of the child during sleep is recommended. Snoring and labored breathing should be noted. Suprasternal retractions and paradoxical rib cage motion are commonly seen when more severe hypopneas and obstructive apneas are present. When complete obstructions are present, respiratory effort will not be accompanied by breath sounds; however, termination of these events may be associated with a gasp, movement, or an awakening.

Physiologic Consequences of OSAS

Hypoxemia

Hypoxemia, defined as arterial oxyhemoglobin saturation (SpO_2) below 92% or 90% is rare in normal infants and children. Marcus et al.[10] performed polysomnography on 50 healthy children aged between 1 and 17 years. They found the mean SpO_2 nadir to be $96 \pm 2\%$, with a single child having a short desaturation to 89% during a central apnea event. Desaturations >4% from baseline value during sleep were found more frequently with a mean rate of 0.3 ± 0.7/h. The maximal oxygen desaturation from peak to nadir value in these children was $4 \pm 2\%$.

Hypoxemia and repetitive significant oxygen desaturation are frequent in most children with OSAS. Stradling et al.[15] found that of 61 children referred for adenotonsillectomy, 61% were noted to be hypoxemic during sleep prior to surgery. Rosen et al.[11] found significant oxygen desaturations to <85% in 19 of 20 children referred for evaluation of OSAS with a relatively low apnea index of 1.9 ± 3.2, suggesting that significant and severe upper airway obstruction in children may not be identified according to the apnea index alone or based on the index as defined in adults. The same authors showed that hypopneas were mostly responsible for gas exchange abnormalities in this group as reported previously by Brouillette et al.[12].

It is not known how the degree and duration of hypoxemia relate to the outcome of children with OSAS with respect to their neurologic or cardiopulmonary status, and what type of events have a reversible versus a permanent effect on these systems. Hypoxemia leading to asphyxia and permanent neurologic disabilities has been reported in children with OSAS[12]. Moreover, infants with apparent life-threatening events (ALTEs) have been reported to have OSAS at the time or soon after these events[26], suggesting an etiology for ALTE or sudden infant death in some infants.

Hypercarbia

Obstructive apnea and hypopnea are usually associated with hypoventilation and can be easily detected by an increase in end-tidal CO_2 ($P_{ET}CO_2$) by capnography in children with OSAS. In healthy children, $P_{ET}CO_2$ is considered a reliable estimate of arterial pCO_2 and thus of alveolar ventilation. In the past, values of $P_{ET}CO_2 > 45$ torr during sleep have been conventionally considered abnormal. More recently, normal sleeping values for $P_{ET}CO_2$ have been suggested for the pediatric age group. Based on data in 50 healthy infants and adolescents, hypoventilation may be described when: peak $P_{ET}CO_2 > 53$ torr, or $P_{ET}CO_2 > 50$ torr more than 8% of sleep time, or when duration of hypoventilation ($P_{ET}CO_2 > 45$ torr) exceeds more than 60% of total sleep time[10].

In earlier reports, daytime hypercarbia in children with OSAS was usually associated with cor pulmonale and cardiorespiratory failure. However, these reports do not reflect current experience since cor pulmonale is not a common complication today and daytime hypercarbia is not frequently seen. However, hypercarbia during sleep in children with OSAS is at least as common as hypoxemia, although the proportion of children with nighttime hypercarbia and the degree of hypercarbia is unknown. Brouillette et al.[12], found hypercarbia (>45 torr) during sleep in 12 of 22 children with OSAS. Rosen et al.[11] found hypercarbia (>50 torr), in 26 of 36 (72%) children who were referred for evaluation of OSAS.

There are several groups who are at high risk for developing hypercarbia and hypoventilation. Hypoventilation is the most common polysomnographic abnormality in children with Down syndrome and OSAS, and was reported in 81% of 16 children studied by Marcus et al.[27]. Obese children with OSAS were also found to develop hypoventilation during sleep. Silvestri et al.[28], who studied 32 obese children, found hypercarbia in 75% of the children. Those who were morbidly obese with an ideal body weight above 200% were at greatest risk for the development of this abnormality.

Sleep and Sleep States

Effects of OSAS on sleep in children are poorly understood. In adults, OSAS is known to cause sleep fragmentation and alterations in sleep architecture due to multiple arousals. As a result, adults with OSAS have less rapid eye movement (REM) sleep and slow wave sleep, and spend more time in light sleep of stages 1 and 2[16]. These alterations in sleep architecture are responsible for the main side effect of OSAS in adults, which is EDS, reported in more than 90%[29].

In children, however, few data exist to support these findings. Several studies have found that children with OSAS have normal amounts of slow wave sleep[18,19,30], and absence of sleep fragmentation was reported in children with hypopneas and OSAS[14]. In contrast, significant alterations in sleep architecture were reported by Guilleminault et al.[4] in all 8 patients presenting with severe OSAS. In these children, normal progression to stages 3–4 non-REM sleep was delayed or pre-empted due to the repetitive apneic events. In a second report on 50 children with primary and secondary OSAS, Guilleminault et al.[8] noted complete disappearance of stage 3 non-REM sleep in 86% of children, a 22% reduction in REM sleep and an increase in percent of stage 1 non-REM sleep compared with controls. Moreover, movement time during sleep was higher in those with OSAS than in controls by as much as 100–250%[8].

Movements/Arousals

Movement is a normal phenomenon during sleep. However, increased motor activity is frequently reported in subjects with OSAS. Movement may range from simple leg jerks to gross movement of extremities and trunk. Movements are usually associated with arousals or with awakenings from sleep. In adults, movement/arousals were found to correlate strongly with the apnea/hypopnea index, and were normalized with the use of CPAP[16].

Mograss et al.[30] described three types of movement/arousals in children with OSAS in a sleep laboratory setting. They studied 15 children aged 2–11 years with a mean respiratory disturbance index (RDI) of 7.5 ± 8.2, and classified movement/arousals as: spontaneous, respiratory, and technician-induced. Of the total movement/arousals studied, spontaneous arousals were the most common and accounted for 51%. Respiratory arousals were found in 29.5% and technician-induced arousal in 19.5%. Nearly all obstructive events were terminated by a movement/arousal and had the effect of re-establishing airway patency in these children. In addition, the respiratory movement/arousal index was directly related to the RDI. However, these authors found that sleep stages were not altered and were similar to those reported in age-matched children. They have speculated that since movement/arousals were usually short (<3 seconds), children may experience fragmented sleep without altering various sleep stages.

In a more recent study, McNamara et al.[31] reported that a minority of the respiratory events in infants and children with OSAS were terminated by an arousal, while the remaining events resolved spontaneously. Fifteen children (1–14 years), aroused to less than 40% of obstructive events and 20 infants (term to 21 weeks) aroused to only 8% of the obstructive events. Therefore, these authors concluded that arousals are not an important mechanism of termination of obstructive events during sleep in children and are even less important in infants.

HIGH-RISK GROUPS FOR DEVELOPING OSAS

As mentioned above OSAS is associated with many pediatric conditions aside from adenotonsillar hypertrophy. These conditions mainly fall into the categories of craniofacial and neurologic disorders affecting upper airway anatomy and patency during sleep (Table 5-2). In addition, other conditions may be associated with high risk for OSAS and are discussed below.

Obesity
Obesity is a major risk factor in adults for developing OSAS, and an increased neck collar size is strongly associated with OSAS in this group[7]. In contrast, the majority of children with OSAS are not obese, many have normal weight, and failure to thrive is a common complication. However, there is evidence that obesity is a risk factor for the existence of OSAS in children. Guilleminault et al.[8] reported that 10% of the 50 children who were diagnosed with OSAS were obese, and a similar finding was reported by Brouillette et al.[12] who studied 22 infants and children. A higher incidence of OSAS was reported when obese children were referred for evaluation of OSAS. Silvestri et al.[28] found partial airway obstruction in 66% and complete airway obstruction in 59% of 32 obese children.

The above studies, however, were all performed on children who were referred for possible OSAS and therefore the prevalence of sleep-disordered breathing may have been overestimated in this group. To evaluate more precisely the prevalence of OSAS in the general obese population, Marcus et al.[22] studied 22 obese children and adolescents age 10 ± 5 years with an ideal body weight of $184 \pm 36\%$ and with no history of sleep-disordered breathing. They found that 10 children (46%) had abnormal polysomnography and in 6 children (27%) abnormalities were moderate to severe. Moreover, a positive correlation between obesity and apnea index was found ($r = 0.47$, $P < 0.05$) as was an inverse relation

between obesity and oxygen saturation nadir ($r = -0.5$, $P < 0.01$). Asymptomatic obese infants also have a higher incidence of obstructive apnea events compared with controls[32], suggesting that OSAS is common in obese children of all ages.

Adenotonsillar hypertrophy is not always the cause for the development of OSAS in obese children[22,28]. Several other reasons may contribute to OSAS in this group. Upper airway narrowing may result from deposition of adipose tissue within the muscles and tissues surrounding the airway and increase pharyngeal resistance[33]. Moreover, obese subjects were shown to have decreased chest wall compliance and displacement of the diaphragm while in the supine position. These physiologic alterations can result in decreased lung volumes and oxygen reserves during sleep and increase the risk for OSAS in this group.

Down Syndrome
Down syndrome (trisomy 21) is the most common genetic cause of developmental disability and mental retardation with an incidence of 1/660 live births. Obstructive sleep apnea is common in this group and is noted in 30–60% of subjects[27,34,35]. Anatomic factors related to the Down syndrome phenotype have been attributed to the causation of OSAS in this group. These include midfacial and mandibular hypoplasia, enlarged tongue, adenoid and tonsillar hypertrophy, laryngotracheal anomalies, and obesity[36]. Reduced neuromuscular tone has also been suspected of having a role in the development of OSAS in these subjects.

Post-adenotonsillectomy
Postoperative respiratory compromise has been reported to occur in 16–27% of children with OSAS. Particularly high-risk children include those younger than 3 years of age, those with severe OSAS, and those with additional complex medical conditions[24,25]. A postoperative polysomnogram 2–3 months following surgery is recommended for patients with additional risk factors for OSAS, or those with a high apnea index, to ensure that additional treatment is not required.

Complications

The cumulative effects of OSAS have adverse sequelae on neurologic and cardiac function, and on growth. Complications may be mild and reversible or become severe and progressive in untreated children. The various complications of childhood OSAS are the result of chronic nocturnal hypoxemia, acidosis, and sleep fragmentation.

Neurobehavioral and Neurocognitive Manifestations
Nocturnal hypoxemia and sleep fragmentation are considered the main causes for the neurobehavioral

sequelae of OSAS. In adults, EDS, decreased ability to perform everyday tasks, impairment in memory and attention, and reduction in general intellectual abilities have been reported[16,29,37,38]. Sleep fragmentation may lead to personality changes that are often first recognized by family members. These include irritability, anxiety, aggression, and depression.

Excessive daytime sleepiness is less common in children with OSAS. However, there are some discrepancies in the prevalence of EDS reported in children with OSAS. Guilleminault et al.[8] reported EDS in 84% of 50 children with OSAS, and in 70% of those cases symptoms were noted by school teachers. However, Brouillette et al.[9], in a controlled study, reported EDS in 33% of 23 children, and Frank et al.[18] reported EDS as a significant problem in only 9% of the 32 children they studied. Carroll et al.[39] reported a similarly low rate of EDS in a pediatric population. It is conceivable that fewer or shorter arousals and a more preserved sleep architecture seen in children with OSAS compared with adults with OSAS results in less daytime sleepiness[18,30]. It is also possible that since EDS is a subjective complaint, it is underdiagnosed in young children who may take daytime naps routinely. The multiple sleep latency test (MSLT), in which patients are studied during four or five 20-minute naps after overnight polysomnography to determine how quickly a patient falls asleep, affords an objective measurement of sleepiness. Although widely used in adults, its applicability in children with OSAS has not been established; such studies could be useful to objectively assess prevalence and degree of EDS in children with OSAS.

Brouillette et al.[12] reported significant neurologic impairment related to OSAS in 7 of 22 children with OSAS. In 5 children dysfunction was reversible with treatment and included EDS, behavioral disturbances, and mild developmental delay. However, 2 children, of whom one had a metabolic disorder, presented with permanent neurologic dysfunction related to asphyxia occurring during obstructive events. Delays in referral and diagnosis were noted in most of these children and were considered the cause for some of the above sequelae. In a second study[9], 33% of children with OSAS had EDS and pathologic shyness/social withdrawal was noted in 22%, rates which were significantly more common than in controls. Other parental reports such as delays in development, morning headaches, hyperactivity, and bizarre behavior were not observed more frequently in these patients.

In another study Guilleminault et al.[8] reported abnormal behavior in 42% of children in elementary school, kindergarten, and in day care centers. The most common behavioral abnormality described was hyperactivity; however, asocial behavior and disciplinary problems were also noted. A small group of patients were reported to have personality changes and bizarre withdrawn behavior suggestive in 2 children of psychosis.

Learning difficulties such as delayed language development and inadequate school performance are commonly reported, although only one report on neurocognitive function in children with OSAS has been published. Rhodes et al.[40] studied 14 obese patients of whom 5 had severe OSAS. The OSAS children demonstrated significantly lower scores for learning, memory, and vocabulary tests. Moreover, severity of OSAS measured by an apnea/hypopnea index, was found to be significantly and inversely correlated with the neurocognitive impairment. Recently, Gozal[41] reported on the effects of adenoid and tonsillar hyperplasia and sleep-disordered breathing on school performance. His study demonstrated that correction of these abnormalities resulted in improved school performance among first- and second-grade students. These findings, although preliminary, may explain reports of lower school performance and developmental delay in children with OSAS. However, it is still unknown whether the neurocognitive deficits result from chronic hypoxemia or sleep fragmentation and whether these deficits accumulate with time or are reversible. The extent to which recovery of functions is possible may depend on the age of onset of OSAS, severity, and chronicity of the disorder. More studies of this type are clearly required to define better the effect of OSAS on neurobehavioral/cognitive function.

Cardiovascular Complications

In adults with OSAS significant cardiovascular complications contribute to morbidity and mortality. These complications are associated with acute and/or chronic effects of hypoxemia, acidosis, and the hemodynamic effect of obstructive apnea on the cardiovascular system. Acute cyclic changes in heart rate, blood pressure, intrathoracic pressures, and oxygen saturations may induce cardiac arrhythmia and various degrees of atrioventricular blocks. Recent evidence suggests that adults with OSAS are at an increased risk for ischemic heart disease and cerebral infarction[42].

In contrast to adults with OSAS, systemic hypertension is reported only anecdotally in children. However, pulmonary hypertension is the main cardiovascular complication described in children with long-standing OSAS[12,43,44].

In 1988 Tal et al.[44] performed cardiac evaluations in 27 children with OSAS between 9 months and 7.5 years of age. A radionuclide heart scan demonstrated a significant reduction in right ventricular ejection fraction in 10 (37%) of the children and normalization of heart function after adenotonsillectomy. A more recent study of 28 children with OSAS has demonstrated hypertrophy involving both the right and the left ventricles and that the degree of left ventricular hypertrophy is related to the degree of severity of OSAS[45]. In addition, cardiac arrythmias during obstructive events have been reported by some investigators[8,46,47].

Children with severe OSAS (SpO$_2$ < 70%, apnea index > 10/hour) should undergo cardiac evaluation prior to adenotonsillectomy. Preoperative and postoperative deaths have been observed in this group. Therefore, a careful cardiac evaluation including physical examination, electrocardiogram, chest radiograph, and echocardiogram should be performed to evaluate for any signs of congestive heart failure or perioperative risks. If these signs or abnormal laboratory findings are present, admission to an intensive care unit for preoperative stabilization is indicated.

Growth Impairment

Growth impairment is one of the unique features of childhood OSAS. Early reports of children with severe OSAS almost always associated the two, especially when another complication such as cor pulmonale was present. Later reports in the 1980s found failure to thrive in 27–56% of the children with OSAS, while obesity in the same population was reported in about 10% of children[8,12].

Adenotonsillectomy in children with OSAS has a significant impact on growth. Brouillette et al.[12] found that relief of airway obstruction resulted in catch-up growth in all 6 children studied with failure to thrive. Moreover, Lind and Lundell[48] described a group of 14 children with OSAS in whom height and weight velocity were normal but significantly increased after adenotonsillectomy. These investigators hypothesized that abnormal release of growth hormone may alter growth in children with OSAS.

Poor caloric intake may also result in inadequate growth. Brouillette et al.[9] reported the presence of poor appetite, difficulty swallowing, and nausea and vomiting more frequently in children with OSAS compared with controls. Potsic et al.[49] reported that 60% of children with OSAS were slow eaters and 37% had trouble swallowing.

Marcus et al.[17] investigated the relation between growth, caloric intake, and energy expenditure during sleep before and after adenotonsillectomy in 14 children age 4 ± 1 years with moderate OSAS. Diagnosis was based upon an apnea index of 6 ± 3, oxygen desaturation to $85 \pm 5\%$, and an increase in P$_{ET}$CO$_2$ during sleep. Caloric intake prior to intervention in these children was normal at 91 ± 30 kcal/kg/day, and remained the same after adenotonsillectomy with resolution of OSAS in all. However, energy expenditure during sleep dropped from 51 ± 6 kcal/kg/day prior to surgery to 46 ± 7 kcal/kg/day after surgery ($P < 0.005$). This finding was associated with a significant increase in weight in all children. These findings suggest that poor growth described in some children with OSAS may be secondary to an increased energy expenditure and increased work of breathing during sleep.

Evaluation

Polysomnography

The gold standard for diagnosing childhood OSAS is polysomnography. This tool enables one to evaluate the breathing quality of the child in addition to objectively quantifying gas exchange, number of apneas and hypopneas, and sleep architecture during the night. Studies should be scored and interpreted using age-appropriate criteria. The American Thoracic Society has published a consensus statement outlining the requirements for pediatric polysomnography[3].

Screening Studies

Questionnaires, physical examination, lateral neck radiographs (Figure 5-4), and nocturnal audiotapes have been shown to have a low sensitivity and specificity for diagnosis[3]. Other screening tests, such as nocturnal videotaping, pulse oximetry, or nap polysomnograms, have limited utility and have a high false-negative rate. Thus, they may be useful for initial testing if polysomnography is not readily available, but polysomnography is recommended if the studies are negative or if the patient has other significant medical conditions.

If suspicion of cor pulmonale from severe or long-standing OSAS exists, cardiologic evaluation is indicated. An electrocardiogram may show evidence of right ventricular hypertrophy. Only after significant right ventricular hypertrophy has occurred will the chest radiograph show evidence of cardiomegaly. Echocardiography is a more sensitive technique and is indicated if more detailed information is needed or if there is suspicion of impaired cardiac function, or if congestive heart failure is present.

Treatment

Adenotonsillectomy should lead to complete resolution of clinical symptoms and polysomnographic abnormalities in most children with OSAS. However, it is important to note that OSAS results from abnormalities in the size and function of the upper airway structure as a whole, rather than from the absolute size of the adenoid and tonsils.

Additional treatment modalities are available for those children who do not respond to adenotonsillectomy or those in whom adenotonsillectomy is not indicated. Noninvasive ventilatory support in the form of CPAP is commonly used and is well tolerated in infants and older children[50,51]. However, behavioral techniques or admission to the hospital to acclimate the child to the use of this modality of treatment is necessary for it to be successful.

Uvulopharyngopalatoplasty has been successful in overcoming airway obstruction in children with oropharyngeal hypotonia, as in children with Down syndrome. More involved craniofacial surgery such as maxillary and

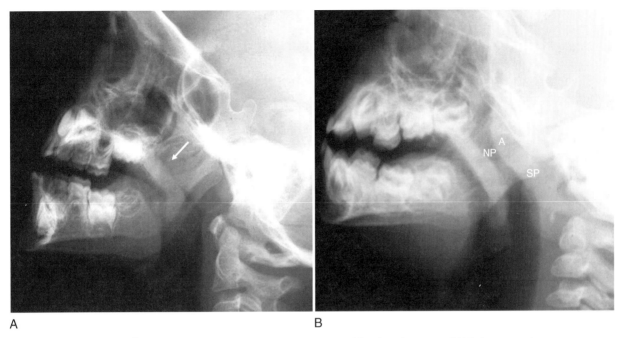

Figure 5-4   (**A**) Lateral neck radiograph of a 2-year-old girl with severe OSAS demonstrating complete occlusion of the nasopharyngeal airway space (white arrow). (**B**) Lateral neck radiograph of a 4-year-old girl with mild OSAS demonstrating a narrowed nasopharyngeal airway space (NP). A, adenoid; SP, soft palate.

mandibular advancement is appropriate for some children with craniofacial anomalies restricting the mid- and lower-face skeleton. Tracheostomy with or without ventilatory support should be considered as a short- or long-term treatment for severe cases when other modalities of therapy have failed. A weight management program should be offered to obese children with OSAS in conjunction with CPAP or non-invasive positive pressure ventilation (NPPV) therapy once evaluation and treatment for adenotonsillar hypertrophy has been completed.

The American Academy of Pediatrics has recently published guidelines for the evaluation and management of OSAS in children[52]. Recommendations include: (1) all children should be screened for snoring; (2) complex high-risk patients should be referred to a specialist; (3) patients with cardiorespiratory failure cannot await elective evaluation; (4) diagnostic evaluation, ideally with polysomnography, is useful in discriminating between primary snoring and OSAS; (5) adenotonsillectomy is the first line of treatment for most children, and CPAP is an option for those who are not candidates for surgery or do not respond to surgery; (6) high-risk patients should be monitored as inpatients postoperatively; and (7) patients should be re-evaluated postoperatively to determine whether or not additional treatment is required.

Outcome

The natural history of children with OSAS is variable. The course is most affected by the etiology of airway

obstruction, degree of obstruction, and chronicity of the disorder. The time elapsed from initial symptoms to diagnosis and management is a significant factor when assessing the outcome of children with long-standing OSAS. Nowadays, when OSAS is more commonly recognized by physicians as well as parents, delays in diagnosis are seen less often. It is difficult to predict the exact outcome of each child with OSAS today. However, in severe cases, and if untreated, children can be expected to progress, as in the past, to develop cor pulmonale and congestive heart failure. Furthermore, they will encounter neurologic deficits that may extend to permanent brain damage due to asphyxia[12].

Only one study has evaluated long-term outcome after intervention. Guilleminault and colleagues[53] re-evaluated adolescents who had been successfully treated with adenotonsillectomy during childhood. Thirteen percent of those evaluated had recurrence of OSAS. This study leads to the hypothesis that children at risk for OSAS, due to such factors as a small pharyngeal airway or decreased upper airway neuromuscular tone, develop OSAS when they reach the age of maximal adenotonsillar hyperplasia. The adenotonsillar hypertrophy results in an increased mechanical load on a marginal upper airway, thus precipitating OSAS.

It is important to mention that most complications described in the pediatric literature, including cor pulmonale, neurobehavioral, and growth impairments were reversible once patients were treated and relieved of airway obstruction. However, it is not known whether neurocognitive deficits will also reverse with treatment. The extent to which recovery of function is possible may depend on the age of onset of OSAS, severity, and chronicity of the disorder.

Some children may present with a mild form of OSAS or upper airway resistance syndrome. These children may have minimal findings by history, clinical examination, and polysomnography. If there are no abnormalities in gas exchange during sleep, complications related to these changes are not expected. However, symptoms related to sleep fragmentation such as alteration in neurobehavioral functions may persist and indicate need for treatment. When no abnormal neurobehavioral symptoms exist, close observation of the child and symptoms is sufficient, since children may experience spontaneous resolution in mild cases.

SLEEP-DISORDERED BREATHING IN PREMATURE INFANTS AND IN INFANTS

Apnea of Prematurity

The association between prematurity and central apnea is well known. It is particularly high in neonates of 24–32 weeks' gestational age. Apnea of prematurity often resolves by 38 weeks postconceptual age but could persist until 42 weeks. The close relationship between age and both the incidence and severity of apnea suggest that immaturity of the respiratory center is a major underlying factor. Others have stressed the causative role of various perinatal factors such as asphyxia, infection, hypoglycemia, thermal instability, seizures, and brain injury. In the majority of preterm infants, however, no clear etiology is found.

Apnea is more common during active sleep, when there is loss of intercostal muscle tone, diminished postinspiratory breaking, reduced upper airway dilator muscle activity, and decreased respiratory drive. Secondary to these physiologic changes there is a 30% reduction in lung volumes, and a slight fall in PaO_2. Both ventilatory responses to hypoxia and sensitivity to carbon dioxide are depressed more in active sleep than quiet sleep. The premature and newborn infant spends 80% of the time asleep, most of which is in active sleep.

All infants considered to be at risk should be monitored continuously for heart rate and respiratory rate using conventional monitoring devices. A pharmacologic approach is also available in the form of caffeine or theophylline to increase respiratory drive. Caffeine has much more stable plasma levels. The drugs may be used on a trial basis for 2 weeks and then stopped, or they may be continued until 52 weeks postconception.

Periodic breathing is another form of apnea consisting of very brief apneas of 5–10 seconds' duration, followed by breathing for 10–15 seconds before the next brief apnea. This pattern is common in premature infants and may be accentuated by high altitude. Periodic breathing responds well to supplemental oxygen and distending airway pressures in the form of CPAP.

In addition, premature infants are predisposed to upper airway obstruction and oxygen desaturations during sleep due to poor airway stability and a highly compliant chest wall. Dransfield et al.[54] found that of 76 premature infants presenting clinically with apnea, 52 (68%) of them had obstructive apnea and 24 (32%) had central apnea only. Milner et al.[55] found that half of the apneic episodes associated with periodic breathing in 8 premature infants were the result of upper airway obstruction and glottic closure. Spontaneous neck flexion was also found to cause upper airway obstruction in premature infants and was suggested to play a role in the pathogenesis of apnea in some preterm infants[56].

Apnea of Infancy

Periodic breathing and apnea during sleep are uncommon in normal term infants during the first few months of life. When prolonged apneas occur, especially if resuscitation is required, apnea of infancy may be diagnosed. Other possible causes of prolonged apnea include: gastroesophageal reflux, pharyngeal incoordination, convulsions, infection, heart disease, congenital central hypoventilation syndrome, metabolic disorders, and brain tumors.

Full-term neonates may also develop OSAS. Neonates are obligate nose-breathers and may develop upper airway obstruction whenever a mild nasal obstruction such as a respiratory infection is present. Central nervous system immaturity, a highly compliant chest wall, and reduced airway stability all predispose newborn infants to gas exchange abnormalities even during brief episodes of OSAS. OSAS in early infancy can coexist with central apnea and sometimes can be mistaken for central apnea. Guilleminault et al.[57] found a peak incidence of obstructive and mixed apnea to occur at 6 weeks of age in 30 healthy infants. These events occur most commonly in non-REM sleep and progressively decline by 6 months to a non-significant amount[57]. Resolution of the events by 6 months may represent improved upper airway stability with growth.

Several reports describe the association between OSAS and apparent life-threatening event (ALTE) during early infancy. ALTE refers to an acute and unexpected change in an infant's appearance or behavior that is frightening to the caregivers and causes them to seek medical attention. Guilleminault et al.[57] reported a higher number of mixed and obstructive sleep apneas in children who had ALTE. Moreover, a later report from the same group described 5 infants with ALTE who subsequently developed severe OSAS. Polysomnography of the infants at the time of the initial ALTE (3 weeks to 6 months old) demonstrated a high index of mixed and obstructive apnea. These infants became progressively more symptomatic by 6–10 months and improved only after adenotonsillectomy[58].

Similar finding have been observed in a few infants who subsequently died of the sudden infant death syndrome (SIDS) and who had polysomnography. When compared with age matched controls, these infants showed a higher number of mixed and obstructive events[57,59]. Kahn et al.[59], in addition, found a lower number of sighs in these infants and postulated that abnormalities in peripheral chemoreceptor function may have led to death in some of these children.

Upper airway obstruction and at times ALTE are reported in infants with severe gastroesophageal reflux. Gastroesophageal reflux may induce symptoms in infants while awake or asleep. Symptoms usually occur after meals in a sequence consisting of sudden cessation of breathing, rigidity and opisthotonic posture, plethora and sudden cyanosis or pallor.

CENTRAL HYPOVENTILATION AND SLEEP

Central alveolar hypoventilation is defined as an increase in $PaCO_2$ due to a decrease in central nervous system ventilatory drive. Its hallmark is elevation of the $PaCO_2$ on arterial blood gas sampling with a normal alveolar–arterial oxygen gradient $[(A–a)DO_2]$. Patients with central hypoventilation fail to ventilate adequately particularly during sleep. Central hypoventilation can be primary as in congenital central hypoventilation syndrome, or secondary to neurologic disorders such as: Arnold–Chiari malformation, hypoxic-ischemic encephalopathy, Leigh's encephalomyelopathy, brainstem and spinal cord tumors, and encephalitis. Other causes include inborn errors of metabolism, hypothyroidism, and drugs.

Congenital Central Hypoventilation Syndrome

Congenital central hypoventilation syndrome (CCHS) is a congenital form of severe central hypoventilation of undetermined etiology. Patients with CCHS usually present with cyanosis, respiratory failure, or occasionally apnea at birth. Rarely, infants present later with ALTEs or cor pulmonale. It is quite possible that some cases of sudden infant death syndrome are actually due to CCHS.

Patients with CCHS have intact voluntary control of ventilation but lack automatic control. Patients usually have a decreased tidal volume and respiratory rate during sleep[60]. Most patients breathe adequately during wakefulness; a subset requires ventilatory support 24 hours a day.

CCHS may be associated with other abnormalities, including Hirschsprung's disease, autonomic dysfunction, and neural crest tumors. The association of CCHS with these disorders has led to the hypothesis that CCHS is due to a defect in neural crest migration. Physiologic studies have shown that children with CCHS have decreased or absent ventilatory chemosensitivity in response to progressive hypoxia and hypercapnia during wakefulness and sleep.

The diagnosis of central hypoventilation is usually based on a high suspicion, clinical findings, and polysomnographic findings of hypoventilation[61]. Evaluation for the cause of hypoventilation should include a cranial magnetic resonance imaging examination. Other etiologies include respiratory muscle weakness and metabolic disorders. The treatment of choice is chronic ventilatory support particularly during sleep, although, as mentioned, a subset of children require ventilatory support 24 hours a day. Various modalities of ventilation are used to treat CCHS including NPPV, diaphragm pacing, and mechanical ventilation via tracheostomy.

OBSTRUCTIVE AND RESTRICTIVE LUNG DISEASES AND SLEEP

Obstructive Lung Diseases

Sleep-disordered breathing including hypoxemia, hypercarbia, and sleep fragmentation has been reported in children with chronic obstructive lung diseases. Mechanisms that can exacerbate sleep-disordered breathing include effects of circadian rhythm on bronchoconstriction, hypoventilation during sleep, and decreased mucociliary clearance during sleep. In addition, cough may further disrupt normal sleep architecture by inducing arousals and awakenings.

Bronchopulmonary Dysplasia

Bronchopulmonary dysplasia (BPD) is a chronic lung disease of infancy that follows acute lung injury in the neonatal period. BPD has been associated with degree of prematurity, barotrauma, oxygen toxicity, and severity of lung inflammation during this period. Infants with BPD have altered lung mechanics with low lung volumes and low compliance in the early stages of the disease, and airway obstruction with air trapping at later stages. Most infants require extended mechanical ventilatory support, oxygen supplementation, diuretics, and bronchodilator therapy. In addition, many of these children have gastroesophageal reflux and swallowing difficulties that could further worsen their underlying lung disease.

Significant hypoxemia during sleep is common in BPD infants[62,63]. These infants have also been reported to have an increased risk of SIDS and ALTE. The reason for this predisposition is unclear but preventing hypoxemia with oxygen supplementation can minimize it. A possible explanation is that chronic hypoxemia and hypercapnia may blunt the development of the normal chemoreceptor and arousal responses to chemical stimuli. Supporting this hypothesis is the study by Garg et al.[64], who have shown diminished arousal responses to hypoxia in a stable group of BPD infants who did not require supplemental oxygen. Although 11 of 12 infants in this study aroused, vigorous stimulation was needed for 2 of 3 of the infants to recover from persistent apnea, bradycardia, and hypoxemia that developed following the challenge.

Asthma

Asthma and persistent wheezing predict sleep-disordered breathing in children[2]. In this context, possible mechanisms for sleep-disordered breathing include increased parasympathetic tone during sleep, circadian variations in plasma levels of cortisol and histamine, reduced lung volumes, gastroesophageal reflux disease, increased airway inflammation and decreased airway clearance, and, finally, abnormalities in chemoreceptor function that can adversely affect respiration during sleep. Patients with life-threatening episodes of asthma have been shown to have impaired peripheral chemoreceptor function[65] and impaired perception of respiratory loads that could lead to a worsening of hypoxemia, as well as abnormal arousal responses to respiratory stimuli.

Cystic Fibrosis

Children with cystic fibrosis (CF) demonstrate abnormalities in gas exchange during sleep, particularly during pulmonary exacerbation and with progression of their lung disease. Allen et al.[66] noted nocturnal hypoxemia during pulmonary exacerbation followed by resolution with treatment. Tepper et al.[67] found that oxygen desaturation in these subjects occurred particularly during REM sleep. In another study of young adults with CF, those with severe disease were found to have significantly more nocturnal hypoxemia, which could explain the development of cor pulmonale in some of these patients.

Alterations in gas exchange may disrupt normal sleep architecture in CF subjects. Spier et al.[67] studied 10 CF adults with severe lung disease, under baseline conditions in the absence of pulmonary exacerbation. They noted low sleep efficiency, significant amount of awakenings, and less time spent in REM stage when compared with healthy adults[68].

Progressive deterioration of lung function in CF patients may lead to significant hypoxemia and hypercapnia, especially during sleep. Therefore, several studies evaluated the use of NPPV versus low-flow oxygen on respiration and sleep parameters in these subjects[69,70]. These studies noted that sleep architecture and arousals remained unchanged during both NPPV and oxygen therapy. However, NPPV markedly improved alveolar ventilation during all sleep states in comparison with low-flow oxygen therapy.

Restrictive Lung Diseases

Chest Wall Deformities

Not much literature exists on the effects of thoracic deformities and respiratory compromise during sleep in children. Several disorders should be considered in this context including idiopathic scoliosis, congenital scoliosis, and congenital malformations involving the spine and chest wall leading to a small thorax.

Adults with severe kyphoscoliosis may experience respiratory failure and cor pulmonale if untreated. Significant hypoventilation and oxyhemoglobin desaturations were documented in these subjects especially during REM sleep. Most children with idiopathic scoliosis are diagnosed and treated early and therefore are not usually at risk for developing sleep-disordered breathing and respiratory failure. However, in congenital forms of scoliosis and when the spinal angle exceeds 70°, sleep-disordered breathing may develop and should be evaluated.

Several chest wall deformities could lead to respiratory insufficiency including congenital deficiency of ribs, thoracic dystrophy, and short limb dwarfism. Congenital diaphragmatic hernia, eventration of diaphragm, and abdominal wall defects such as omphalocele and prune belly syndrome, should also be considered in this context. Respiratory symptoms may be mild to severe, even during wakefulness. Few data on breathing during sleep exist in these patients, although it would be anticipated that desaturations and hypercapnia would be worse during sleep. One group that has been studied is children with achondroplasia. These children are prone to develop both central apnea due to a small foramen magnum with potential brainstem compression, and obstructive sleep apnea due to mid-facial hypoplasia. In addition, short flare ribs lead to a small rib cage and significant restrictive lung disease. Mogayzel et al.[71] noted that of 88 children with this disorder, 48% had sleep-disordered breathing, and 44% had at least one episode of desaturation to <90%.

Ventilatory Muscle Weakness

Sleep disorders may occur in children with neuromuscular disorders associated with respiratory muscle weakness. Most studies of children and adolescents with ventilatory muscle weakness have focused on patients with Duchenne muscular dystrophy (DMD).

The disorder presents with proximal muscle weakness at 2–4 years of age. The patient usually becomes confined to a wheelchair around 10–12 years of age, invariably dying prematurely before the age of 30 years. Respiratory muscle weakness evolves as the disease progresses and this leads to more serious secondary problems such as scoliosis, thoracic mechanical abnormalities, widespread microatelectasis with reduced lung compliance, a weak cough with retained secretions, and ventilation–perfusion imbalance. Lyager and coworkers[72] reported that patients with DMD are at risk for respiratory failure if vital capacity is less than 1.2 liters (or forced vital capacity <30% predicted). Hypercapnea results when vital capacity falls below 55% of predicted values, and later becomes progressive. The risk of pulmonary morbidity and mortality from acute respiratory failure correlates with increasing hypercapnea.

The first significant blood–gas abnormality seen in older children with DMD occurs during REM sleep as short periods of hypercapnea and eventually hypoxemia[73]. These were observed in non-ambulatory patients who complained of frequent awakenings and need for repositioning in bed during sleep several years prior to the study. Smith and coworkers[74] described that in patients with advanced DMD, nocturnal hypoventilation often occurs with profound oxygen desaturations during REM sleep despite normal wakeful ventilation. In a recent prospective study Phillips and coworkers[75] reported that the age of onset of sleep-disordered breathing was 16.5 years and the incidence was broadly spread across the population above this age group.

Given the background of progressive neuromuscular weakness and consequent restrictive lung disease, patients with DMD are potentially at risk for sleep hypopnea syndrome. Early diagnosis and treatment of this syndrome is important and can prevent long-term complications[76,77].

There have been fewer investigations in other forms of neuromuscular diseases such as spinal muscular atrophy, nemaline myopathy, and myotonic dystrophy, documenting nocturnal desaturation and apnea in these children[78,79]. Affected individuals were chronically symptomatic with morning headaches and excessive sleepiness or acutely ill with respiratory failure and cor pulmonale.

Treatment

Supportive Therapy

Supportive therapy is important for children with obstructive or restrictive lung disease and chronic respiratory failure. Medical management should include, where appropriate, bronchodilators, steroids, diuretics, etc. Nutritional needs of these children should be addressed and treated by experts. In patients with ventilatory muscle weakness, chest physical therapy and modalities to enhance mucociliary clearance should be introduced in order to prevent lung infections.

Supplemental Oxygen During Sleep

Supplemental oxygen should be prescribed when nocturnal hypoxemia is present, although such guidelines have not been developed for children. Supplemental oxygen has been demonstrated to improve growth in infants with BPD who are hypoxemic. It has been suggested that SpO_2 be maintained at >92–93% for BPD children as well as for children with chronic lung diseases[64].

Supplemental oxygen is frequently prescribed for patients with CF and nocturnal hypoxemia[80], although large controlled studies are not available to show the efficacy of this treatment on morbidity or mortality.

Non-invasive Positive-Pressure Ventilation

Non-invasive positive-pressure ventilation (NPPV) has become available in recent years to children with a wide range of disorders that lead to respiratory failure[81]. NPPV is being used for children with advanced obstructive lung disease such as CF[82], as well as restrictive lung disease due to respiratory muscle weakness, such as DMD and spinal muscular atrophy[81,83]. Moreover, nocturnal use of NPPV was shown in the latter group to improve gas exchange further during spontaneous breathing while awake[84] as well as sleep architecture[85]. For DMD patients, NPPV has been shown to improve quality of life, reduce number of hospitalizations and improve mortality[81,86].

Some children with ventilatory muscle weakness will eventually require a tracheostomy and positive-pressure ventilatory support throughout the day and night. Such a decision should be made after in-depth discussion with the family and patient when appropriate, when signs of daytime hypoventilation develop and/or when such support could enhance airway clearance.

SUMMARY

Sleep is an active process and has significant physiologic impact on healthy children as well as on children with underlying respiratory disorders. Significant advancement in the field of pediatric sleep medicine occurred since the first description by Guilleminault et al.[4] of 8 children with OSAS. Although many questions remain unanswered, especially in regard to the long-term effects of sleep-disordered breathing on the neurocognitive development of children, many other questions have been answered and are well documented. For most sleep-related breathing disorders treatment is available today. This treatment can prevent most known complications if instituted early. An ever-growing variety of diagnostic tools and technological solutions for the care of these children is available.

MAJOR POINTS

1. Obstructive sleep apnea syndrome during childhood differs significantly from the disorder in adults in terms of pathophysiology and treatment.
2. Both anatomic and physiologic abnormalities are suspected to play a significant role in the

Continued

MAJOR POINTS—Cont'd

pathophysiology of obstructive sleep apnea syndrome (OSAS) in children.

3. Long-standing obstructive sleep apnea syndrome can lead to significant end-organ injury and negatively affect the cardiovascular system, neurocognitive function, and behavior of children.

4. Children with underlying craniofacial syndromes and neurologic disorders affecting their muscular tone are at particular risk for obstructive sleep apnea syndrome.

5. The "gold standard" tool for diagnosis of children with sleep-disordered breathing and particularly for obstructive sleep apnea is polysomnography.

6. Treatment for obstructive sleep apnea syndrome in most cases is surgical (adenotonsillectomy) and is a definite solution for the majority of children.

REFERENCES

1. Ali NJ, Pitson DJ, Stradling JR. Snoring, sleep disturbance, and behaviour in 4-5 year olds. Arch Dis Child 68: 360-366, 1993.

2. Redline S, Tishler PV, Schluchter M, et al. Risk factors for sleep-disordered breathing in children. Associations with obesity, race, and respiratory problems. Am J Respir Crit Care Med 159:1527-1532, 1999.

3. American Thoracic Society. Standards and indications for cardiopulmonary sleep studies in children. Am J Respir Crit Care Med 153:866-878, 1996.

4. Guilleminault C, Eldridge FL, Simmons B, et al. Sleep apnea in eight children. Pediatrics 58:23-30, 1976.

5. Guilleminault C, Pelayo R, Leger D, et al. Recognition of sleep-disordered breathing in children. Pediatrics 98:871-882, 1996.

6. Corbo GM, Fuciarelli F, Foresi A, et al. Snoring in children: association with respiratory symptoms and passive smoking. BMJ 299:1491-1494, 1989.

7. Redline S, Tishler PV, Hans MG, et al. Racial differences in sleep-disordered breathing in African-Americans and Caucasians. Am J Respir Crit Care Med 155:186-192, 1997.

8. Guilleminault C, Korobkin R, Winkle R. A review of 50 children with obstructive sleep apnea syndrome. Lung 159:275-287, 1981.

9. Brouillette R, Hanson D, David R, et al. A diagnostic approach to suspected obstructive sleep apnea in children. J Pediatr 105:10-14, 1984.

10. Marcus CL, Omlin KJ, Basinki DJ, et al. Normal polysomnographic values for children and adolescents. Am Rev Respir Dis 146:1235-1239, 1992.

11. Rosen CL, D'andrea L, Haddad GG. Adult criteria for obstructive sleep apnea do not identify children with serious obstruction. Am Rev Respir Dis 146:1231-1234, 1992.

12. Brouillette RT, Fernbach SK, Hunt CE. Obstructive sleep apnea in infants and children. J Pediatr 100:31-40, 1982.

13. Guilleminault C, Stoohs R, Clerk A, et al. A cause of excessive daytime sleepiness. The upper airway resistance syndrome. Chest 104:781-787, 1993.

14. Guilleminault C, Winkle R, Korobkin R, et al. Children and nocturnal snoring: evaluation of the effects of sleep related respiratory resistive load and daytime functioning. Eur J Pediatr 139:165-171, 1982.

15. Stradling JR, Thomas G, Warley AR, et al. Effect of adenotonsillectomy on nocturnal hypoxaemia, sleep disturbance, and symptoms in snoring children. Lancet 335:249-253, 1990.

16. Collard P, Dury M, Delguste P, et al. Movement arousals and sleep-related disordered breathing in adults. Am J Respir Crit Care Med 154:454-459, 1996.

17. Marcus CL, Carroll JL, Koerner CB, et al. Determinants of growth in children with the obstructive sleep apnea syndrome. J Pediatr 125:556-562, 1994.

18. Frank Y, Kravath RE, Pollak CP, et al. Obstructive sleep apnea and its therapy: clinical and polysomnographic manifestations. Pediatrics 71:737-742, 1983.

19. Weider DJ, Sateia MJ, West RP. Nocturnal enuresis in children with upper airway obstruction. Otolaryngol Head Neck Surg 105:427-432, 1991.

20. Baruzzi A, Riva R, Cirignotta F, et al. Atrial natriuretic peptide and catecholamines in obstructive sleep apnea syndrome. Sleep 14:83-86, 1991.

21. Pasterkamp H, Cardoso ER, Booth FA. Obstructive sleep apnea leading to increased intracranial pressure in a patient with hydrocephalus and syringomyelia. Chest 95:1064-1067, 1989.

22. Marcus CL, Curtis S, Koerner CB, et al. Evaluation of pulmonary function and polysomnography in obese children and adolescents. Pediatr Pulmonol 21:176-183, 1996.

23. Brodsky L. Modern assessment of tonsils and adenoids. Pediatr Clin North Am 36:1551-1569, 1989.

24. McColley SA, April MM, Carroll JL, et al. Respiratory compromise after adenotonsillectomy in children with obstructive sleep apnea. Arch Otolaryngol Head Neck Surg 118:940-943, 1992.

25. Rosen GM, Muckle RP, Mahowald MW, et al. Postoperative respiratory compromise in children with obstructive sleep apnea syndrome: can it be anticipated? Pediatrics 93:784-788, 1994.

26. Guilleminault C, Heldt G, Powell N, et al. Small upper airway in near-miss sudden infant death syndrome infants and their families. Lancet 1:402-407, 1986.

27. Marcus CL, Keens TG, Bautista DB, et al. Obstructive sleep apnea in children with Down syndrome. Pediatrics 88:132-139, 1991.

28. Silvestri JM, Weese-Mayer DE, Bass MT, et al. Polysomnography in obese children with a history of

sleep-associated breathing disorders. Pediatr Pulmonol 16:124–129, 1993.

29. Partinen M, Guilleminault C. Daytime sleepiness and vascular morbidity at seven-year follow-up in obstructive sleep apnea patients. Chest 97:27–32, 1990.

30. Mograss MA, Ducharme FM, Brouillette RT. Movement/arousals. Description, classification, and relationship to sleep apnea in children. Am J Respir Crit Care Med 150:1690–1696, 1994.

31. McNamara F, Issa FG, Sullivan CE. Arousal pattern following central and obstructive breathing abnormalities in infants and children. J Appl Physiol 81:2651–2657, 1996.

32. Kahn A, Mozin MJ, Rebuffat E, et al. Sleep pattern alterations and brief airway obstructions in overweight infants. Sleep 12:430–438, 1989.

33. Horner RL, Mohiaddin RH, Lowell DG, et al. Sites and sizes of fat deposits around the pharynx in obese patients with obstructive sleep apnoea and weight matched controls. Eur Respir J 2:613–622, 1989.

34. Southall DP, Stebbens VA, Mirza R, et al. Upper airway obstruction with hypoxaemia and sleep disruption in Down syndrome. Dev Med Child Neurol 29:734–742, 1987.

35. Stebbens VA, Dennis J, Samuels MP, et al. Sleep related upper airway obstruction in a cohort with Down's syndrome. Arch Dis Child 66:1333–1338, 1991.

36. Jacobs IN, Gray RF, Todd NW. Upper airway obstruction in children with Down syndrome. Arch Otolaryngol Head Neck Surg 122:945–950, 1996.

37. Findley LJ, Barth JT, Powers DC, et al. Cognitive impairment in patients with obstructive sleep apnea and associated hypoxemia. Chest 90:686–690, 1986.

38. Greenberg GD, Watson RK, Deptula D. Neuropsychological dysfunction in sleep apnea. Sleep 10:254–262, 1987.

39. Carroll JL, McColley SA, Marcus CL, et al. Inability of clinical history to distinguish primary snoring from obstructive sleep apnea syndrome in children. Chest 108:610–618, 1995.

40. Rhodes SK, Shimoda KC, Waid LR, et al. Neurocognitive deficits in morbidly obese children with obstructive sleep apnea. J Pediatr 127:741–744, 1995.

41. Gozal D. Sleep-disordered breathing and school performance in children. Pediatrics 102:616–620, 1998.

42. Shahar E, Whitney CW, Redline S, et al. Sleep-disordered breathing and cardiovascular disease: cross-sectional results of the Sleep Heart Health Study. Am J Respir Crit Care Med 163:19–25, 2001.

43. Perkin RM, Anas NG. Pulmonary hypertension in pediatric patients. J Pediatr 105:511–522, 1984.

44. Tal A, Leiberman A, Margulis G, et al. Ventricular dysfunction in children with obstructive sleep apnea: radionuclide assessment. Pediatr Pulmonol 4:139–143, 1988.

45. Amin RS, Kimball TR, Bean JA, et al. Left ventricular hypertrophy and abnormal ventricular geometry in children and adolescents with obstructive sleep apnea. Am J Respir Crit Care Med 165:1395–1399, 2002.

46. D'andrea L A, Rosen CL, Haddad GG. Severe hypoxemia in children with upper airway obstruction during sleep does not lead to significant changes in heart rate. Pediatr Pulmonol 16:362–369, 1993.

47. Aljadeff G, Gozal D, Schechtman VL, et al. Heart rate variability in children with obstructive sleep apnea. Sleep 20:151–157, 1997.

48. Lind MG, Lundell BP. Tonsillar hyperplasia in children. A cause of obstructive sleep apneas, CO_2 retention, and retarded growth. Arch Otolaryngol 108:650–654, 1982.

49. Potsic WP, Pasquariello PS, Baranak CC, et al. Relief of upper airway obstruction by adenotonsillectomy. Otolaryngol Head Neck Surg 94:476–480, 1986.

50. Marcus CL, Ward SL, Mallory GB, et al. Use of nasal continuous positive airway pressure as treatment of childhood obstructive sleep apnea. J Pediatr 127:88–94, 1995.

51. Waters KA, Everett FM, Bruderer JW, et al. Obstructive sleep apnea: the use of nasal CPAP in 80 children. Am J Respir Crit Care Med 152:780–785, 1995.

52. Clinical practice guideline: diagnosis and management of childhood obstructive sleep apnea syndrome. Pediatrics 109:704–712, 2002.

53. Guilleminault C, Partinen M, Praud JP, et al. Morphometric facial changes and obstructive sleep apnea in adolescents. J Pediatr 114:997–999, 1989.

54. Dransfield DA, Spitzer AR, Fox WW. Episodic airway obstruction in premature infants. Am J Dis Child 137:441–443, 1983.

55. Milner AD, Boon AW, Saunders RA, et al. Upper airways obstruction and apnoea in preterm babies. Arch Dis Child 55:22–25, 1980.

56. Thach BT, Stark AR. Spontaneous neck flexion and airway obstruction during apneic spells in preterm infants. J Pediatr 94:275–281, 1979.

57. Guilleminault C, Ariagno R, Korobkin R, et al. Mixed and obstructive sleep apnea and near miss for sudden infant death syndrome. 1. Report of an infant with sudden death. 2. Comparison of near miss and normal control infants by age. Pediatrics 64:837–843, 882–891, 1979.

58. Guilleminault C, Souquet M, Ariagno RL, et al. Five cases of near-miss sudden infant death syndrome and development of obstructive sleep apnea syndrome. Pediatrics 73:71–78, 1984.

59. Kahn A, Blum D, Rebuffat E, et al. Polysomnographic studies of infants who subsequently died of sudden infant death syndrome. Pediatrics 82:721–727, 1988.

60. Fleming PJ, Cade D, Bryan MH, et al. Congenital central hypoventilation and sleep state. Pediatrics 66:425–428, 1980.

61. Weese-Mayer DE, Silvestri JM, Menzies LJ, et al. Congenital central hypoventilation syndrome: diagnosis, management, and long-term outcome in thirty-two children. J Pediatr 120:381–387, 1992.

62. Garg M, Kurzner SI, Bautista DB, et al.1988 Clinically unsuspected hypoxia during sleep and feeding in infants with bronchopulmonary dysplasia. Pediatrics 81:635–642, 1983.

63. Moyer-Mileur LJ, Nielson DW, Pfeffer KD, et al. Eliminating sleep-associated hypoxemia improves growth in infants with bronchopulmonary dysplasia. Pediatrics 98:779-783, 1996.

64. Garg M, Kurzner SI, Bautista D, et al. Hypoxic arousal responses in infants with bronchopulmonary dysplasia. Pediatrics 82:59-63, 1988.

65. Kikuchi Y, Okabe S, Tamura G, et al. Chemosensitivity and perception of dyspnea in patients with a history of near-fatal asthma. N Engl J Med 330:1329-1334, 1994.

66. Allen MB, Mellon AF, Simmonds EJ, et al. Changes in nocturnal oximetry after treatment of exacerbations in cystic fibrosis. Arch Dis Child 69:197-201, 1993.

67. Tepper RS, Skatrud JB, Dempsey JA. Ventilation and oxygenation changes during sleep in cystic fibrosis. Chest 84:388-393, 1983.

68. Spier S, Rivlin J, Hughes D, et al. The effect of oxygen on sleep, blood gases, and ventilation in cystic fibrosis. Am Rev Respir Dis 129:712-718, 1984.

69. Gozal D.1997 Nocturnal ventilatory support in patients with cystic fibrosis: comparison with supplemental oxygen. Eur Respir J 10:1999-2003, 1983.

70. Milross MA, Piper AJ, Norman M, et al. Low-flow oxygen and bilevel ventilatory support: effects on ventilation during sleep in cystic fibrosis. Am J Respir Crit Care Med 163:129-134, 2001.

71. Mogayzel PJ Jr., Carroll JL, Loughlin GM, et al. Sleep-disordered breathing in children with achondroplasia. J Pediatr 132:667-671, 1998.

72. Lyager S, Steffensen B, Juhl B. Indicators of need for mechanical ventilation in Duchenne muscular dystrophy and spinal muscular atrophy. Chest 108:779-785, 1995.

73. Redding GJ, Okamoto GA, Guthrie RD, et al. Sleep patterns in nonambulatory boys with Duchenne muscular dystrophy. Arch Phys Med Rehabil 66:818-821, 1985.

74. Smith PE, Edwards RH, Calverley PM. Ventilation and breathing pattern during sleep in Duchenne muscular dystrophy. Chest 96:1346-1351, 1989.

75. Phillips MF, Smith PE, Carroll N, et al. Nocturnal oxygenation and prognosis in Duchenne muscular dystrophy. Am J Respir Crit Care Med 160:198-202, 1999.

76. Barbe F, Quera-Salva MA, Mccann C, et al. Sleep-related respiratory disturbances in patients with Duchenne muscular dystrophy. Eur Respir J 7:1403-1408, 1994.

77. Barthlen GM. Nocturnal respiratory failure as an indication of noninvasive ventilation in the patient with neuromuscular disease. Respiration 64(Suppl 1):35-38, 1997.

78. Manni R, Cerveri I, Ottolini A, et al. Sleep related breathing patterns in patients with spinal muscular atrophy. Ital J Neurol Sci 14:565-569, 1993.

79. Labanowski M, Schmidt-Nowara W, Guilleminault C. Sleep and neuromuscular disease: frequency of sleep-disordered breathing in a neuromuscular disease clinic population. Neurology 47:1173-1180, 1996.

80. Zinman R, Corey M, Coates AL, et al. Nocturnal home oxygen in the treatment of hypoxemic cystic fibrosis patients. J Pediatr 114:368-377, 1989.

81. Padman R, Lawless S, Von Nessen S. Use of BiPAP by nasal mask in the treatment of respiratory insufficiency in pediatric patients: preliminary investigation. Pediatr Pulmonol 17:119-123, 1994.

82. Granton JT, Shapiro C, Kesten S. Noninvasive nocturnal ventilatory support in advanced lung disease from cystic fibrosis. Respir Care 47:675-681, 2002.

83. Bach JR, Wang TG. Noninvasive long-term ventilatory support for individuals with spinal muscular atrophy and functional bulbar musculature. Arch Phys Med Rehabil 76:213-217, 1995.

84. Hukins CA, Hillman DR. Daytime predictors of sleep hypoventilation in Duchenne muscular dystrophy. Am J Respir Crit Care Med 161:166-170, 2000.

85. Barbe F, Quera-Salva MA, De Lattre J, et al. Long-term effects of nasal intermittent positive-pressure ventilation on pulmonary function and sleep architecture in patients with neuromuscular diseases. Chest 110:1179-1183, 1996.

86. Vianello A, Bevilacqua M, Salvador V, et al. Long-term nasal intermittent positive pressure ventilation in advanced Duchenne's muscular dystrophy. Chest 105:445-448, 1994.

Asthma

HAVIVA VELER, M.D.
RUSSELL G. CLAYTON, Sr., D.O.

In 63 AD, Aretaeus the Cappadocian wrote, "If from running, gymnastic exercises, or any other work, the breathing becomes difficult, it is called Asthma." Almost two thousand years later, our scientific understanding of asthma has grown, yet this entity is still defined using similar clinical constructs. A working definition from the current guidelines for the diagnosis and treatment of asthma states that asthma is a chronic inflammatory disease of the airways, and this inflammation causes an increase in (a) bronchial hyper-responsiveness to a variety of stimuli and (b) recurrent episodes of wheezing, breathlessness, chest tightness, and coughing usually associated with widespread but variable (c) airflow obstruction that is often reversible. This definition provides the basis for both diagnostic criteria and treatment of the disorder[1].

There is a wide variety of symptom expression and severity in people with asthma, reflecting the heterogeneous nature of the disease. It is unclear whether this heterogeneity is due to extreme differences in phenotypic variability or the possibility that what we call asthma may represent a collection of similar airway diseases that we have yet to appreciate. This variability can cause confusion in relation to the diagnosis, assessment, and treatment of the child with asthma. This confusion is amplified by "synonym" diagnoses such as reactive airways disease or wheezy bronchitis and by the assignment of "types" of asthma, such as "bronchial" asthma, cough-variant asthma, intrinsic or extrinsic asthma, and allergic or nonallergic asthma. While this expanded nomenclature may serve the individual who evokes this terminology, there is neither a physiologic basis nor broad acceptance of these terms. An individual who fulfills diagnostic criteria has asthma, and the diagnosis should only be modified by classification of severity.

Asthma is the most common chronic disease in childhood, affecting over 5 million children in the United States. It is one of the leading causes of emergency room utilization and hospitalizations in children and adults, although the rate of hospitalization is higher in children. There is no racial, ethnic, or socioeconomic predisposition to the development of asthma, but the rate of hospitalization is higher among African-Americans and urban lower-income groups. The rate of death from asthma has increased steadily over the last 10 years, despite a growing understanding of the disease and the initiation of aggressive disease management programs. Death from asthma in children occurs regardless of disease severity[2].

ETIOLOGY OF ASTHMA

The prevalence of asthma has been increasing, particularly among children. The observance of this phenomenon has led to much speculation and attempts to identify the reason behind the rising prevalence. Factors ranging from increased numbers of immunizations to increased air pollution have been suggested, but subsequent analysis has failed to provide supporting evidence to implicate most of these possibilities. However, a concept known as the hygiene hypothesis has gained some support from epidemiologic studies. This hypothesis is based on the relative decrease in microbial exposure in environments of modernized countries in relation to early immune development, and states that children with increased microbial exposure are less likely to develop asthma[3].

Observations of birth cohorts have suggested that young children who have increased numbers of upper respiratory and gastrointestinal infections are less likely to develop asthma or allergic disease later in life. Similar studies involving farm/non-farm cohorts demonstrated that children exposed to relatively higher amounts of bacterial endotoxin were less likely to develop asthma or atopic disease. In addition, children with animal contact from a young age seem to be less likely to develop asthma, possibly related to higher environmental levels of bacterial endotoxin associated with animals. While the evidence supporting the hygiene hypothesis is compelling, there are other studies that implicate certain viral infections, inhalant allergens, and ambient bacterial endotoxin as possible causes for the development of asthma. At this time, the reason or reasons for the increased prevalence of asthma remains unclear.

There is also ambiguity shadowing the factors leading to the development of asthma in the individual. In many cases asthma seems to be an inherited disease. Often the parents or siblings of children with asthma also have the disease, or there is at least some family history of asthma[4]. However, the variability of presumed inheritance and the heterogeneous expression of the disease suggest a complex inheritance pattern that may involve several genes on several different chromosomes in variable degrees of expression. Numerous genome-wide screens searching for links to atopy and asthma have led to the identification of possible active regions of almost every chromosome. Despite intense effort, however, few genes have been linked to asthma with any degree of certainty. Hence, there is presently no "genetic test" for asthma. Most of the chromosome regions identified are associated with genes encoding for inflammatory mediators or beta$_2$-adrenergic receptors. While these discoveries have yet to yield clinically relevant information, their sum in time will probably yield important insight into the genotypic and phenotypic variations of asthma.

Viruses have been implicated in the development of asthma. Animal studies have provided the basis for direct causal evidence for this mechanism, while human clinical studies have been inferential at best. The strongest epidemiologic evidence supporting a causal relationship between viral infection and asthma comes from longitudinal studies following children infected with the respiratory syncytial virus (RSV). RSV is a common cause of bronchiolitis in infants, and is also a common precipitant of asthma exacerbations in all age groups. Infants hospitalized with RSV bronchiolitis have been observed to be more likely to have recurrent wheezing episodes or asthma, but a direct cause and effect relationship has yet to be established. Since young children with asthma can develop exacerbations from common respiratory viruses, it is unclear as to whether those hospitalized infants may have asthma triggered by the RSV infection[5].

Animal models likewise support the potential for the induction of asthma as a result of exposure and sensitization to common inhaled antigens. In these studies, subsequent sensitization to common indoor allergens (dust mite, mold, cat dander, dog dander, cockroach) resulted in clinical and histologic changes consistent with asthma[6]. Data from human studies also suggest that sensitized children exposed to common allergens have greater asthma severity. However, the specific relationship between the development of allergen sensitivity and the development of asthma remains unclear.

In addition, other environmental exposures, specifically particulate matter, have been linked to the development of asthma in children. Passive exposure to tobacco smoke is most predictive of the subsequent development of asthma in children above all other environmental exposures. Epidemiologic studies have linked exposure to tobacco in utero to the subsequent development of asthma. Tobacco-exposed infants also have lower lung function that persists throughout life[7]. There also appears to be a relationship between tobacco exposure and worsening asthma severity. While the precise mechanisms governing these relationships have not been fully uncovered, the effect of tobacco smoke on the development of asthma and its severity is undeniable.

It is most likely that the development of asthma, as well as the severity of the disease, is multi-factorial. The potentially complex interaction of the various factors may itself explain the heterogeneous nature of asthma. While most individuals with asthma experience the onset of symptoms in childhood, the age of onset can vary from infancy to senescence. Similarly, asthma severity can worsen or lessen over time. These observations suggest that asthma occurs in individuals with some degree of genetic susceptibility who are further influenced by various environmental exposures, and the severity is influenced by genetics, environmental exposure, and the "life history" of the airways. Without a clearly identified etiology or group of causative factors, asthma prevention, identification of the pre-symptom individual with asthma, or precise prediction of prognosis is impossible. However, insight into the natural history of asthma may provide some degree of accurate prognostication in children.

Consistent with the theme of heterogeneity, the natural history of asthma in children is variable. This variability has caused considerable controversy, particularly with regard to the infant and toddler with asthma. However, data from large epidemiologic studies continue to provide greater understanding of the natural history of asthma[8].

Although asthma can present at any age, the peak ages of presentation for males are during the first 3 years of life and then at school age. The peak ages for females are again during the first 3 years of life and then at puberty or adolescence. It is not clear why the second peak occurs earlier in males. However, studies in respiratory system development suggest that the average airway caliber is smaller relative to body size in infant and pre-pubescent males than in females of the same age. After puberty, airway caliber is generally smaller in females than in males[9].

In population studies, nearly half of all infants and toddlers exhibit recurrent asthma symptoms. However, only a small percentage of these children have persistence of symptoms or evidence of bronchial hyper-reactivity beyond the sixth year of life. While it is impossible to predict which children will have persistent asthma, some general characteristics have been identified[10]. Children under 3 years of age who have evidence of atopy, who wheeze in between viral respiratory infections, or whose parents have asthma, are more likely to have persistence of symptoms beyond age 6. In contrast, young children who do not have these risk factors and wheeze only with viral respiratory infections are less likely to have asthma symptoms or bronchial hyper-reactivity later in life. Overall, there is approximately a 50% likelihood that a young child with recurrent wheezing will go on to have asthma after age 6.

The high prevalence of asthma symptoms in this youngest age group and the potential marked difference in outcomes in preschool children and infants have raised the question of whether or not children in this age group should be diagnosed with asthma or if different terminology should be used. As there is no uniform agreement on this topic at present, the term asthma should be used for children who fit diagnostic criteria. In most cases the child should receive therapy commensurate with the level of disease severity, and symptom occurrence should be closely monitored over the first 3–6 years of life. If the child is symptom-free for a period of time despite exposure to known triggers, an observed trial off therapy is warranted.

Older children, adolescents, or adults with asthma may enter a period of time when they do not seem to have symptoms even when they are not taking controller medication. Although it appears that they no longer have asthma, bronchial challenge testing reveals that they still have airway hyper-responsiveness. Little is known about this remission period. It may last only a year or two before symptoms return, or it may continue for the rest of the individual's life. Children and adolescents with an established diagnosis of asthma who are in remission should continue to have quick-relief medication available and should be monitored at regular intervals in case the asthma again becomes active.

For most children who have asthma, symptoms remain present indefinitely if not properly treated. With the exception of infants and toddlers, there is no evidence that supports the notion that children "outgrow" asthma. To the contrary, longitudinal population studies confirm the persistence of airway hyper-responsiveness into adulthood. However, the severity of asthma can change in either direction. This may occur in response to therapy or with withdrawal of therapy, with a change in environment, during periods of hormonal change, or for no identifiable reason.

PATHOPHYSIOLOGY OF ASTHMA

The classic description of the pathology of asthma includes a mucosa that is thickened and infiltrated with inflammatory cells, presence of smooth muscle hypertrophy, and alteration of the epithelium of the bronchi and bronchioles[11]. The airway caliber is smaller, and the lumen contains mucus mixed with debris. Neutrophils and eosinophils may be abundant within the airways, and the degradation of the latter gives rise to Charcot-laden crystals. Mucus casts of smaller airways, referred to as Curschman's spirals, are also present in extreme cases. This classic description arose mostly from post-mortem specimens from individuals who succumbed to asthma. In contrast, biopsy specimens from airways of patients with asthma have yielded a spectrum of pathologic findings, ranging from normal airway histology to that seen in fatal asthma. However, consistent findings among these specimens include mucosal thickening with cellular infiltration, disorganization of the epithelium, and submucosal alteration[12].

This last observation, seen in some but not all patients, has given rise to a theory that asthma, over time, causes remodeling of the airway. Airway remodeling, while not yet a proven concept, is supported by longitudinal observations of declining lung function in some children with asthma, along with a more rapid decline of lung function in adults with asthma relative to the normal decline in healthy non-smokers. This alteration is thought to occur secondary to prolonged exposure of airway tissue to inflammation, leading to destruction of normal airway tissue and deposition of fibrin. It is important to note that these changes have been observed in patients in all classes of severity, including patients with mild and less frequent symptoms. It is unclear whether airway remodeling (a) is preventable, (b) is reversible, and (c) potentially can occur in all patients with asthma or is limited to a yet unspecified subset of patients.

A variety of chemical inflammatory mediators have also been identified in the airways of patients with asthma.

Interleukins, kinins, and leukotrienes have been isolated in significantly elevated concentrations in specimens obtained by bronchial lavage. These findings, along with the discovery of inflammatory cells, have given rise to the idea that a complex cascade of pro-inflammatory events potentially takes place within the airways of patients with asthma. Despite intense research, no single predominant inflammatory pathway has been identified. Furthermore, it is difficult to discern which pathways are important in a given individual patient, reinforcing the concept of asthma as a heterogeneous disease. Finally, since there is poor correlation between inflammatory mediators found in the lung and serum or urine markers, a laboratory test to confirm the diagnosis of asthma does not yet exist[13].

Inflammation of the airway mucosa and constriction of airway smooth muscle are the key pathophysiologic features of asthma. Airway inflammation gives rise to epithelial irritation, excess mucus production and cellular damage that in turn gives rise to cough. The inflammation also causes mucosal swelling, leading to a narrowed airway lumen. The airway caliber is further reduced by airway smooth muscle constriction that is presumably triggered by inflammatory mediators. Debris in the airway causes additional obstruction, and during exacerbations of asthma the increased numbers of polymorphonuclear leukocytes increase the viscosity of airway secretions. The resultant airway obstruction causes increased resistance to airflow, particularly during expiration. As ventilation continues through the narrowed bronchial tree, gas is trapped in the lung, and hyperinflation of the chest ensues. The increase in residual volume must be balanced by a decrease in vital capacity, inspiratory capacity, and ultimately tidal volume.

The patient with intrathoracic airway obstruction attempts to compensate by employing a prolonged and active expiratory phase. To maintain minute ventilation, the respiratory rate increases, limiting the total expiratory time. If the obstruction is not relieved, the patient is maintained in a constant state of respiratory compromise. The decrease in vital capacity limits the respiratory reserve available, so that minute ventilation cannot increase in response to activity. Progressive decrease in tidal volume and respiratory muscle fatigue can lead to respiratory failure.

CLINICAL PRESENTATION

In the absence of laboratory tests or genetic markers for asthma, the diagnosis of asthma is made with clinical information (Table 6-1). A detailed history of the child's symptoms provides most, if not all, of the information necessary to make a diagnosis. The four common symptoms of asthma are cough, wheeze, chest discomfort, and labored breathing[14]. Some children may experience all

Table 6-1 Diagnostic Findings in Asthma

Symptoms	Signs	Investigations
Cough	Wheeze	Pulmonary function test
Prolonged	Retractions	Chest radiograph
"Deep, hacking"	Prolonged	Pulse oximetry
After exertion	expiration	
After exposure to trigger	Tachypnea	
During sleep		
Wheeze		
With colds		
With exertion		
After exposure to trigger		
Chest discomfort		
With exertion		
Labored breathing		
With colds		
With exertion		
After exposure to trigger		

Symptom should be *recurrent*, in *response* to a trigger, and *reversible* with asthma medications

four symptoms, while others exhibit only one. A precise initial history will usually reveal that the patient has experienced more than one symptom, but there may not be a clear temporal relationship between the symptoms. In any case, it is critical to establish a pattern of recurrence or persistence of these symptoms to support a diagnosis of asthma. It is also important to investigate patterns in the recurrences that suggest potential triggers, as these patterns support the characteristic of airway hyper-responsiveness. Finally, the symptoms should diminish or disappear when a bronchodilator or anti-inflammatory medication is administered to the child.

Cough occurs naturally as a defense mechanism in response to airway irritation. In asthma, it probably reflects the hypersensitive state of the mucosa of inflamed airways. Cough is the most common symptom in children with asthma, but it is also ubiquitous and non-specific in the pediatric population. Therefore, it is important to establish a chronic or recurrent pattern in order to decrease the number of diagnostic possibilities. However, there are qualitative and chronologic features of this symptom that are more consistent with a diagnosis of asthma.

In most cases of asthma, the cough is described as "dry," "tight," or non-productive, particularly when the cough is episodic or in the early stages of an exacerbation. It is not unusual for the cough to become "wet," "loose," or productive as an asthma exacerbation evolves. However, a recurrent or persistent productive cough suggests alternative conditions, such as postnasal drip or cystic fibrosis. Parents may also use other descriptors, such as a "deep," "hacking," or "chest" cough. These qualities are consistent with cough in asthma, but can suggest alternative diagnoses as well. The cough is usually not paroxysmal, but children may have "coughing fits" during asthma exacerbations.

The timing of the occurrence of cough is often helpful. In a child with asthma, a cough will start or increase in frequency or severity after exposure to a potential allergen (e.g., an animal, pollen, or mold) or irritant (e.g., smoke, fumes, or cold air). This can occur from within a few minutes to 12–24 hours after exposure. Further, the cough may abate shortly after the child is removed from the stimulus or can continue or even worsen despite separation of the child and the trigger. The duration and severity of the cough in this case is usually related to the severity of the asthma, but can also be a reflection of the degree of underlying airway inflammation. Cough may also occur after several minutes of sustained exercise. In this case, the cough probably is a manifestation of airway irritation from cooler, drier air introduced into the airways as tidal volume increases, rather than of the exercise itself.

Children with asthma will often manifest cough during sleep. However, it is important to be precise when establishing the chronology of the cough during sleep. Typically, children with asthma will cough several hours into sleep. In contrast, cough from gastroesophageal reflux tends to occur soon after lying down, as well as throughout the night. Cough from postnasal drip also occurs soon after lying down, but also around the time of waking. Usually the cough will not wake the child, but will wake other members of the household. Therefore, it is helpful to question not only the parents but also the siblings or other members of the household.

A wheeze is a continuous, musical sound that is produced by turbulent flow that occurs in the bronchi. In asthma, this turbulence is produced by partial airway obstruction, or narrowing, from mucosal inflammation, airway debris, and contraction of airway smooth muscle. During exhalation, lung volume decreases and intrathoracic pressure increases, resulting in decreased airway caliber throughout the lung. Therefore, wheezing usually occurs exclusively during the expiratory phase of breathing. However, airway narrowing present in some children may also result in wheezing during the inspiratory phase as well. A continuous musical sound that occurs only during inhalation is usually termed stridor and reflects extrathoracic airflow obstruction.

A further clarification regarding the terminology of wheezing is necessary. Wheezing can be polyphonic (or heterophonous) or it can be monophonic (or homophonous). Like a pipe organ, heterophonous sounds are produced by forcing air through tubes of different calibers. Therefore, a heterophonous wheeze reflects gradations of airway narrowing throughout the bronchial tree and is the more common type of wheeze heard in asthma. In contrast, a homophonous wheeze occurs when air is forced through tubes with similar calibers. A homophonous wheeze, for example, may occur from a partial obstruction in a fixed segment of the intrathoracic airway, or if several bronchi approximate a similar caliber. Although a homophonous wheeze usually suggests a condition other than asthma, it can occur in children with asthma, especially during the recovery phase of an exacerbation.

A reliable history of wheezing is difficult to obtain, particularly since children may make a variety of noises during breathing. Parents may interpret other noises as a wheeze. On the other hand, the wheeze may be present but unappreciated without a stethoscope. Therefore, probing questions requiring detailed answers are required to validate a history of wheezing. Astute historians will associate the wheeze with exhalation, or be able to describe or mimic the sound. Parents or children may also describe a "chest rattle" or perceived chest "congestion." Older children and adolescents may also report that they hear themselves wheeze, or that they can "feel" the wheeze in their chest. Again, precise questioning and thoughtful consideration of the answers are required to establish a true history of wheeze.

Once a history of wheeze has been elicited, the timing of the wheezing occurrences should be ascertained. Similar to cough, the wheeze in asthma should be recurrent and follow exposure to an identifiable trigger. The perception of wheeze in children is usually episodic. Reports of a continuous, ever-present wheeze suggest other causes of partial intrathoracic airflow obstruction. Wheezing may get louder as airflow obstruction worsens, but it may also become louder during times of increased tidal volume, such as during excitement or during or after periods of exertion. Conversely, wheezing may become inaudible during sleep or as severely narrowed airways limit airflow. Wheezing from asthma should diminish to some extent after bronchodilator or anti-inflammatory treatment. If these therapies do not decrease wheezing when administered, alternative diagnoses should be considered.

Labored breathing can be a symptom by itself, but in this context represents a category of "observed symptoms" that are most often reported by a caregiver in infants and younger children with asthma. Parents have a sense of their child's labored breathing but have difficulty describing the observations that prompt that feeling. An increased respiratory rate is an early sign of respiratory compromise, but in asthma this can occur gradually and therefore be too subtle for the parent to notice until the breathing rate is very high. Similarly, thoraco-abdominal asynchrony can occur in asthma, particularly in infants and toddlers, but it is often unnoticed by an untrained observer unless there is serious respiratory compromise. Therefore, these representative observations of labored breathing in young children with asthma are usually noticed only during exacerbations, along with subcostal and intercostal retractions. Occasionally, an astute caregiver may notice a prolonged expiratory phase.

Older children and adolescents with asthma may describe a vague sense of difficulty breathing during inspiration, although some may articulate that they have difficulty getting air out. In this age group, this symptom usually occurs during exacerbations or as part of a complaint of exercise intolerance. The latter situation is common in patients with asthma, but can also occur with other conditions. Children with asthma should be able to exercise for a few minutes before experiencing dyspnea, unless their asthma is severe or they are in the midst of an exacerbation. Dyspnea within the first minute of exertion is less likely due to asthma, and alternative etiologies should be considered. Also, the patient should be able to distinguish between dyspnea and fatigue. In asthma, dyspnea may occur after a few minutes of exercise, but fatigue should not be present unless the exertion continues in the face of impaired breathing. Alternative diagnoses should be sought if fatigue occurs prior to or simultaneous with dyspnea during exertion.

Chest discomfort, or tightness, is sometimes mistaken as dyspnea, but is a separate and distinct symptom that is characteristic of asthma. The precise physiologic basis for this complaint is not known, although the sensation probably reflects the hyperexpansion of the pleura or thoracic cage. Although the sensation is uncomfortable, it should be distinguished from chest pain, a symptom that suggests other conditions.

Older children and adolescents with asthma present with chest tightness as a chief complaint or offer this symptom without solicitation. However, even verbal preschool children may articulate this symptom if asked in age-appropriate language. Like the other symptoms of asthma, chest tightness can occur by itself or in association with other symptoms, and its historical occurrence should establish a pattern of recurrence and a temporal relationship with potential triggers. Chest tightness can occur at any time in patients with asthma, but most often it is experienced during exacerbations and with exercise. To be consistent with a diagnosis of asthma, both labored breathing and chest tightness should diminish with bronchodilator or anti-inflammatory therapy. However, when these symptoms are associated with exertion, they may also resolve with rest.

A family history of asthma, particularly in the parents or siblings, is not part of the diagnostic criteria for asthma. However, it is supportive of the diagnosis if present. A history of eczema or allergic rhinoconjunctivitis also is supportive of the diagnosis, since these conditions often coexist with asthma. The review of systems is important in excluding alternative diagnoses and identifying comorbid conditions.

Unless the patient is experiencing an exacerbation, there may be no physical findings consistent with the diagnosis of asthma on presentation, even if symptoms were present within the previous 24 hours. Many of the physical findings of asthma, such as tachypnea and subcostal retractions, are non-specific and reflect pulmonary compromise in general. Other signs, such as wheeze and a prolonged expiratory phase, are more specific to intrathoracic airway obstruction, but are not exclusive to asthma. Furthermore, wheezing may be missed during quiet breathing, or if the patient is so compromised that there is inadequate airflow to produce a wheeze. To avoid missing a wheeze, the patient should be encouraged to take a slow deep breath in and then exhale forcefully. In a young or uncooperative child, the examiner can compress the thorax anteroposteriorly to mimic a forced exhalation. It is important to note that while there are physical findings that are supportive of a diagnosis of asthma, these findings do not confirm the diagnosis. However, an observed improvement in these findings by the examiner after bronchodilator administration demonstrates reversibility of airflow obstruction, a key component of the diagnostic criteria. Findings on physical examination that are not consistent with a diagnosis of asthma should lead to an investigation of alternative diagnoses or comorbid conditions.

Laboratory Evaluation

Laboratory investigations of the patient with asthma may support the diagnosis, but no investigation can independently confirm the diagnosis of asthma. Blood eosinophilia can be found in patients with asthma, but is neither a universal nor a specific finding. Some patients with asthma may have an elevated serum immunoglobulin E (IgE), but this finding is also non-specific. Although patients with asthma often have atopy, RAST or skin testing may be negative; alternatively, demonstration of sensitivity does not confirm a diagnosis of asthma.

Chest radiographic findings also are non-specific. These include hyperinflation, peribronchial thickening, and atelectasis, but the study can be normal as well (Figure 6-1). Radiographic examination is useful to rule out complications of asthma when suspected, such as pneumothorax, pneumomediastinum, or large areas of atelectasis.

School-age children and adolescents who can execute a forced expiratory maneuver can perform spirometry at baseline and following bronchodilator administration[15]. While some patients with asthma will exhibit airflow obstruction at baseline, spirometry is within accepted reference limits in most children with asthma unless they are in the midst of an exacerbation[16]. A significant increase in flows following bronchodilator administration demonstrates full or partial reversal of airflow obstruction, but this finding represents only one component of the diagnostic criteria (Figure 6-2). Moreover, some patients with asthma and airflow obstruction may not demonstrate reversal of the obstruction with the

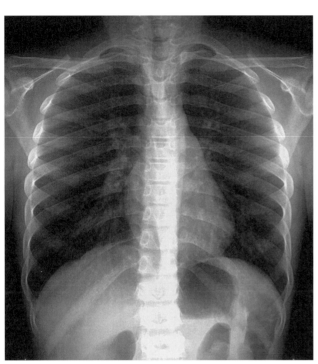
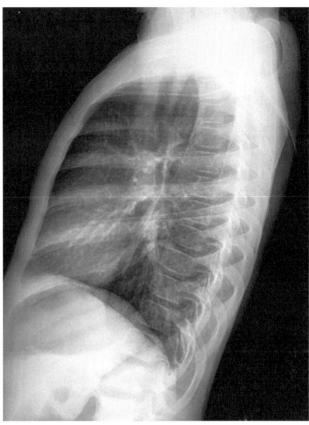

A   B

Figure 6-1   (**A**) Posterior-anterior chest radiograph of an 11-year-old boy with asthma during an acute exacerbation. The interstitial markings are mildly increased. The cardiothymic silhouette is normal. (**B**) Lateral view, demonstrating mild hyperinflation with flattening of the diaphragm and an increase in the retrosternal air space. (Radiographs courtesy of Avrum Pollock, M.D.)

standard dose of bronchodilator used in pulmonary function laboratories.

When airway hyper-responsiveness cannot be established by history in a patient suspected of having asthma, an airway provocation test can be performed[17]. This test uses a physical stimulus (exercise, inhaled cold air, or hypertonic saline) or pharmacologic stimulus (inhaled methacholine or histamine) to assess airway sensitivity (Figure 6-3). After baseline spirometry is performed, the stimulus is applied and titrated either by accumulated time that the stimulus is applied (e.g., cold dry air) or by increasing dose (e.g., methacholine). Spirometry is performed again after the stimulus, and a significant decrease in flows indicates airway hyper-responsiveness. Usually a bronchodilator is administered after the last spirometry to assess the reversibility of the airflow obstruction. Widely accepted standards exist for the performance and interpretation of commonly used provocative tests.

Airway provocation tests are usually employed when some of the clinical diagnostic criteria are present, suggesting the diagnosis of asthma, but a degree of

uncertainty exists. Provocative tests provide two of the three criteria for diagnosis: airway hyper-responsiveness (abnormal decrease in expiratory flow following exposure to the stimulus) and reversibility of airflow obstruction (expiratory airflow returns to baseline, exceeds baseline, or at least improves significantly when a bronchodilator is administered following a decrease in airflow provoked by a stimulus). Within a population suspected of having asthma, the sensitivity and specificity of provocative testing are both above 90%. However, this high sensitivity and specificity is dependent on the proper performance of the test on an appropriate patient and correct interpretation of the results.

Patients without asthma who have allergic rhinitis, respiratory infections, or other airway diseases (bronchopulmonary dysplasia, cystic fibrosis) may have "positive" provocative tests on either a transient or a recurrent basis. It is therefore important to use provocative testing as a confirmatory test in patients with a history of chronic or recurrent symptoms of asthma. It is impractical to use provocative testing as a screening tool for asthma in the clinical setting because of the time and expense of the test

Spirometry

		Ref	Pre meas	Pre % ref	Post meas	Post % ref	Post % change
FVC	Liters	2.45	2.66	109	3.09	126	16
FEV1	Liters	2.13	1.48	70	2.28	107	54
FEV1/FVC	%	87	56		74		
FEF25–75%	L/sec	2.89	0.41	14	1.67	58	305
PEF	L/sec	6.02	5.29	88	7.33	122	39
FEF/FIF50			0.27		0.67		143
FET100%	Sec		16.02		10.05		−37
FEV.5	Liters		1.11		1.80		62

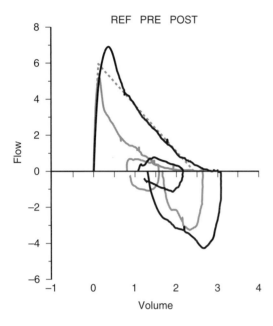

REF PRE POST

(Plot: Flow vs Volume)

Figure 6-2 Spirogram obtained from a 16-year-old girl with severe persistent asthma during an acute exacerbation. At baseline (smaller curve) there is significant reduction in flows through small airways, reflected by a markedly decreased value for Forced Expiratory Flows between 25 and 75% of the vital capacity (FEF$_{25-75\%}$). There is a dramatic increase in forced expiratory flows at all lung volumes after inhalation of albuterol and ipratropium (larger curve). Note that peak expiratory flows are normal both before and after bronchodilator administration, despite the obvious reversible small airway obstruction. The triangle represents reference values for gender and height.

and the lack of information on the significance of the test in asymptomatic individuals.

What constitutes a significant decrease after provocation or increase after bronchodilator administration varies according to the provocative stimulus or bronchodilator used and the type of measurement employed. Accordingly, normal values and significant changes in airflow are often determined by the testing laboratories based on accepted standards and modified as needed to reflect the individual laboratory testing conditions and experience with the local population. In general, a 15–20% decline in the forced expiratory volume in the first second (FEV$_1$) is considered to be a significant decrease after provocation, while a 12–15% rise in FEV$_1$ after bronchodilator inhalation constitutes a significant increase.

Any form of lung function testing should be performed by trained and experienced personnel using high-quality calibrated equipment. Testers should have demonstrated proficiency working with the age group being tested, and the testing laboratory should have documented testing procedure, quality assurance, and infection control practices that conform to accepted standards. Suboptimal testing, including poor performance by the patient, yields results that have little diagnostic value.

Likewise, interpretation of test results should be performed by individuals with expertise in lung function test analysis. In particular, provocative testing should be administered and interpreted by qualified persons because of added safety concerns inherent in the test and the complex nature of the data generated.

Some experts advocate the widespread use of peak expiratory flow (PEF) monitoring. A variety of simple and inexpensive peak flow meters are available for measuring PEF, but values from one device are not interchangeable with those of another. Proper use of a peak flow meter requires a period of 1–2 weeks of twice-daily use and recording of values to establish the patient's "personal best." Both the absolute value and degree of diurnal variability are used to determine the presence of bronchospasm or airway hyper-reactivity. A maximal effort is mandatory to obtain information that accurately reflects the underlying condition of the airways. This high degree of effort dependence, and the fact that PEF measurements are fairly insensitive to changes in small airway caliber (Figure 6-2), limit the usefulness of routine PEF monitoring. PEF monitoring is poorly reproducible in school children[18], and several studies show that it adds little to programs of asthma education that stress symptom

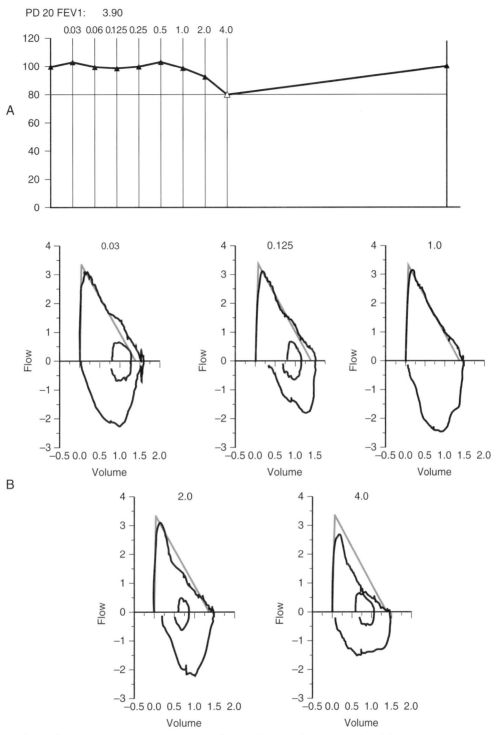

Figure 6-3 Methacholine challenge in a 6-year-old boy with exercise-related dyspnea. Spirometry is performed after which a methacholine aerosol is administered. Spirometry is repeated after each dose of methacholine administered, and the dose is doubled until the forced expiratory volume in the first second (FEV_1) falls by 20% or a maximum dose of methacholine is administered. (**A**) The FEV_1 as a percent of the baseline value before and after each doubling dose of methacholine. The FEV_1 began to fall at 1 mg methacholine, and fell below the targeted range with the 4 mg dose. The dose of methacholine causing a 20% drop in the FEV_1 was calculated to be 3.9 mg. Bronchodilator administration returned the FEV_1 to its pre-challenge level. (**B**) Progression from a normal, convex expiratory flow-volume loop at 0.03 mg, 0.125 mg and 1.0 mg methacholine, to a concave shape at 2.0 and 4.0 mg methacholine, reflecting small airway obstruction. The curve shape reverted to normal after administration of albuterol (not shown).

recognition by patient or caregiver. The greatest utility of PEF monitoring, then, is for the subset of patients who are not sensitive enough to recognize chest tightness or shortness of breath when symptoms begin to escalate. Such patients might benefit from routine PEF testing to identify early signs of an acute exacerbation in order to initiate therapy early.

DIFFERENTIAL DIAGNOSIS

There are several conditions that mimic asthma by producing similar chronic or recurrent symptoms, or exist as comorbid conditions. These conditions are presented in Table 6-2. In most cases, there is little or no relief from bronchodilator administration, and pulmonary function tests are in the normal range. However, in many cases patients may report a substantial subjective relief after bronchodilator use, and some conditions can be associated with spirometric abnormalities.

Sinusitis and other rhinosinal diseases can result in cough from postnasal drip[19]. However, these disorders by themselves are not associated with wheezing, chest discomfort, or difficulty breathing. The cough associated with postnasal drip is usually most prominent upon lying down, and again first thing in the morning, but is not associated with cough during exertion. There is usually no relief after bronchodilator use, and spirometry is normal in patients without lower airway disease. Symptoms of nasal disease are usually elicited, and nasal and pharyngeal discharge and irritation can be found. Identifying rhinosinal disease, however, does not rule out asthma. Indeed, untreated sinusitis or rhinitis can act as a symptom trigger in patients with asthma, complicating treatment.

Gastroesophageal reflux (GER) can also mimic asthma, causing cough, wheeze, chest discomfort, and a perception of labored breathing[20]. These symptoms can result from microaspiration of refluxate, or can also occur due to afferent stimulation of the esophagus from stomach acid. Most patients with GER, when questioned, will complain of burning, dyspepsia, or other symptoms of gastroesophageal reflux disease (GERD). However, some patients may have "silent reflux" and deny overt symptoms, and have no evidence of esophageal irritation on endoscopy. Respiratory symptoms from GER typically occur after eating or upon lying down, but can also occur at random times. Furthermore, patients with GER may report decreased symptoms with bronchodilator use, and may exhibit subtle abnormalities on spirometry. Consequently, it can be extremely difficult to differentiate asthma from GER. Diagnostic testing, such as gastric radionuclide scans or sustained esophageal pH recordings, may demonstrate that the patient has GER, but such testing does not prove a link between the GER and respiratory symptoms. Therefore, a trial of antacid therapy of at least 4–6 weeks may be necessary to determine whether the symptoms can be attributed to GER. Even if symptoms decrease over time with antacid therapy, the patient can still have asthma that is being exacerbated by GER.

Although foreign body aspiration usually presents with acute onset of symptoms, unwitnessed inhalation of a relatively small foreign object can result in more indolent symptoms of cough and wheeze that can be mistaken for asthma. Although the aspiration event itself might not be identified, the parent can usually pinpoint the precise day symptoms started. In addition, unlike asthma, the symptom intensity in the patient with foreign body aspiration usually is high initially, and stays the same or even decreases slightly over time. The wheeze, if present, will usually be homophonous and can often be localized. There is minimal relief after bronchodilator use, and if the child is old enough to perform spirometry, a fixed expiratory airflow obstruction might be present. If foreign body aspiration is being considered, thorough airway endoscopy should be performed.

Chronic aspiration due to swallowing dysfunction can also produce cough and wheeze, resulting in an erroneous diagnosis of asthma. Although typically occurring in patients with underlying neurologic disease or subtle upper airway anatomic abnormalities, swallowing dysfunction can also occur in an otherwise normal child. In most cases, the symptoms occur only during oral feeding, and are otherwise absent. However, symptoms may occur from aspiration of oral or nasopharyngeal secretions or from gastric refluxate. This latter scenario is mostly limited to patients with neurodevelopmental challenges. Patients with suspected swallowing dysfunction should be evaluated by a speech therapist in conjunction with swallowing videoradiography. Gastric radionuclide scan might show aspiration of gastric refluxate, but usually only massive aspiration will be detected with this test. Aspiration of oropharyngeal secretions is demonstrated by a radionuclide salivagram.

Patients with intrinsic intrathoracic airway abnormalities can present with wheezing and difficulty breathing. These abnormalities, ranging from tracheobronchomalacia

Table 6-2 Differential Diagnosis

Disease	Diagnosis
Rhinitis	Clinical
Sinusitis	CT of sinuses
Gastroesophageal reflux	Radionuclide scan, pH probe
Foreign body	Endoscopy
Chronic aspiration	Swallowing study, salivagram
Airway compression	Endoscopy, CT, MRI
Cystic fibrosis	Sweat test

to bronchial stenosis, can be congenital or acquired. Characteristically the wheeze is homophonous, and the difficulty in breathing occurs during respiratory challenges such as with exercise and during respiratory tract infections. There is no relief with bronchodilator administration, and wheezing can increase after bronchodilator use in patients with tracheomalacia or bronchomalacia. Spirometry in these patients reveals fixed airflow obstruction. Classically, airway endoscopy has been used to characterize the airway abnormality. More recently, fixed-caliber airway abnormalities have been evaluated using high-resolution computed tomography, while dynamic airway collapse has been demonstrated using cine-computed tomography.

Extrinsic intrathoracic airway compression can also mimic asthma, and presents with the same characteristics as intrinsic airway abnormalities. The airways in these cases are usually compressed either by an aberrant vessel or by a mediastinal tumor. The compressed area can be visualized by airway endoscopy, but this approach will not definitively identify the compressing object. Computed tomography with intravenous contrast is the investigation of choice if airway compression is suspected.

Cystic fibrosis may be mistaken for asthma, particularly in younger children or in CF patients who have mild disease. Symptoms can be identical, and relief may occur after bronchodilator therapy. Spirometry can be normal, or airflow obstruction can be present and possibly reversible with bronchodilator administration. Non-specific triggers, such as exercise or fumes, may exacerbate symptoms. Pathognomonic productive cough and failure to thrive may be subtle or absent. Although cystic fibrosis occurs most commonly in Caucasians, it is found in patients of all ethnic backgrounds. A sweat test or genetic testing for cystic fibrosis should be strongly considered when evaluating a child with cough, wheeze, and labored breathing, especially if symptoms are present from early childhood and digital clubbing is present.

CLASSIFICATION OF ASTHMA SEVERITY

Once the diagnosis of asthma is confirmed, the severity of disease should be classified in order to guide therapy. National guidelines provide an outline for the assessment of severity[1]. Similar to the diagnostic criteria for asthma, severity is mainly assessed by report of symptoms, and the classification is therefore limited by the accuracy of the reporter. Information solicited for classification of severity includes the frequency of symptom occurrence within a defined period and the subjective assessment of the impact of these symptoms on activities of daily living. Spirometry is also used for classification for those patients who can reliably perform pulmonary function testing.

To minimize inaccuracy that may result from memory limitations, the frequency and severity of symptoms are recounted by the historian within a defined 2–4 week time period.

The initial publication of the National Institutes of Health Guidelines for the Diagnosis and Treatment of Asthma identified four categories of severity[1]: mild intermittent, mild persistent, moderate persistent, and severe persistent. These categories of severity, along with treatment recommendations, are summarized in Table 6-3. The word "persistent" actually refers to the persistence

---

Table 6-3   Classification of Asthma Severity

Severity	Symptom Frequency	Lung Function (% predicted)	Recommended Therapy
Mild intermittent	< 2 days/week < 2 nights/month <3 episodes/year	$FEV_1 \geq 80\%$	Short-acting beta-agonist (SABA) PRN
Mild persistent	≥ 2 days/week ≥ 2 nights/month ≥ 3 episodes/year	$FEV_1 > 80\%$	Low-dose inhaled corticosteroid (ICS) Leukotriene modifier Cromones Methylxanthines

Moderate persistent	Daily
	1 night/week
		FEV_1 80–60%	Moderate-dose ICS
			or
			Combination ICS plus:
			    (a) long-acting beta-agonist (LABA) or
			    (b) leukotriene modifier

Severe persistent	Continuous during day
	Every night
		$FEV_1 < 60\%$	Combination high-dose ICS or oral corticosteroid
			    plus long-acting beta-agonist (LABA),
			    leukotriene modifier, methylxanthine

of symptoms, rather than the persistence of the severity or of the disease. Therefore, patients with mild persistent asthma have fewer symptoms that affect activities of daily living to a lesser degree than those with moderate asthma. As symptom frequency and activity limitation increase, the severity escalates to moderate or severe. However, a patient with mild persistent asthma can still have a severe exacerbation. In fact, a study of asthma mortality revealed that a third of patients who died from asthma were classified as having mild asthma[21].

The classification of mild intermittent asthma provides for an interesting paradox. As a chronic disease, asthma is always present in an affected individual, yet the disease may be quiescent and produce no symptoms for months. However, the potential for onset of symptoms, or even an asthma exacerbation, exists even for patients with very intermittent symptoms. In addition, airway inflammation can be present at low levels, below the threshold that would cause discernible symptoms or measurable changes in lung function, in patients with so-called intermittent asthma. Therefore, this term is somewhat misleading, since it is not possible to discern easily whether it is the disease process that is present only intermittently or the symptoms.

So-called exercise-induced asthma exists as a sub-classification of mild intermittent asthma[22]. This term is also misleading, since exercise does not confer asthma on the would-be athlete, but rather brings out the symptoms of asthma. In these cases exercise by itself is not a trigger in the usual sense. Exercise of all but the briefest duration causes an increase in minute ventilation, and this increase overwhelms the normal heating and humidification process in the upper respiratory system and allows cooler, drier air into the lower airways. In theory, the cooler, drier air irritates the bronchial airways of the person with asthma, and asthma symptoms arise. This effect is more intense in an individual experiencing an asthma exacerbation, and leads to speculation that asthma symptoms during exercise may be an indicator of the relative degree of inflammation of the airway. If this theory is true, it suggests that patients with exercise-induced asthma have persistent airway inflammation, and therefore should receive daily anti-inflammatory therapy. Indeed, in many patients who present with complaints of asthma symptoms only with exercise, a careful history reveals that they also have asthma symptoms at other times. However, it should be noted that while anti-inflammatory therapies decrease the degree of airway compromise, as measured by exercise testing, they do not completely ablate the reduction in expiratory flow observed in patients with asthma.

Since asthma can be highly variable from day to day, season to season, and year to year, patients may move from one classification to another independent of medical intervention. Asthma symptoms also episodically worsen, and this should be termed an asthma exacerbation. The popular term "asthma attack" should be avoided, since it describes the patient as a victim, and the disease as an episodic aggressor. Asthma exacerbations can vary widely in severity, and there is no uniform classification. The term "status asthmaticus" is still employed to describe a serious asthma exacerbation. Classically, this term was used when a patient with obvious respiratory compromise did not improve significantly after three subcutaneous injections of a sympathomimetic, and implied that the patient was at risk to develop respiratory failure and would require intensive inpatient therapy. Presently, the term is sometimes applied in a similar fashion, but more often describes a patient who is not wheeze-free after three consecutive treatments with an inhaled bronchodilator. While this term does imply a serious condition that warrants at least inpatient therapy, it has less precision in describing the actual condition of the patient.

THERAPY FOR ASTHMA

Pharmacologic Therapy

The overall objective of therapy for the child with asthma is to maintain disease control. The specific goals of therapy are:

- Minimal (ideally no) chronic symptoms, including nocturnal symptoms
- Minimal (infrequent) exacerbations
- No emergency visits
- Minimal (ideally no) use of as-needed beta$_2$-agonist
- No limitations on activities, including exercise
- Near-normal pulmonary function test
- Minimal (or no) adverse effects of medication.

Asthma therapies can be categorized in three ways: as chronic and acute therapy, as inhalation and systemic therapy, and as anti-inflammatory and bronchodilator therapy. While it is helpful to consider the available asthma therapies within these classification schemes, there is overlap in each grouping. For example, anti-inflammatory medications are the mainstays of chronic therapy but are also used in acute therapy. Similarly, the systemic availability of inhaled medications is dose-dependent, and some anti-inflammatory medications may also cause some degree of bronchodilation. Therefore, the classification of asthma therapy is helpful in understanding the application of the therapy in the context of treating a patient with asthma, but not as a way of describing the inherent properties of the medications.

Since asthma is confined to the airways, inhalation therapy is employed as a kind of "topical" therapy in order to limit drug exposure to the target organ and to avoid systemic side effects. This elegant concept, however, is fraught with practical difficulties. First, medications need to be developed into a formulation that can be safely and effectively inhaled. This limits the medications to those that are completely soluble in aqueous solutions with a neutral pH. Second, the respiratory system is designed to circulate gas in and out of the airways while filtering out particulate matter. Therefore, the size of the medication particles has to be in the "respirable range" (0.5-5 μm); that is, not so large that they get trapped in the upper airway and not so small that they get exhaled without settling on the airway. Finally, while chemical absorption occurs to a lesser degree along the airways than in the alveoli, substantial drug absorption can still take place through the bronchial mucous membranes. Medications should therefore be active at the airway surface, but should either be poorly absorbed into the circulation or be systemically inactive. Considering these limitations, effective inhalation therapy is difficult to achieve.

Inhaled medications are mostly delivered either by nebulization or with metered-dose inhalers. Nebulization is a process by which energy is applied to a solid or liquid to produce a vapor. The earliest nebulization therapy involved applying heat to a liquid to produce steam or burning a substance to produce smoke. Modern nebulization techniques utilize either vibration or jet streams of gas to produce a vapor. Ultrasonic nebulizers work by providing vibrational energy to a discrete amount of liquid. While this method can nebulize a large amount of fluid within a short time, the resultant vapor particles are large and tend to settle out on the upper airway surfaces. Jet nebulizers utilize a high-velocity gas stream, provided either by a compressed gas source or by a compressor, to broach a gas-liquid interface and "drag" the liquid particles into the stream, producing a vapor. Jet nebulizers take longer to aerosolize a discrete amount of liquid, but produce more particles that are within the respirable range.

While jet nebulizers seem easy to use, they are inefficient as drug delivery devices. Inhalation of the vapor discharged in the vicinity of the nose and mouth, the so-called blow by technique, delivers less than 10% of the nebulized medication into the lower airways. Using a mask over the nose and mouth at the point of delivery improves this percentage to about 15%. In the best-case scenario, in which the patient receives the vapor using a mouthpiece while sitting or standing, inhaling slowly and deeply, and holding the breath for 5-10 seconds, delivery can be improved to 25-30%. Furthermore, medication delivery using jet nebulizers is time-consuming. Depending on the power of the compressor, it usually takes 5-15 minutes to nebulize 3 ml of liquid fully. In addition, the bulkiness of the compressor and the need for a power source limit the portability of this therapy.

Considering the inefficiency and use limitations of this delivery method, it should be used only if the medication cannot be delivered safely and effectively by any other means.

Metered-dose inhalers (MDIs) are available in two forms: as pressurized canisters (pMDIs) and as dry powder inhalers (DPIs). Both devices deliver a discrete quantity of medication per administration cycle, hence "metered-dose," and therefore an MDI contains a set number of doses. Medication in the pMDI is discharged from the canister by actuating the inhaler. In most cases, this is achieved by compressing a triggering device, although some pMDI are breath-actuated and are triggered by the patient inhaling at the mouthpiece. Medication from a DPI is delivered by active inhalation from the patient.

MDIs are portable, less expensive, and more efficient at medication delivery than nebulizers, but are more difficult to use correctly. Medication from a pMDI is discharged at a high initial velocity. If a patient discharges a pMDI while the mouthpiece is at the lips, much of the medication will impact the oropharyngeal structures and will be swallowed, thereby decreasing the amount of medication delivered to the airways. Even in a well-coordinated individual, only 15-25% of the medication will reach the lower airways by this method.

Efficiency increases if the patient uses a spacer, which is a conduit that provides a set distance between the pMDI and the lips. Medication delivery can be further optimized using a fixed-volume holding chamber. This device is a spacer modified with valves that hold the medication in the chamber until the patient inhales. Both spacers and holding chambers can be fitted with either a mouthpiece, or a mask for infants and children who cannot use a mouthpiece. When using these devices, the patient should actuate the inhaler then either take a slow deep breath and hold the breath for 5-10 seconds, or take 6-10 normal breaths while the mask or mouthpiece is in place.

To use a DPI, patients must initiate an inhalation that is above a set minimum flow rate. This forceful and sustained inhalation is necessary to extract the medication from the inhaler. Therefore, this device should not be used by infants or children who cannot generate the required inspiratory flow rate. Once the inhalation is completed, the patient should hold his or her breath for 5-10 seconds.

While asthma is a chronic disease, there are episodic exacerbations that can occur, regardless of the severity. Therefore, both chronic and acute therapies are needed. The primary goals of long-term asthma therapy, referred to as controller therapy, include preventing exacerbations, decreasing or eliminating symptoms, and optimizing lung function. Achieving these goals should result in an improved quality of life, as long as the therapies imposed do not negatively impact the patient. The therapies, therefore, should be maximally effective but easy to implement and free of adverse experiences. Since the pathophysiology of asthma is caused by airway inflammation and bronchoconstriction, asthma treatment should reduce and prevent inflammation and relax airway smooth muscle. The goals of acute therapy are to reverse the progression of an exacerbation and provide for a rapid recovery to control of disease at baseline.

Controller Therapy

Inhaled Corticosteroids

Inhaled corticosteroids (ICSs) provide the most effective anti-inflammatory therapy that can be used long term with relative safety. ICSs are available in formulations for nebulization and in pMDIs and DPIs.

Corticosteroids enter the cell and bind to glucocorticoid receptors at the nucleus. ICSs inhibit a broad spectrum of inflammatory processes in the airway. ICSs also upregulate beta-agonist receptors, theoretically increasing the effectiveness of bronchodilators that stimulate these receptors. However, ICSs also have the potential of causing side effects attributed to glucocorticoids. For this reason, the daily dose of ICS should be as low as possible while achieving the therapeutic goals.

Generally, therapeutic effectiveness and side effects are dose-dependent. However, topical potency and systemic bioavailability are two properties of ICSs that further dictate the relative benefits and risks of their use. Topical potency describes the degree of inflammatory wheal reduction achieved by a specified dose of the glucocorticoid, so that an ICS with a high topical potency can reduce inflammation at a lower dose. Systemic bioavailability defines the amount of circulating glucocorticoid that results from a fixed inhaled dose, so that an ICS with a low systemic bioavailability will result in a minimal amount of glucocorticoid in the systemic circulation. Therefore, the ideal ICS will have a high topical potency and low systemic bioavailability.

In children with asthma, daily use of ICS decreases symptom and exacerbation frequency and improves pulmonary function and exercise tolerance. Although some patients may exhibit a "first dose" effect, usually patients will not show improvement in symptom control until they have received at least 1 week of daily therapy. The starting dose of ICS is based on the severity classification of the patient at the time of evaluation, and should be adequate to effect a significant reduction in symptoms within 2 weeks. In most cases, the therapeutic effect will plateau in 6–8 weeks, and at this point the dose may be decreased in a stepwise fashion. However, it is prudent to maintain the initial dose of ICS until the patient has contact with some of the usual asthma triggers or weathers an exacerbation, in order to judge the effectiveness

of the dose in preventing symptoms and decreasing the severity of exacerbations. If the patient demonstrates tolerance to trigger exposure with few or no symptoms or has a shorter or less severe exacerbation, the dose may be decreased.

With each change in dose, the patient should be re-evaluated at regular intervals, and symptom and exacerbation frequency and severity should be reviewed. Pulmonary function tests should also be performed at each follow-up visit. An increase in symptom or exacerbation frequency or severity, or a decline in lung function, may indicate that the ICS dose should be increased. In an individual patient, the ICS dose may be titrated up or down over time, and periodic re-evaluation is critical to determine the lowest dose of ICS that will achieve the therapeutic goals.

Since the majority of children have mild asthma, symptom control will be achieved at the lowest possible daily dose, and caregivers or health care providers are often tempted to discontinue ICS therapy, either for a season ("medication holiday") or indefinitely. In children who have had persistent asthma symptoms over the age of 4 years this practice usually results in a relapse of symptoms, or even an exacerbation. If ICS therapy is discontinued on a trial basis, an ICS, along with the means to administer it, should be readily available. Therapy should be reinitiated at the first indication that symptoms have returned. Such patients should be evaluated yearly for a return of asthma symptoms, and pulmonary function tests should be obtained. ICS therapy should be reinstituted if there is a report of asthma symptoms, decreased exercise tolerance, or if there is a decline in lung function.

There are no data from placebo-controlled studies that demonstrate a benefit from the use of ICS as a short-term therapy for exacerbations of asthma. However, observations from a few case-control studies suggest that increasing the dose of ICS at the beginning of an exacerbation may decrease the need for systemic corticosteroid use.

There are potential local and systemic side effects related to ICS use. The most common side effect of ICS use is oropharyngeal candidiasis. This side effect can usually be avoided by having the patient rinse the oropharyngeal cavity after ICS use and by the use of a spacer or holding chamber to minimize oropharyngeal deposition. Occasionally, dysphonia and reflex cough are associated with ICS use, and are more common in patients who do not use a holding chamber during administration. Evidence to date suggests that chronic use of ICS does not cause alterations in dental enamel or respiratory tract mucosa and does not predispose the user to dental caries or bacterial and viral infections.

Systemic side effects of chronic ICS use involve bone metabolism and possible adrenal suppression. In the first year of use of some ICSs a small reduction in growth velocity has been demonstrated. However, longer-term studies of ICS use in children, as well as follow-up studies, suggest that there is no difference in ultimate height between patients who use ICS as children and controls[23]. Biochemical evidence of bone resorption has been observed in both adults and children during ICS use. However, changes in bone mineral density have not been detected in patients using ICSs in daily doses less than 500 µg. Treatment with high doses of ICS has been associated with suppression of the hypothalamic-pituitary-adrenal (HPA) axis in children, but doses less than 400 µg daily are not normally associated with any significant suppression. Rarely, posterior subcapsular cataracts have been associated with high-dose ICS use, but have not been reported at doses of ICS under 400 µg per day.

Systemic Glucocorticoids

In patients with severe asthma or those who have allergic bronchopulmonary aspergillosis, chronic systemic glucocorticoid therapy may be necessary. In these patients, therapy is initiated at a dose that will control symptoms, and then the dose is gradually tapered to the lowest dose that will still control symptoms. Often, the dose can be reduced to once every other day. Despite the use of low, alternate-day dosing, serious side effects of chronic glucocorticoid use can still occur. At the onset of chronic systemic glucocorticoid use, blood pressure and height should be measured. Baseline bone densitometry and an ophthalmologic evaluation should also be performed, and repeated annually. Patients requiring chronic systemic glucocorticoid use should be evaluated frequently, and blood pressure and height should be carefully tracked at each visit.

Cromolyn Sodium and Nedocromil

Cromolyn sodium and nedocromil (cromones) are non-steroidal inhaled anti-inflammatory medications that are available as a nebulized formulation (cromolyn) and as pMDIs. Their mechanism appears to involve the blockade of chloride channels, and it is speculated that these drugs modulate mast cell mediator release and eosinophil recruitment to provide long-term control of symptoms. Their anti-inflammatory effect is moderate compared with ICSs and therefore they are not usually recommended as monotherapy. They are also less convenient to use than are ICS, because they must be used several times throughout the day for maximum effectiveness. However, these medications have an excellent safety profile.

Leukotriene Modifiers

Leukotriene modifiers (LMs) block the effects of leukotrienes, biochemical mediators released from mast cells, eosinophils, and basophils. Leukotrienes have been demonstrated to contract airway smooth muscle, increase vascular permeability, increase mucus secretion, and attract and activate other inflammatory cells in the airways of patients with asthma[24]. LMs are available as oral medications and are prescribed once or twice daily. Data from studies to date suggest that while LMs work well to control asthma symptoms in some patients, they are not effective in others. LMs are considered to be alternative therapy to ICSs, and are generally considered to be effective as monotherapy only in patients with mild asthma. However, the concomitant use of LMs with ICSs often allows for a reduction of the ICS dose while maintaining the same degree of symptom control. LMs should not be used as quick-relief agents. LMs also have a benign side effect profile.

Methylxanthines

Methylxanthines are relatively weak bronchodilators that are administered systemically. They have been used for treatment of acute exacerbations as well as for long-term control of asthma symptoms. The most common methylxanthine used for asthma treatment is theophylline. In addition to its bronchodilator effects, theophylline has also been shown to increase respiratory drive and sensitivity to blood pCO_2, and to increase diaphragmatic contractility. These latter effects make theophylline a useful drug for patients with asthma who are in impending respiratory failure.

Because of their variable absorption and high side effect profile, methylxanthines are presently considered less favorable for daily use. In addition, drug levels must be monitored to assure that they are within the therapeutic range, especially because metabolism can be affected by simultaneous use of other medications or viral infections, and toxic levels are associated with serious side effects, such as seizures and cardiac arrhythmias.

Long-Acting Beta-Agonists

Long-acting beta-agonists (LABAs) have both a longer onset of action (about 20 minutes) and a longer duration of action (up to 12 hours) compared with short-acting $beta_2$-agonists. Presently, all are available in the United States only as DPIs, although an MDI form of salmeterol is available in Europe and Canada. Side effects, such as tachycardia and jitteriness, are much less common with LABAs than with short-acting beta-agonists, provided that the LABA is not overused. LABAs should only be used in conjunction with ICS therapy when asthma symptoms are incompletely controlled by ICSs alone. Their use has been shown to permit a significant reduction in the dose of ICS required for symptom control[25]. LABAs are especially useful for children with persistent nocturnal symptoms or exercise-induced asthma (EIA). Because their onset of action is relatively long, LABAs should not be used as quick-relief medication for treatment of acute exacerbations.

Anti-immunoglobulin E

Anti-immunoglobulin E therapy has been shown to decrease the frequency of asthma exacerbations and to allow for a decrease in ICS daily dose. Anti-IgE reduces free serum IgE levels and therefore averts inflammatory cell degranulation by preventing the binding of IgE to its high-affinity receptor. Anti-IgE is administered by injection and is given monthly. Because of the cost and complexity of this therapy, its use is generally confined to patients with moderate or severe asthma.

The assessment of the severity of disease determines the plan of maintenance therapy for a patient. As disease severity increases, the daily dose of ICS increases, and other medications can be used in conjunction with ICSs to maintain disease control. When initiating therapy, the philosophy of treatment is to gain control then "step down." Therefore, initial therapy will utilize the regimen that will most likely achieve disease control, and subsequent therapy should be judiciously reduced to establish the lowest amount of medication required to maintain control. The National Institutes of Health Guidelines for the Diagnosis and Treatment of Asthma[1,26] recommends a stepwise approach to the pharmacologic management of asthma. These recommendations are summarized in Table 6-3.

Since the mainstay of asthma management is daily use of controller medications over many years, concerns about the medications' effects and side effects should be explored and addressed to assure adherence[27]. This is especially true regarding ICS use. Many families and patients are reluctant to use steroids at all, let alone for a long period of time. Therefore, patients and caregivers should be educated about the benefits of ICS use as well as the common side effects and how to minimize or prevent them.

Acute Therapy

Short-Acting Beta-Agonists

Short-acting beta-agonists (SABAs) have been the mainstay of acute asthma treatment in children for many years. These drugs are by far the most effective "quick-relief" bronchodilators available and therefore are the first-line treatment for acute asthma exacerbations. Although earlier preparations of beta-agonists stimulated both beta-1 and beta-2 receptors (i.e., isoproterenol, isoetharine), more recent preparations are considered "selective" because they stimulate primarily beta-2 receptors. As such, they cause fewer extrapulmonary symptoms such as tachycardia, although side effects are experienced with frequent or higher doses. These drugs are available in oral tablet or liquid, inhaled MDI, DPI or nebulizer solution, or intravenous preparation. Rapid-acting beta$_2$-agonists preferably should be given via inhalation to maximize efficacy and minimize side effects. However, delivery of inhaled medication may be suboptimal in patients with acute respiratory distress and airway narrowing. In these clinical situations, subcutaneous or intravenous administration of beta-agonist may be more effective than inhaled therapy.

Onset of action of short-acting beta$_2$-agonists is usually within 5 minutes when given by inhalation. The typical duration of bronchodilation produced by a single dose of rapid-acting inhaled beta$_2$-agonist in children is 1–5 hours. Side effects of beta$_2$-agonists include tremors, tachycardia, "hyperactivity," and hypokalemia. During frequent or continuous administration of beta-agonists during acute exacerbations, patients should be observed for these side effects, and the dose should be decreased in amount and frequency as tolerated as quickly as possible.

Beta$_2$-agonists should always be prescribed as quick-relief therapy for all patients with asthma unless the patient has a well-defined intolerance for any form of the drug. The patient should use the beta$_2$-agonist as needed for symptom relief. Sporadic use of beta$_2$-agonist generally signifies good disease control, whereas patients who are using their beta$_2$-agonist frequently probably require additional controller therapy. For patients with exercise-related symptoms, inhalation of beta$_2$-agonists can offer significant protection against exercise-induced symptoms[28].

Anticholinergic agents have a limited role in the treatment of children with asthma. Like beta-agonists, they cause relaxation of airway smooth muscle, but by the cholinergic, not adrenergic, pathway. There is some evidence that concomitant use of anticholinergic agents with inhaled beta$_2$-agonists provides additive benefit in severe asthma exacerbations[29]. Their effectiveness in long-term management of asthma has not been demonstrated. Anticholinergics are available in formulation for nebulization as well as in pMDI for inhalation.

Systemic Glucocorticoids

Systemic glucocorticoids are often required to treat asthma exacerbations. Oral glucocorticoids should be used in patients who develop asthma symptoms that do not fully diminish with the use of short-acting beta-agonists. Intravenous glucocorticoids may be administered in patients who cannot tolerate oral medications, but there are no data demonstrating that intravenous administration is superior to oral dosing in terms of efficacy.

In general, prednisone or prednisolone in doses of 1–2 mg/kg per day should be prescribed for a duration of 3–7 days. Therapy of longer duration may be necessary in patients with severe disease or in patients who have experienced an exacerbation in the recent past. There is no evidence to suggest that twice-daily dosing is superior to once-daily dosing, and morning administration of glucocorticoid will decrease the incidence of sleep disruption experienced by some patients. There is no need to taper the dose of glucocorticoid unless the course of therapy is longer than 7 days, the patient recently finished a course of systemic steroid therapy, or the patient receives chronic systemic glucocorticoid therapy. Side effects of short-term systemic glucocorticoid therapy include water retention, mood changes, and increased appetite.

Asthma exacerbations can occur at any time, but they occur less frequently in patients whose disease is well controlled. An exacerbation can develop quickly, usually as a result of exposure to a trigger such as a viral infection or an allergen that causes airway inflammation. However, an exacerbation can also develop slowly, with a more gradual pattern of deterioration that may reflect failure of long-term management to control airway inflammation adequately.

It is important to recognize the asthmatics who are at increased risk for severe or even fatal asthma. Patients with a history of near-fatal asthma requiring intubation and mechanical ventilation have a 19-fold increased risk of needing intubation during subsequent exacerbations. Other risk factors include: patients who have had a hospitalization or emergency care visit for asthma in the past year; patients who are not currently using inhaled glucocorticosteroids or who are dependent only, or mostly, on rapid-acting inhaled beta$_2$-agonists; and patients with a history of non-adherence with an asthma medication plan. In addition, significant morbidity and mortality are most often associated with failure to recognize the severity of the exacerbation[30].

Initiation of appropriate therapy at the earliest possible signs of deteriorating control of asthma is important in the successful management of asthma exacerbations[31,32]. Initial treatment of an asthma exacerbation should start at home. Parents and patients should be instructed to start acute relief medication, i.e., short-acting beta$_2$-agonists, with the first signs or symptoms of an asthma exacerbation. There is some evidence that increasing the dose of ICSs, together with recurrent doses of short-acting beta$_2$-agonist, can resolve an acute asthma exacerbation faster compared with inhaled beta$_2$-agonist use alone. Studies have also suggested that increasing ICS therapy at the first signs of upper respiratory infection can prevent an asthma exacerbation[33]. Failure to respond to these initial measures should prompt further evaluation and treatment by medical caregivers. Medical attention should be sought if the patient is at a high risk for asthma-related death, the response to the bronchodilator is not prompt and sustained for at least 3 hours, or there is no improvement or even deterioration 2–6 hours after glucocorticosteroid treatment is started.

The primary therapy for an asthma exacerbation in a medical facility is the repetitive administration of rapid-acting inhaled beta$_2$-agonist and the early introduction of systemic glucocorticosteroids. The patient should be closely monitored, since children with asthma may deteriorate rapidly. Oxyhemoglobin saturation should also be assessed to insure that there is adequate oxygen saturation. Patients who are hypoxemic should receive supplemental oxygen[34]. Along with the increase in inflammation and airway swelling, small areas of atelectasis form secondary to mucous plugging. These areas

lead to ventilation perfusion ($\dot{V}/\dot{Q}$) imbalances, which in turn cause a decrease in oxygen saturation. Occasionally, the oxygen saturation will drop as inhaled beta-agonist is given. This phenomenon is thought to reflect an increase in $\dot{V}/\dot{Q}$ mismatch due to the vasodilatory effect of albuterol. Persistent oxyhemoglobin desaturation often suggests a potential severe exacerbation, and patients with low oxygen saturation in room air should be considered for admission to the hospital. If blood gas tensions are measured in a patient with an asthma exacerbation, the pCO$_2$ should be below 40 torr. A normal or high pCO$_2$ in this clinical scenario at best suggests a severe exacerbation and may signify impending respiratory failure.

Addition of an anticholinergic drug might be considered if the improvement following recurrent doses of albuterol is not satisfactory. Ipratropium bromide can be added to the beta-agonist, as some studies showed an added benefit of the practice in acute settings. If little or no improvement is seen following initial intensive management, the patient will probably require continued aggressive therapy and expert monitoring, with admission to the hospital.

Hospital management of the patient with asthma should provide continuous therapy that is modulated based on frequent assessment. In addition to assessing vital signs and oxyhemoglobin saturation, work of breathing and gas excursion should be taken into account in tandem. The presence or absence of wheeze is less relevant, since wheeze may be present in a patient who is nearly fully recovered and may be absent in a patient with impending respiratory failure.

Frequent or continuous beta-agonist inhalation should be administered, along with systemic glucocorticoid therapy. Supplemental oxygen should be administered if needed, and intravenous fluids should be provided if the patient cannot maintain adequate oral hydration. As the patient improves, bronchodilator therapy can be reduced. Patients who fail to improve despite therapy should be assessed for comorbidities, and patients whose condition worsens should be transferred to an intensive care setting. In some cases, patients appear to improve in terms of decreased work of breathing but continue to have low oxyhemoglobin saturation. It is likely that atelectasis has occurred in these patients, and airway clearance and increased activity out of bed will hasten the resolution of this comorbidity.

It should be noted that full recovery from the exacerbation is often gradual, and medications for the exacerbation may need to be continued for several days to sustain relief of symptoms and improvement in pulmonary function.

Non-Pharmacologic Therapy

As with any chronic disease, the cornerstone of successful asthma therapy lies with patient education.

In order to insure adherence with therapy and proper medication administration, the patient and caregivers should have a thorough knowledge of asthma and asthma therapy. It is important that patients and caregivers understand what asthma is and that it is a chronic disease that is constantly present, regardless of the presence or absence of symptoms.

Education should start at the time of diagnosis and should be incorporated into each visit[35]. The key facts that should be repeatedly assessed are the patient's and family's understanding of the basic facts about asthma, the role of medications, correct technique of inhaler use, environmental control measures, and when and how to take rescue medications[36].

All patients should have a written management plan that outlines the patient's daily therapy, how to recognize signs of deterioration and assess the severity of symptoms, and when to modify or augment treatment, or obtain more specialized care if appropriate (Figure 6-4). This treatment plan should be devised with the specific knowledge of the patient's and caregiver's lifestyle and means, and ideally it is done in partnership with the patient and caregiver. Developing an asthma action plan together with the patient and caregiver involves the patients (or the family) in their own management plan. A "joint effort" will increase the probability that the plan can be carried out successfully in terms of daily schedule and the amount of medications. The final written management plan should be shared with all potential caregivers, including day care providers and school health care workers.

Each asthma patient has triggers that can lead to an acute exacerbation. It is important for each patient to sort out each precipitating factor and try to avoid them as much as possible. Such factors include allergens (environmental and household), air pollutants (cigarette smoking), respiratory infections, exercise and hyperventilation, weather changes, sulfur dioxide, foods and drugs, and extreme emotional expression.

One of the most common exacerbating factors in asthma is allergic sensitization. To eliminate these external factors one must first attempt to determine the patient's exposure to allergens. This can be done mostly by reviewing the patient's exposure history or by using skin testing. If an allergen is not found, but there is a strong clinical suspicion for an allergic component of asthma, or if there is an allergen that cannot be completely avoided (e.g., grass, trees), a trial of antihistamine medication, with or without nasal steroid preparation, should be instituted with a goal of symptom control. In some patients, immunotherapy (allergy vaccines or "shots") is warranted.

COMPLICATING FACTORS

Once a diagnosis of asthma is made, the severity classified, and the appropriate treatment plan is given and explained, a reasonable control of symptoms should be expected. However, in some cases the patient's symptoms do not diminish despite what seems to be appropriate therapy. This often gives rise to so-called steroid-dependent asthma patients. Although there are a few patients who do require low-dose systemic steroids to control their disease, this condition is rare in pediatrics. In such cases there is often a complicating factor that has not been discovered or properly treated.

The most common pitfall in asthma management is poor adherence to the asthma management plan. Reasons for poor adherence include a lack of understanding of disease chronicity, the patient's poor perception of his or her asthma severity, concerns about the safety and efficacy of medication, and low treatment expectations. Good patient education that includes explanation of the disease and its pathophysiology, as well as the medications' mechanisms of action and side effects, increases the patient's understanding and acceptance of treatment. Reassessment of the patient's or family's perception of the disease and the treatment plan, with recurrent exploration of treatment barriers, will assure better adherence and cooperation.

Another common reason for treatment failure is the incorrect use of inhaled medications. Errors in inhaled medication administration include using an inhaler that no longer contains medication, improper operation of the device, and failure to actuate the inhaler, inhale the medication properly, or use a holding chamber. At each visit the correct use of MDI, DPI or nebulizer should be assessed, and the correct method for determining the refill time of the device should be confirmed.

Continued exposure to triggers is another cause for incomplete symptom control. Questions about exposure to animals or tobacco smoke should be asked in relation to all venues the child may visit. If trigger avoidance has been maximized, an evaluation for allergic triggers and candidacy for immunotherapy should be considered.

Comorbid conditions, such as rhinitis, sinusitis[37], and gastroesophageal reflux[38], should be considered in patients who do not respond fully to appropriate controller therapy. Rhinitis or sinusitis may cause (through inflammation or infection) continuous irritation of the sinopulmonary tree. Allergic rhinitis should be treated with antihistamines and intranasal steroids, while rhinitis should be treated with decongestants. Sinusitis should be treated with a suitable antibiotic regimen, along with decongestants to allow drainage of the sinuses.

Gastroesophageal reflux (GER) has frequently been shown to coexist with asthma. Often, uncontrolled asthma can, in turn, worsen GER through hyperinflation and increased intra-abdominal pressure. An assessment for GER should always be considered in a patient whose asthma is uncontrolled despite therapy.

Allergic bronchopulmonary aspergillosis (ABPA), an extreme sensitivity to the mold *Aspergillus fumigatus*,

AMP-999 Rev 7/04

The Children's Hospital of Philadelphia Asthma Care plan
Name: John Wheezer , Date: 12/30/2004
MRN: 123456, DOB: 1/1/01

Take these medicines everyday:

Give these **controller (anti-inflammatory)** medicines everyday, to prevent problems. Even when you/your child is well!

Medicine	How much?	How often?
Flovent Inhaler 44 mcg with a spacer	2 puffs	2 times a day

GREEN ZONE   REMEMBER TO RINSE YOUR MOUTH OUT AFTER TAKING INHALED MEDICINES!!!

Take these medicines if you have trouble breathing with exercise:

Albuterol inhaler with a spacer	2 puffs	15-30 minutes before exercise

Take these medicines when symptoms start:

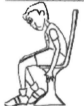

For cough, wheeze, shortness of breath or chest tightness use a **quick-relief (bronchodilator)** medicine:

Albuterol inhaler with a spacer	2 puffs	up to every 4 hours as needed

YELLOW ZONE   IF QUICK-RELIEF MEDICINE IS NEEDED MORE THAN ONCE A DAY FOR YOUR ASTHMA SYMPTOMS, A FLARE MAY BE STARTING!

Take these medicines for Flares

For cough, wheeze, shortness of breath or chest tightness:
1. Continue to use your **quick-relief (bronchodilator)** medicines for **UP TO 7 DAYS** :

Albuterol inhaler with a spacer	2 puffs	up to every 4 hours as needed

2. Give extra **controller (anti-inflammatory)** medicine:

Flovent Inhaler 44mcg with a spacer	4 puffs	2 times a day FOR 7 DAYS

- Call your doctor's office if the symptoms don't improve in 2 days OR IF THE FLARE lasts for longer than 7 days .
- If the flare ends by the 7 days day go back to Green Zone and take everyday medications as instructed

RED ZONE:
IF asthma symptoms are getting worse, breathing is hard and fast and your child cannot talk:
Take Albuterol one vial by nebulizer or 4 puffs with spacer **AND** call _____

IF YOU CANNOT REACH ANYONE GO TO NEAREST EMERGENCY ROOM!!

Provider: _____
Service:

Figure 6-4   Typical asthma action plan, detailing prescription for controller (every day) medications and steps to be taken in case of an escalation of asthma symptoms. (Courtesy of The CHOP Asthma Initiative.)

and aspirin sensitivity are rare entities in children with asthma. However, these conditions can also result in poor asthma control. The diagnosis for ABPA is usually centered on a very high serum IgE level, while the diagnosis of aspirin sensitivity is discovered by careful history. Since the evaluation and treatment of these entities is complex, patients suspected of having these disorders should be evaluated by an asthma specialist.

Finally, a consideration of misdiagnosis or incomplete evaluation must be considered in the pediatric patient with asthma who fails to demonstrate improvement despite what seems to be proper therapy. Referral to an asthma specialist should be considered in cases where the patient is not meeting the goals of therapy after suitable interventions have taken place or if the patient requires specialty testing, has severe asthma, or has a history of life-threatening exacerbations.

MAJOR POINTS

- Asthma is a common, chronic disease that affects infants, children, adolescents, and adults, and its severity, course, and progression are variable both among patients and within an individual patient.
- The precise etiology of asthma is not known, although there appear to be both genetic and environmental factors involved.
- The diagnosis of asthma is made primarily by history of symptoms that are *recurrent*, occur in *response* to a trigger, and are *reversible* with asthma medications; the most common symptom is cough.
- A successful treatment plan for asthma includes daily controller therapy, availability of reliever therapy, and thorough patient education.
- When patients with asthma fail to improve despite the proper prescription of controller therapy, an investigation of potential complicating factors should be performed.

REFERENCES

1. National Heart, Lung, and Blood Institute. National Asthma Education Program. Expert Panel Report. Guidelines for the diagnosis and management of asthma. J Allergy Clin Immunol 88:425-534, 1991.
2. The International Study of Asthma and Allergies in Childhood (ISAAC). Worldwide variations in the prevalence of asthma symptoms. Eur Respir J 12:315-335, 1998.
3. Ramsey CD, Celedon JC. The hygiene hypothesis and asthma. Curr Opin Pulm Med 11:14-20, 2005.
4. Holgate ST. Genetic and environmental interaction in allergy and asthma. J Allergy Clin Immunol 104:1139-1146, 1999.
5. Tuffaha A, Gern JE, Lemanske RF Jr. The role of respiratory viruses in acute and chronic asthma. Clin Chest Med 21:289-300, 2000.
6. Djukanovic R, Feather I, Gratziou C, Walls A, Peroni D, Bradding P, et al. Effect of natural allergen exposure during the grass pollen season on airways inflammatory cells and asthma symptoms. Thorax 51:575-581, 1996.
7. Nafstad P, Kongerud J, Botten G, Hagen JA, Jaakkola JJ. The role of passive smoking in the development of bronchial obstruction during the first 2 years of life. Epidemiology 8:293-297, 1997.
8. Guilbert TW, Morgan WJ, Zeiger RS, Bacharier LB, Boehmer SJ, Krawiec M, et al. Atopic characteristics of children with recurrent wheezing at high risk for the development of childhood asthma. J Allergy Clin Immunol 114:1282-1287, 2004.
9. Martinez FD, Helms PJ. Types of asthma and wheezing. Eur Respir J Suppl 27:3s-8s, 1998.
10. Guilbert TW, Morgan WJ, Krawiec M, Lemanske RF, Jr., Sorkness C, Szefler SJ, et al. The Prevention of Early Asthma in Kids study: design, rationale and methods for the Childhood Asthma Research and Education network. Control Clin Trials 25:286-310, 2004.
11. Dunnill MS. The pathology of asthma, with special reference to changes in the bronchial mucosa. J Clin Pathol 13:27-33, 1960.
12. Jacoby DB, Costello RM, Fryer AD. Eosinophil recruitment to the airway nerves. J Allergy Clin Immunol 107:211-218, 2001.
13. Bousquet J, Jeffery PK, Busse WW, Johnson M, Vignola AM. Asthma. From bronchoconstriction to airways inflammation and remodeling. Am J Respir Crit Care Med 161:1720-1745, 2000.
14. Abramson MJ, Hensley MJ, Saunders NA, Wlodarczyk JH. Evaluation of a new asthma questionnaire. J Asthma 28:129-139, 1991.
15. Bye MR, Kerstein D, Barsh E. The importance of spirometry in the assessment of childhood asthma. Am J Dis Child 146:977-978, 1992.
16. American Thoracic Society. Standardization of spirometry, 1994 update. Am J Respir Crit Care Med 152:1107-1136, 1995.
17. Cockcroft DW, Hargreave FE. Airway hyperresponsiveness. Relevance of random population data to clinical usefulness. Am Rev Respir Dis 142:497-500, 1990.
18. Frischer T, Meinert R, Urbanek R, Kuehr J. Variability of peak expiratory flow rate in children: short and long term reproducibility. Thorax 50:35-39, 1995.
19. Leynaert B, Bousquet J, Neukirch C, Liard R, Neukirch F. Perennial rhinitis: an independent risk factor for asthma in nonatopic subjects: results from the European Community Respiratory Health Survey. J Allergy Clin Immunol 104:301-304, 1999.
20. Field SK. Gastroesophageal reflux and asthma: are they related? J Asthma 36:631-644, 1999.

21. Turner MO, Noertjojo K, Vedal S, Bai T, Crump S, Fitzgerald JM. Risk factors for near-fatal asthma. A case-control study in hospitalized patients with asthma. Am J Respir Crit Care Med 157:1804–1809, 1998.

22. Randolph C. Exercise-induced asthma: update on pathophysiology, clinical diagnosis, and treatment. Curr Probl Pediatr 27:53–77, 1997.

23. The Childhood Asthma Management Program Research Group. Long-term effects of budesonide or nedocromil in children with asthma. N Engl J Med 343:1054–1063, 2000.

24. Szefler SJ. Current concepts in asthma treatment in children. Curr Opin Pediatr 16:299–304, 2004.

25. Lazarus SC, Boushey HA, Fahy JV, Chinchilli VM, Lemanske RF Jr., Sorkness CA, et al. Long-acting beta2-agonist monotherapy vs continued therapy with inhaled corticosteroids in patients with persistent asthma: a randomized controlled trial. JAMA 285:2583–2593, 2001.

26. National Asthma Education and Prevention Program. Expert Panel Report. Guidelines for the diagnosis and management of asthma: update on selected topics 2002. J Allergy Clin Immunol 110(5 Suppl):S141–219, 2002.

27. Suissa S, Ernst P, Benayoun S, Baltzan M, Cai B. Low-dose inhaled corticosteroids and the prevention of death from asthma. N Engl J Med 343:332–336, 2000.

28. Sears MR, Taylor DR, Print CG, Lake DC, Li QQ, Flannery EM, et al. Regular inhaled beta-agonist treatment in bronchial asthma. Lancet 336:1391–1396, 1990.

29. Rebuck AS, Chapman KR, Abboud R, Pare PD, Kreisman H, Wolkove N, et al. Nebulized anticholinergic and sympathomimetic treatment of asthma and chronic obstructive airways disease in the emergency room. Am J Med 82:59–64, 1987.

30. Rodrigo G, Rodrigo C. Assessment of the patient with acute asthma in the emergency department. A factor analytic study. Chest 104:1325–1328, 1993.

31. Cowie RL, Revitt SG, Underwood MF, Field SK. The effect of a peak flow-based action plan in the prevention of exacerbations of asthma. Chest 112:1534–1538, 1997.

32. Jones KP, Mullee MA, Middleton M, Chapman E, Holgate ST. Peak flow based asthma self-management: a randomised controlled study in general practice. British Thoracic Society Research Committee. Thorax 50:851–857, 1995.

33. Ververeli K, Chipps B. Oral corticosteroid-sparing effects of inhaled corticosteroids in the treatment of persistent and acute asthma. Ann Allergy Asthma Immunol 92:512–522, 2004.

34. Lipworth BJ, Clark RA, Dhillon DP, Brown RA, McDevitt DG. Beta-adrenoceptor responses to high doses of inhaled salbutamol in patients with bronchial asthma. Br J Clin Pharmacol 26:527–533, 1988.

35. Wasilewski Y, Clark NM, Evans D, Levison MJ, Levin B, Mellins RB. Factors associated with emergency department visits by children with asthma: implications for health education. Am J Public Health 86:1410–1415, 1996.

36. Evans D. To help patients control asthma the clinician must be a good listener and teacher. Thorax 48:685–687, 1993.

37. Watson WT, Becker AB, Simons FE. Treatment of allergic rhinitis with intranasal corticosteroids in patients with mild asthma: effect on lower airway responsiveness. J Allergy Clin Immunol 91:97–101, 1993.

38. Nelson HS. Gastroesophageal reflux and pulmonary disease. J Allergy Clin Immunol 73:547–556, 1984.

CHAPTER 7

Cystic Fibrosis

JUDITH A. VOYNOW, M.D.

THOMAS F. SCANLIN, M.D.

DEFINITION

Cystic fibrosis (CF) is an autosomal recessive disorder caused by mutations in a gene that encodes for a chloride channel and ion conductance regulator, the cystic fibrosis transmembrane conductance regulator (CFTR). This disease occurs predominantly in Caucasians and is ultimately lethal with a median survival of approximately 31 years. The disorder affects exocrine glands with the major manifestations involving the gastrointestinal and respiratory tracts. The primary manifestations of the disease include protein and fat malabsorption, and recurrent bronchitis with organisms such as *Pseudomonas aeruginosa* leading to bronchiectasis and, ultimately, respiratory failure. Another cardinal feature of the disease is excessive chloride concentrations in sweat, which is the basis for the first diagnostic test for the disease. CF is difficult to diagnose and manage due to the great variability in its presentation and clinical course. Since the identification of the CFTR gene in 1989, there have been significant advances in our understanding of the pathogenesis of the disease, which have spurred the development of new molecular approaches to therapy. This chapter will review the latest information on the genetic, molecular, and cellular basis of the disease, and then focus primarily on the clinical manifestations, complications, diagnosis, and current management of CF.

GENETICS

Cystic fibrosis is inherited as an autosomal recessive trait. In the United States, the incidence of disease in Caucasians is approximately 1 in 3300, and in African-Americans, 1 in 15,000. The frequency of unaffected heterozygote Caucasian carriers is 1 in 25 (reviewed in Welsh et al.[1] and Robinson and Scanlin[2]).

As mentioned above, CF is caused by mutations in the gene encoding a protein called the cystic fibrosis transmembrane conductance regulator (CFTR). This gene was first identified in 1989[3] as a candidate gene for CF because of the linkage between the most common mutation of the gene and disease-affected individuals in large family cohorts. Complementation studies demonstrated that transfection of the normal CFTR gene into native CF cells corrected a major physiologic abnormality in CF cells, abnormal chloride ion transport[4]. This provided the formal proof that mutations in the CFTR gene are responsible for CF.

The CF gene is located on chromosome 7, and is a 230 kb gene containing 27 exons. The most common mutation, a three-base pair deletion in exon 10, results in deletion of phenylalanine at position 508 (ΔF508). The ΔF508 mutation accounts for approximately 66% of allelic mutations causing CF. To date, more than 1000 mutations have been reported[1]; however, only five other mutations— G542X, G551D, W1282X, N1303K, R553X—occur at greater than 1% frequency. CF mutations are localized throughout the CFTR gene but fall into five major categories of CFTR dysfunction[5] (Figure 7-1). Class I mutations, including nonsense mutations such as G542X and W1282X, result in failure to transcribe mRNA and, thus, cause absence of CFTR protein. Class II mutations, including the most common mutation, DF508, cause abnormal protein folding, aberrant trafficking and, subsequently, protein degradation. Class III mutations, including G551D, permit proper protein processing and localization but cause loss of ion channel function. Class IV mutations, such as R117H and R334W, allow normal protein processing and localization but reduce normal ion conduction properties. Class V mutations, including mutations in the CFTR gene promoter and introns, affect transcription, translation, or protein processing, and may result in mild CF disease or isolated disorders such as congenital bilateral absence of the vas deferens[6] or idiopathic pancreatitis[7].

Manifestations of CF disease may be affected by modifier genes independent of CFTR gene mutations. For example, a modifier locus on chromosome 19 segregates with patients who have meconium ileus[8]. Another striking example is the correlation between mutations in the mannose-binding lectin gene and increased severity of CF lung disease[9].

PATHOPHYSIOLOGY

The CF gene encodes an integral membrane glycoprotein containing 1480 amino acids. The protein structure includes two transmembrane domains, two nucleotide-binding fold domains with sites for ATP binding, and a

Molecular Consequences of CFTR Mutations

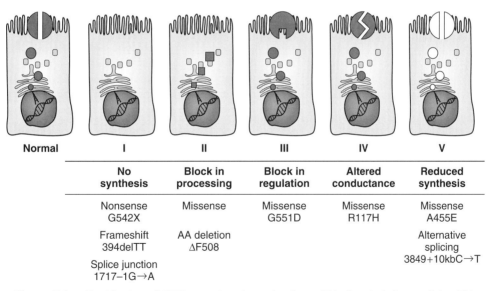

	Normal	No synthesis	Block in processing	Block in regulation	Altered conductance	Reduced synthesis
		I	II	III	IV	V
		Nonsense G542X	Missense	Missense G551D	Missense R117H	Missense A455E
		Frameshift 394delTT	AA deletion ΔF508			Alternative splicing 3849+10kbC→T
		Splice junction 1717–1G→A				

Figure 7-1   Classification of CFTR mutations by molecular and biochemical abnormalities. This schematic depicts the effect of different classes of CFTR mutations on expression and function in the cell. Class I mutations block mRNA transcription. Class II mutations prevent normal CFTR protein processing and localization. Class III mutations permit CFTR localization at the apical membrane but inhibit chloride channel conductance. Class IV mutations result in partial chloride channel conductance. Class V mutations affect transcription, translation or protein processing resulting in reduced CFTR expression at the apical membrane. Examples of mutations in each class are depicted below the cell models. Epithelial cell models with finger-like projections depict cilia at the apical surface. Fully processed CFTR protein is depicted by the grey circles embedded among the cilia at the apical surface of the cells.

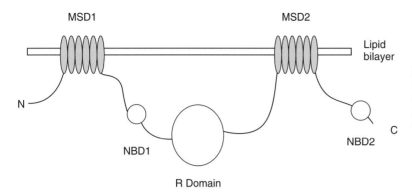

Figure 7-2   Map of CFTR functional peptide domains. CFTR peptide domains within a lipid bilayer are depicted. MSD, membrane spanning domains; NBD, nucleotide binding domains; R domain, regulatory domain.

large regulatory or R domain that has several consensus sites for protein kinase A- or C-mediated phosphorylation (Figure 7-2). CFTR is localized to the apical compartment of epithelial cells in the respiratory, gastrointestinal and genitourinary tracts, and sweat and salivary ducts. CFTR functions as an apical chloride channel; normal function requires correct protein localization to the apical membrane of the cell, as well as both nucleotide binding and phosphorylation. In addition to chloride transport, CFTR regulates other epithelial ion channels including an outwardly-rectifying chloride channel, an apical sodium channel, a potassium channel, and a chloride/bicarbonate exchanger[1]. CFTR may also regulate intra- and extracellular protein transport, and regulate post-translational processing of glycoproteins which would explain the observation that CF glycoproteins have greater fucose content and less sialic acid content than glycoproteins from normal epithelial cells[2,10].

The absence of CFTR function alters the balance of fluid and protein, and the composition of glycoproteins in exocrine gland secretions. These alterations result in abnormal biochemical properties of the secretions that impair mucociliary clearance in the lungs, promote colonization with pathogenic organisms in the airways, and impede normal flow in biliary and pancreatic ducts, leading to the manifestations of the disease.

Respiratory Tract

Although the airways appear normal morphologically at birth, impaired mucociliary clearance, early colonization with pathogenic bacteria, and a robust neutrophilic inflammatory response occur early in infancy. The earliest pathologic findings involve inflammation and mucus obstruction of the distal bronchioles. Within mucus plugs, pathogenic organisms tend to colonize and proliferate. Patients are colonized early with *Staphylococcus aureus*, *Haemophilus influenzae*, *Escherichia coli*, and *Klebsiella* sp. In later stages of the disease, *Pseudomonas aeruginosa* and other Gram-negative organisms predominate; these organisms create large supercolonies within mucus plugs called biofilms that protect them from phagocytosis.

In response to chronic bacterial colonization, neutrophilic inflammation is established. Neutrophil phagocytosis of *Pseudomonas aeruginosa* is inefficient, and the large load of neutrophils in the airway is not cleared, leading to neutrophil necrosis and release of mediators and cellular debris. Neutrophil inflammatory products such as protease and neutrophil elastase injure airway epithelium and activate increased mucin production[11] and excessive mucus secretion[12]. Furthermore, neutrophil DNA[13] and filamentous actin[14] significantly increase mucus viscosity.

Gradually, the increases in mucus volume and viscosity promote further bacterial proliferation and neutrophil-predominant inflammation. Following viral infections, these changes occur more acutely. Patients then experience an exacerbation of bronchitis, usually manifested by increases in respiratory rate, inspiratory intercostal and supraclavicular retractions, and diffuse, coarse, inspiratory crackles. Leukocytosis is common. The chest radiograph demonstrates worsening hyperinflation, peribronchiolar thickening, and nodular or cystic densities. Pulmonary function tests usually decline with decreases in forced expiratory flows and forced expiratory volumes, and increases in air trapping. With recurrent cycles of bronchitis, mucus obstruction, and neutrophilic inflammation, bronchiectasis results. This usually occurs first in the upper lobes and progresses throughout the lungs. In advanced disease, severe diffuse mucus obstruction of bronchiectatic airways causes ventilation–perfusion mismatching and hypoxemia. If untreated, chronic hypoxemia triggers pulmonary hypertension and cor pulmonale. Bronchiectasis also increases the risk of other complications including pneumothorax and hemoptysis. Late in the course, as the lung disease progresses, the bronchiectatic airways obstruct airflow to parenchymal tissue leading to acute and chronic hypercapnia, and respiratory failure.

The upper respiratory tract is also involved in CF. Patients can develop nasal polyposis or chronic sinusitis reflecting increased mucus production and stasis. Indeed, since allergic polyps are rare in the pediatric age group, nasal polyposis is an indication to evaluate for CF.

Gastrointestinal Tract

Many mutations of CFTR result in viscous secretions that obstruct the pancreatic exocrine ducts and result in failure to secrete proteases such as chymotrypsin and trypsin, lipases, amylases, and bicarbonate into the duodenum. Secretion of bicarbonate is an important element of pancreatic function since it neutralizes stomach acid and thus permits activation of pancreatic enzymes. A cycle of destruction and obliteration of the exocrine pancreatic ducts leads to cystic dilatation of the ducts and fibrosis of the pancreatic parenchyma. In advanced stages of disease, the islet of Langerhans cells are destroyed causing insulin-dependent diabetes mellitus. CF patients may also develop acute inflammation of the pancreas, precipitating pancreatitis. This occurs more commonly in those patients whose pancreatic function is better preserved.

In most CF patients, pancreatic exocrine insufficiency is present early in the course of the disease. Ten to twenty percent of newborns with CF present with meconium ileus, an obstruction of the intestine caused by sticky, viscous meconium stool. Approximately 14% of newborns with CF will have meconium plug syndrome, a syndrome of delayed meconium passage due to a meconium plug or cast in the sigmoid or descending colon. This is usually diagnosed and cleared by gastrograffin enema[15]. Infants lack the ability to digest fat and protein in their diet, and present with failure to thrive and frequent, bulky, greasy stools. Abnormal bulky stools may result in rectal prolapse, or partial or total obstruction of the distal ileum resulting in distal intestinal obstructive syndrome (DIOS). DIOS presents with abdominal cramping, distension, and sometimes vomiting. If left untreated, patients can be at risk for abdominal perforation and life-threatening peritonitis. In addition to precipitating DIOS, a fecal impaction can become a lead point within the intestines to induce intussusception.

In the last 10 years, fibrosing colonopathy, a condition associated with ingestion of high (>6000 units lipase/kg per meal) concentrations of pancreatic enzymes has been described. Patients complain of abdominal pain, often bloody diarrhea, and poor weight gain. The colonic wall becomes thickened and non-distensible, and in its most advanced state, local or generalized strictures occur. When present, surgical excision of the stricture is usually required. Careful monitoring of enzyme dosing will avoid most cases of fibrosing colonopathy.

The biliary tract of the liver and the gall bladder are also affected in CF. The primary mechanism of liver disease is inspissated secretions obstructing biliary ducts. The earliest pathologic findings are focal biliary cirrhosis with prolonged obstructive jaundice starting at 2–8 weeks of age. Infants with significant hepatic involvement thus demonstrate prolonged *direct* hyperbilirubinemia. In some patients, focal cirrhosis progresses to diffuse cirrhosis and portal hypertension. Occasionally, progression of hepatic disease is marked by elevated liver enzymes, but often this progression is silent. With advanced portal hypertension, splenic enlargement follows with platelet sequestration. An ominous finding is hematemesis, which is likely due to development of esophageal or gastric varices. Hepatic failure may ensue, associated with ascites, hyperammonemia, encephalopathy, and loss of hepatic synthetic function. Approximately 5% of patients die of liver failure.

Stasis of bile flow and abnormal bile acid composition cause gall bladder complications including cholelithiasis, and cholecystitis.

Sweat Glands

The sweat glands appear morphologically normal, but the ability of the sweat duct to absorb chloride is impaired in CF due to loss of CFTR function. This abnormality results in hypertonic sweat with increased chloride and sodium concentrations. Salt losses can increase dramatically from increased perspiration due to high ambient temperature during the summer, increased exertion, or fever. Excessive sweat sodium and chloride losses increase the risk for dehydration with hypochloremic/hyponatremic metabolic alkalosis.

Reproductive Organs

In female patients, cervical mucus has increased viscosity. However, mucus changes do not appear to affect fertility, as a significant number of women with CF are able to conceive and carry pregnancies to term. The major factors affecting outcome of pregnancy are general health and nutritional status of the mother[16]. In contrast, male infertility is common in CF (greater than 98% of male patients). This is due to obstruction of the vas deferens in utero resulting in atresia or absence at birth. Spermatogenesis and testicular development are normal in males.

DIAGNOSIS

Because of the heterogeneity and variability of presentations associated with CF, the physician must have a high index of suspicion for the disease. Patients with a family history of CF, or with symptoms or signs consistent with CF, should have a diagnostic evaluation for

Table 7-1   Symptoms and Signs Classified by Age of Presentation

Infancy	Childhood	Adolescence/Adulthood
Meconium ileus	Failure to thrive	Delayed sexual development
Obstructive jaundice	Steatorrhea	Obstructive azoospermia
Failure to thrive	Heat prostration with hypoelectrolytemia	Chronic bronchitis with *Pseudomonas aeruginosa*
Edema with hypoproteinemia and anemia	"Atypical" asthma with clubbing, bronchiectasis	Pansinusitis
Recurrent pneumonia/bronchiolitis	Nasal polyps	Chronic abdominal pain, idiopathic pancreatitis, cirrhosis
Rectal prolapse	Rectal prolapse	Hemoptysis, pneumothorax
Salty-tasting skin	Salty-tasting skin	

the disease. Symptoms may be classified by usual age of presentation[2] (Table 7-1).

Chronic pulmonary symptoms suggestive of CF include chronic or productive cough, chronic wheezing, or pneumonia with *Staphylococcus aureus* or Gram-negative bacilli (particularly the mucoid form of *Pseudomonas aeruginosa*). Gastrointestinal symptoms consistent with CF include meconium ileus or meconium plug, failure to thrive, bulky, greasy or foul-smelling stools, rectal prolapse, or prolonged jaundice as an infant. Other historical findings suggestive of CF are excessively salty sweat or a salty taste when a child is kissed, chronic sinusitis, and delayed puberty associated with poor nutritional status.

Clinical findings suggestive of CF include several respiratory and gastrointestinal physical findings. Respiratory tract findings include frequent cough, particularly if productive of mucopurulent sputum, rhonchi, wheezes, crackles, increased anteroposterior chest diameter, nasal polyposis, and digital clubbing. Gastrointestinal signs include hepatosplenomegaly, jaundice, fecal masses, rectal prolapse, failure to thrive, and hypoproteinemic edema.

As part of the evaluation of CF, laboratory findings may be helpful both to support the diagnosis in atypical cases and as an initial evaluation of organ function. Sputum or throat swab cultures should be obtained to assess for pathogenic organisms such as *S. aureus* and *P. aeruginosa*. Chest radiographs should be evaluated to detect early signs consistent with bronchiectasis. In patients with chronic cough or wheeze, pulmonary function tests are helpful in determining whether airway obstruction is present and whether the obstruction is reversible with bronchodilators. Laboratory evaluations of nutritional status, pancreatic sufficiency, and liver functions are important corollary information for establishing the diagnosis of CF (Tables 7-2 and 7-3).

In the context of historical, physical, or laboratory findings associated with CF, the diagnosis is confirmed by the demonstration of an elevated sweat chloride concentration by the quantitative pilocarpine iontophoresis sweat test[17]. This technically demanding test should only be performed at approved CF Centers. It provides a quantitative measure of sweat chloride under conditions of adequate sweat flow. A sweat test is positive if the chloride concentration is greater than 60 mEq/L; borderline values are between 40–60 mEq/L. At least two positive sweat tests with positive historical, physical, and/or laboratory findings are required to confirm the diagnosis. Several factors can affect interpretation of the test. Sweat chloride levels increase with age. Conditions other than CF can cause increased concentrations of sweat chloride including malnutrition, adrenal insufficiency, hereditary nephrogenic diabetes insipidus, ectodermal dysplasia, hypogammaglobulinemia, and fucosidosis[18]. Alternatively, it is important to recognize that false negative sweat tests may be due to edema in CF patients with hypoproteinemia.

Genetic analysis may also be used to confirm the diagnosis of CF. Two alleles with CF mutations must be identified to confirm the diagnosis. Screening for 32 of the most common alleles yields an overall sensitivity of 90% in diagnosing CF. Therefore, a negative genetic analysis does not rule out a diagnosis of CF in an atypical patient.

The serum immunoreactive assay for trypsinogen is used in two states as a screening test for CF in newborns. Serum levels of trypsinogen are often abnormally high in CF due to pancreatic duct obstruction and pancreatic inflammation. However, this test is associated with both false positives and negatives; all positive patients must have a sweat test or genotyping performed to confirm the diagnosis. The CFF Consensus Committee recommended that the diagnosis of CF should be based on the presence of one or more characteristic phenotypic features (Table 7-1) or a history of CF in a sibling, plus laboratory evidence of a CFTR abnormality as documented by elevated sweat chloride concentrations, or identification of two CF mutations, or in vivo demonstration of characteristic abnormalities in ion transport across the nasal epithelium[18].

Table 7-2 Diagnostic Evaluation of Respiratory Tract Disease

Laboratory Studies	Results Consistent with CF Lung Disease
Sputum or throat swab culture	*S. aureus, H. influenzae, P. aeruginosa, B. cepacia, S. maltophilia*; *Aspergillus*; atypical mycobacteria
Chest radiograph/CT scan	Hyperinflation, peribronchiolar thickening; late findings: cysts and nodules consistent with bronchiectasis
Pulmonary function tests	+/− Reversible small airways obstruction, mild air trapping; late findings: severe irreversible large airways obstruction, severe air trapping
Blood gas/oximetry	+/− Mild hypoxemia with pulmonary exacerbations; late findings: persistent severe hypoxemia, hypercapnia, compensated respiratory acidosis

CLINICAL EVALUATION

The goal of the clinical assessment of CF patients is to evaluate the function of the lungs (Table 7-2), the gastrointestinal tract (Table 7-3), and the reproductive tract. This evaluation includes pulmonary function tests, sputum microbiology, chest radiography, nutritional status, liver and pancreatic function tests, and reproductive function.

Pulmonary Function Tests

Patients perform pulmonary function tests, spirometry and plethysmography, at regular intervals during routine visits to follow the overall course of the disease, and more frequently during exacerbations of bronchitis to follow the course of therapy. The earliest deficits found are in the forced expiratory flows between 25% and 75% of the vital capacity (FEF_{25-75}) and at low lung volumes (i.e., at 75% of the vital capacity, FEF_{75}). Decreases in FEF_{25-75} and FEF_{75} correlate with obstruction of small bronchioles.

With more advanced disease, obstruction of large airways becomes predominant with diminished forced expiratory volume at 1 second (FEV_1) and reduced FEV_1: forced vital capacity (FVC) ratio (Figure 7-3). In concert with increasing airway obstruction, air trapping progresses: as measured by plethysmography, hyperinflation related to small airway disease is reflected in elevated ratios of residual volume to total lung capacity (RV/TLC). Treatment of acute exacerbations of bronchitis usually results in improvements in pulmonary function. However, over time, CF causes a relentless deterioration of pulmonary function.

A major challenge in evaluating the pulmonary function of CF patients is that pulmonary function tests are very effort-dependent, and thus children younger than 4–5 years of age cannot reliably perform them. Recently, a procedure for performing pulmonary function tests has been standardized for infants with CF and the equipment is now commercially available. This technique is limited for routine usage because it requires sedation of the infant. This infant pulmonary function test uses passive inflation to a preset pressure (30 cm H_2O)

Table 7-3 Diagnostic Evaluation of Gastrointestinal Tract Disease

Laboratory Studies	Results Consistent with CF Gastrointestinal Disease
72 h Stool fat, absorption of *N*-benzoyl-L-tyrosyl-*p*-amino benzoic acid	Measures of pancreatic exocrine sufficiency: if malabsorption present: stool fat >7% of oral fat intake, decreased *N*-benzoyl-L-tyrosyl-*p*-amino benzoic acid absorption
Serum vitamins A and E	Measures of adequate supplementation
Liver function tests: gamma glutamyl transferase, aspartate transaminase, alkaline phosphatase	Measures of liver inflammation: normal or transiently elevated
Serum total protein, prealbumin, prothrombin time	Measures of nutrition and liver function: may be abnormal
Gastrograffin enema	Indicated for symptoms of DIOS, intussusception
Ultrasound	Indicated to evaluate for cholelithiasis, cirrhosis, volvulus
Serum glucose	Elevated random glucose suggests diabetes mellitus
Electrolytes	Screen for salt wasting

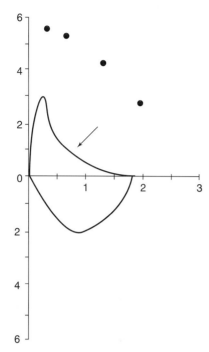

Figure 7-3 Pulmonary function tests in CF. A flow–volume curve obtained by spirometry is depicted. Ordinate values are flows and abscissa values are volumes. Normal values are presented as dots. Note that the flows are decreased at all volumes with a concave pattern of the expiratory loop (arrow) demonstrating small airways obstruction.

to achieve a lung volume near total lung capacity, and then applies a squeeze to the chest during exhalation to recreate a forced vital capacity maneuver[19]. The total test resembles the pulmonary function tests used for older subjects and therefore makes interpretations of results easier to perform and compare with standards. This infant pulmonary function test should be useful to assess early changes in pulmonary function and response to new therapies.

The arterial blood gas reveals abnormal gas exchange during severe exacerbations of bronchitis or in patients with chronic, end-stage lung disease. Early in the course of the disease, ventilation–perfusion abnormalities result in widening of the alveolar–arterial gradient. This abnormality reflects inhomogeneities in alveolar ventilation. With disease progression, ventilation–perfusion mismatching increases and results in progressive hypoxemia. Hypoxemia occurs first during exacerbations of bronchitis, then during sleep, and finally chronically. With chronic hypoxemic respiratory failure, patients are at risk to develop the complications of pulmonary hypertension and cor pulmonale. Initially, ventilation is spared, but with end-stage lung involvement, airway obstruction is so severe that ventilation is impaired and patients develop hypercapnia and respiratory acidosis.

Oxyhemoglobin saturation monitoring is a useful indicator of respiratory function for patients with underlying severe lung disease because it is non-invasive and practical for prolonged observation. During exacerbations of bronchitis in patients with severe airway obstruction, oxyhemoglobin saturations are monitored to detect nighttime or exercise-induced hypoxemia, and to titrate oxygen therapy.

Sputum Microbiology

Sputum samples are routinely assessed for bacterial identity and antibiotic sensitivities. These data are important for selecting antimicrobial therapy during acute exacerbations. Either expectorated sputum or throat swabs during a cough are used for microbiology cultures. Early in the course of CF, *S. aureus*, *H. influenzae*, and *E. coli* are identified. Often within the first few years, *P. aeruginosa* is detected in sputum or throat swab cultures. Once *P. aeruginosa* is detected in the sputum, it is very difficult to eradicate. As patients develop progressive bronchiectasis, other opportunistic organisms may colonize the airways including Gram-negative rods such as *Burkholderia cepacia* and *Stenotrophomonas maltophilia,* molds such as *Aspergillus fumigatus,* and atypical mycobacteria. Expectorated sputum is evaluated for the presence of these opportunistic organisms using specialized culture media, as these organisms induce exacerbations of bronchitis, and accelerate disease progression.

Antibiotic sensitivities are routinely determined using single antibiotics. However, at least two centers offer antibiotic synergy studies[20] for Gram-negative organisms to determine whether synergy exists for bacterial killing using combinations of two or three antibiotics.

Chest Radiography

Chest radiographs obtained yearly are a useful measure to detect subtle changes of airway involvement. Chest radiographs are also obtained at the time of acute exacerbations of bronchitis to evaluate for areas of atelectasis due to mucus plugging. In patients with minimal or no respiratory tract symptoms, the X-ray film may be normal or have mild findings of peribronchiolar thickening or hyperinflation. With more advanced disease, increased linear markings, cystic changes or nodules are present that are consistent with bronchiectasis (Figure 7-4). These findings usually are seen initially in the upper lobes and then progress throughout the lungs. Atelectasis and/or severe hyperinflation with increased anteroposterior diameter are also present in advanced disease.

High-resolution chest computed tomography (CT) scanning is a very sensitive method for detecting bronchiectasis. The signet ring sign, a bronchial airway larger than its associated blood vessel, is the earliest sign of bronchiectasis on CT (Figure 7-5). The high resolution

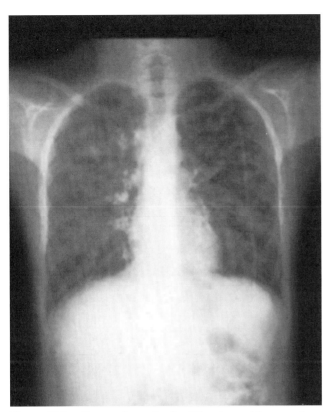

Figure 7-4 Chest radiograph of a CF patient with severe lung disease reveals ring shadows, cystic lesions, and nodular densities consistent with diffuse bronchiectasis.

CT scan is more sensitive than plain radiographs for detecting bronchiectasis[21]. Furthermore, the other major test of pulmonary status, pulmonary function measurements, may not deteriorate until multiple lobes of the lung are injured. Therefore, periodic evaluation of bronchiectasis by CT scan provides the most sensitive

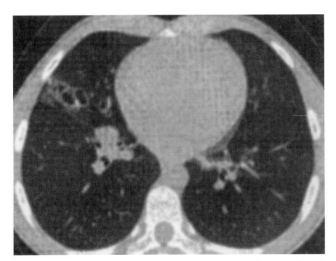

Figure 7-5 Chest CT scan of a CF patient with normal pulmonary function reveals early bronchiectasis with "signet ring" sign, airway thickening, and atelectasis.

measure of disease progression. With the availability of high-speed CT scans, this modality is now available for use in young children without sedation.

Nutrition

The evaluation of pancreatic function is a key element in establishing the diagnosis of CF since almost 90% of patients have pancreatic insufficiency. Furthermore, regular evaluation of nutritional status and sufficiency of pancreatic enzyme replacement are of critical importance because nutritional status correlates directly with pulmonary function and prognosis[22]. Pancreatic insufficiency is suggested by a history of failure to thrive, or frequent, greasy stools. In older children, a history of bulky, malodorous stools, often associated with a voracious appetite, can be elicited. The gold standard measure to evaluate for pancreatic enzyme insufficiency is quantitation of fat malabsorption. Stool is collected for 72 hours and fat content is quantified and compared with total fat intake during the same time period. At least 100 g of fat must be ingested during the collection period, and a malabsorption coefficient of greater than 7% is considered abnormal. In addition to this measure, serum levels of fat-soluble vitamins, A, D and E, are helpful to determine whether fat malabsorption is present, and also whether supplementation of these vitamins is adequate. Another approach to assess pancreatic exocrine function is based on measurements of urinary metabolic products of N-benzoyl-L-tyrosyl-p-aminobenzoic acid, a compound that is ingested orally, hydrolyzed and absorbed by the small intestine in the presence of pancreatic enzymes, and then secreted into the urine.

Evaluation of liver function tests is a standard part of the routine annual evaluation of CF patients. Especially in infancy, there may be transient increase in bilirubin or transaminase levels that reflects focal biliary obstruction. Unfortunately, progression of biliary cirrhosis can be silent, and patients may present with signs of advanced cirrhosis as an incidental finding on an ultrasound scan. Cirrhosis and portal hypertension precede the development of esophageal and gastric varices; a potentially life-threatening complication of varices is hematemesis. Patients with hematemesis are evaluated and treated by endoscopy and banding or sclerosis of varices. The presence of portal hypertension can be confirmed by ultrasound to evaluate the direction of portal and splenic vein flow.

Abdominal pain is a serious complication of CF and can be due to a plethora of etiologies (Table 7-4). Patients with abdominal pain that is sharp or cramping and localized to the right lower quadrant may have DIOS and require a series of abdominal radiographs to confirm the diagnosis and rule out other causes of obstruction. If a patient presents with intermittent abdominal pain, heme-positive stools, and/or an acute abdomen, the patient

Table 7-4   Differential Diagnosis of Abdominal Pain

Distal intestinal obstructive syndrome
Gastroesophageal reflux
Pancreatitis
Cholecystitis
Cholelithiasis
Fibrosing colonopathy
Intussusception
Volvulus
Abdominal muscle pain related to coughing
Referred pain related to basilar pneumonia
Other causes of acute abdomen, for example, appendicitis

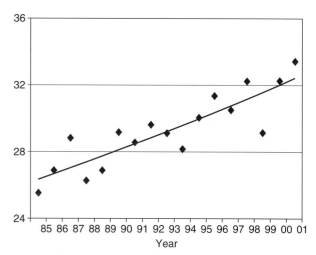

Figure 7-6   Graph of predicted survival age for CF patients, 1985–2001.

should be evaluated by ultrasound to rule out volvulus, fibrosing colonopathy, or intussusception. Severe abdominal pain that radiates to the back and is exacerbated by eating high-fat foods is consistent with acute pancreatitis; abnormal serum amylase and lipase would confirm this diagnosis. Finally, pain localized to the right upper quadrant may be due to gall bladder complications such as cholecystitis or cholelithiasis; these diagnoses would be confirmed by ultrasound.

In CF, development of insulin-dependent diabetes mellitus follows from chronic pancreatic inflammation. Five to six percent of pediatric CF patients develop diabetes. The frequency of diabetes increases with age to an occurrence rate of approximately 50% of adult CF patients. CF-related diabetes may be insidious in onset and may take several years for overt symptoms to develop. All patients are screened annually with a random serum glucose level. If this is elevated (>200 mg/dl) or if patients present with symptoms consistent with diabetes, then a fasting blood glucose level is obtained to confirm the diagnosis[23]. For patients who are pregnant or who have unexplained symptoms consistent with diabetes such as polydipsia, polyuria, poor growth or delayed puberty, a glucose tolerance test is indicated to rule out diabetes.

Reproductive Function

A high percentage of men with CF have infertility due to congenital absence of the vas deferens. Thus, a semen analysis should be performed for adult men with CF. Because of the high association of CF mutations with male infertility[6], men who present with infertility as a primary diagnosis should have a complete evaluation for CF.

THERAPY

Intensive and comprehensive therapy for CF has resulted in a significant improvement in life expectancy

and quality of life over the past 50 years[24] (Figure 7-6). Although there is no question that comprehensive care has dramatically changed the course of the disease, there are limited data supporting specific components of therapy. At present, the best approach appears to be an individualized therapy program determined by the degree of organ dysfunction for each patient. An important aspect of CF care is the network of 100 CF centers that exist throughout the United States. Most centers use a team approach with physicians, nurses, physical therapists, respiratory therapists, nutritionists, genetic counselors, and social workers, to provide a comprehensive approach to the management of each patient.

Management of Pulmonary Disease

The goals of treatment are to prevent mucus obstruction of airways and to reduce the burden of bacteria and inflammation. Several components of therapy are applied simultaneously to achieve these goals[25] (Table 7-5).

Mucociliary Clearance

All treatment programs for CF include a strategy to clear the airways of viscid, sticky secretions. Mucociliary clearance is a mainstay of innate immunity; it reduces bacterial load in the airways and diminishes the associated neutrophilic inflammation. This clearance is accomplished by a combination of techniques to reduce the viscosity of secretions, and to enhance cough clearance of secretions.

Two mucolytic agents, administered by nebulization, are available to reduce sputum viscosity in CF: *N*-acetylcysteine, and recombinant human DNase (Pulmozyme). *N*-acetylcysteine reduces disulfide bonds and decreases sputum viscosity in vitro. It also has activity as an antioxidant agent which may be of benefit in the inflamed milieu of the CF airway. Its use has been limited by

Table 7-5   Components of Therapy for Pulmonary Disease

Chest physiotherapy
  Percussion and postural drainage
  High-frequency chest wall oscillator (ThAIRapy)
  Oscillating positive expiratory pressure device (Flutter or Acapella)
  Intrapulmonary percussive ventilation
  Active cycle breathing techniques
  Aerobic exercise
Mucolytic therapy (nebulized)
  Recombinant human DNase (Pulmozyme)
  N-acetylcysteine (Mucomyst)
Antibiotic therapy

Bacteria	Oral	Intravenous	Inhaled
S. aureus	Amoxicillin + Clavulinic acid	Nafcillin; if resistant, vancomycin	
P. aeruginosa	Ciprofloxacin	Aminoglycoside + ceftazidime or ticarcillin	Tobramycin, colistin
Resistant *P. aeruginosa*		Aztreonam, piperacillin, imipenem, meropenem	

Bronchodilator therapy

reports of airway bronchospasm. This problem can be mitigated if it is administered as a dilute preparation in concert with a bronchodilator. Nebulized *N*-acetylcysteine has not been adequately evaluated in a prospective, controlled trial in CF[26]. However, its mucolytic and antioxidant properties, and its low cost support a trial of its use in selected patients. Its use remains an integral part of ongoing comprehensive respiratory care in several large CF centers.

Pulmozyme cleaves neutrophil DNA in sputum that is a major factor contributing to sputum viscosity. Pulmozyme was approved for use in the United States in 1994 following a large prospective, controlled trial demonstrating that following 1 year of Pulmozyme therapy, patients had mildly improved pulmonary function tests, reduced exacerbations of bronchitis, and reduced days of hospitalization[13]. However, questions regarding patient selection, timing and duration of use of this expensive drug remain unanswered. There is currently intense investigation to discover new therapeutic agents that will reduce mucus secretion or alter mucus–epithelial interactions as adjunctive therapy to reduce mucus obstruction of airways in CF.

Chest Physiotherapy

Chest physiotherapy is a mainstay of CF therapy. The goal of this therapy is to enhance cough clearance of airway secretions. A prospective, controlled study has demonstrated that regular, daily chest physiotherapy maintains pulmonary function better over 3 years compared with deep breathing and cough alone[27]. Thus, chest physiotherapy is prescribed routinely twice per day, with an increased frequency during exacerbations of bronchitis. The most widely prescribed method is percussion and

postural drainage. Alternative methods include a percussion vest that delivers high-frequency chest wall compression; the Flutter or Acapella devices, pipe-like instruments with interrupter structures that produce high frequency, low amplitude vibrations throughout the airways during forced exhalation; autogenic drainage breathing exercises designed to move secretions from distal to proximal airways; positive expiratory pressure devices; aerobic exercise; and forced cough maneuvers (reviewed in Prasad and Main[28]).

Antibiotics

Antibiotics are a key element responsible for increased survival in CF. However, antibiotic regimens are not standardized, and there are many unanswered questions concerning antibiotic choices and duration of therapy. A reasonable approach is to use antibiotic therapy to treat an acute exacerbation of bronchitis when signs and symptoms are consistent with worsening infection (Table 7-6). In early exacerbations, chest physiotherapy is increased and oral antibiotics are initiated. If outpatient therapy fails to resolve signs or symptoms, or if symptoms progress despite therapy, then intravenous antibiotic therapy is initiated.

Useful oral antibiotic agents for treatment of staphylococcal infections include dicloxacillin, cephalexin, amoxicillin/clavulinic acid, and chloramphenicol. For *Pseudomonas* strains, oral antibiotics including trimethoprim-sulfamethoxazole, tetracycline, or chloramphenicol may provide some efficacy early in the course of disease. A quinolone derivative, ciprofloxacin, is effective against many strains of *Pseudomonas*. A major disadvantage of ciprofloxacin is that *Pseudomonas* strains develop resistance to it following prolonged use.

Table 7-6   Criteria for Exacerbation of Bronchitis

Symptoms
Increased cough
Persistent wheezing
Increased sputum production
Change in sputum color
Hemoptysis
Dyspnea on exertion
Chest pain

Signs
Weight loss
Changes on chest examination: crackles, wheezes, or decreased
    air movement
Tachypnea
Retractions
Use of accessory muscles
Decline in pulmonary function tests
New infiltrate or increased peribronchiolar thickening on
    chest radiograph

For severe exacerbations of bronchitis, or exacerbations that fail to respond to oral antibiotics, there is an arsenal of intravenous antibiotics that are used as the next line of therapy. For *Staphylococcus aureus*, oxacillin, or nafcillin are useful agents. If *S. aureus* is resistant to penicillins, then vancomycin is the agent of choice. For *Pseudomonas* infections, at least two agents, usually including an aminoglycoside, are used to provide synergy of antibiotic therapy. Aminoglycosides are titrated to provide higher serum peak concentrations (8–12 μg/ml) than those used for non-CF patients in order to achieve adequate concentrations in such viscous airway secretions. In addition to gentamicin or tobramycin, a third-generation cephalosporin (ceftazidime) or a third-generation penicillin (ticarcillin or piperacillin) are used. Other antibiotics that are used particularly in the case of resistant organisms include amikacin, colimycin, aztreonam, meropenem, or imipenem. If *S. aureus* and *Pseudomonas aeruginosa* are both present, ticarcillin with clavulinic acid, or piperacillin with tazobactam, are used in combination with an aminoglycoside. Usually intravenous antibiotics are used for 10 days up to 2–3 weeks of total therapy. The goals of therapy are to reduce symptoms to the best premorbid level, to reverse any decrement in pulmonary function, and to clear any chest radiographic changes. Once their presence is established, it is usually not possible to eradicate *S. aureus* and *P. aeruginosa* from the airway. Currently, a large prospective, randomized, controlled trial is being initiated under the auspices of the U.S. Cystic Fibrosis Foundation to assess attempts to clear *Pseudomonas* from the airway after it is first detected, and to prolong the time until chronic colonization is established.

Two recent studies suggest that antibiotics may be useful as maintenance therapy in patients colonized with *P. aeruginosa* to maintain pulmonary function and reduce the frequency and severity of bronchitis exacerbations. In a placebo-controlled, randomized, prospective trial over 6 months[29], inhaled preservative-free tobramycin, 300 mg twice per day for alternate months, was shown to maintain pulmonary function. In a 3 month, prospective, placebo-controlled trial[30], therapy with oral azithromycin, 250 mg daily, maintained pulmonary function, reduced measures of inflammation and improved quality of life. Further investigations are currently under way to determine the optimal use of these agents in CF.

For the special circumstance of allergic bronchopulmonary aspergillosis, oral antifungal therapy in concert with corticosteroid therapy is useful for reducing airway inflammation and reactivity[31]. Atypical mycobacteria present a special challenge for patients and clinicians. It is difficult to determine when these organisms are contributing to airway infection and inflammation. If sick patients are not responding to antibiotic therapy, or if they have fever, night sweats, or cachexia, and chest CT scan reveals nodules and sputum stain reveals a high concentration of acid-fast bacilli[32], then these patients may have an active mycobacterial infection and require multi-drug antimycobacterial therapy. Atypical mycobacterial infections are also extremely difficult to treat as they require multiple antibiotics for prolonged courses and the bacteria develop resistance to antibiotics.

Bronchodilators and Anti-inflammatory Therapy
Bronchodilators, such as short-acting inhaled β$_2$-agonists, may be useful for CF patients with reversible airway obstruction; their use can promote improved mucociliary clearance[25]. However, some patients with bronchiectasis may worsen with bronchodilator therapy because these agents will make the central airways more collapsible and so "paradoxically" decrease airway caliber, especially during cough. Therefore, their use should be individualized and monitored over time.

Corticosteroids are a useful therapy for patients with severe airway reactivity associated with exacerbations of CF bronchitis, or for patients with allergic bronchopulmonary aspergillosis. A recent prospective controlled study over 4 years[33], demonstrated that alternate-day corticosteroids (1 mg/kg/day) significantly improved pulmonary function compared with placebo-control. However, the study group had diminished linear growth after 1 year, precluding a general recommendation for chronic steroid therapy in CF.

A more targeted anti-inflammatory agent, ibuprofen, was studied in a 4 year, controlled, prospective trial[34]. High-dose ibuprofen reduced the deterioration in pulmonary function that occurred in the control group; it was particularly beneficial for the subgroup of teenagers colonized with *Pseudomonas*. Since the original publication, concerns have been raised about side effects associated with this therapy including gastric ulcers and decreased glomerular filtration rate, limiting its widespread acceptance.

With the promise of improved pulmonary outcomes but the limitations due to side effects, the current anti-inflammatory agents have limited use. However, other anti-inflammatory agents such as montelukast are currently being evaluated in CF.

Oxygen and Non-invasive Assisted Ventilation

With progressive respiratory failure, and the development of persistent hypoxemia, patients have an increased risk of secondary pulmonary hypertension and cor pulmonale. To prevent these complications, supplemental oxygen therapy is initiated by nasal cannulae. Once hypoxemia or hypercapnia is detected and becomes chronic, patients have 50% mortality at 2 years[35]. Non-invasive assisted ventilation with bilevel positive airway pressure (B_LPAP) is a useful temporary modality to support patients' ventilation while they are awaiting lung transplantation.

Lung Transplantation

For patients with impending respiratory failure, lung transplantation offers a last resort as a therapy. The two most common approaches for transplant are double lung cadaveric transplant, or transplantation of two living related donor lobes. The current criteria for consideration of lung transplantation include progressive pulmonary impairment manifested by FEV_1 <30% predicted, increasing functional impairment including increasing frequency of hospitalizations, and major life-threatening complications such as massive hemoptysis[36]. The current waiting time for transplant surgery in the United States is 2–3 years, depending on the recipient's blood type. Although the immediate outcome results have significantly improved, with 80% survival at 1 year, the long-term complications of chronic rejection still limit long-term success with survival rates of approximately 50% at 5 years.

Management of Nutrition and Gastrointestinal Disease

CF patients require therapy to replace missing exocrine enzymes, enhance nutrition, replete wasted salt, and to treat intestinal complications (Table 7-7).

Nutritional Support

Patients with CF require an initial evaluation and then re-evaluation over time to assess their pancreatic exocrine function. As most patients have some degree of pancreatic exocrine insufficiency, supplemental enzymes are ingested with food. The enzyme preparations are enteric-coated capsules with microspheres

Table 7-7 Components of Therapy for Gastrointestinal Disease

Nutrition
  Supplemental fat-soluble vitamins (ADEK)
    Pancreatic exocrine enzymes (protease, lipase, amylase)
    High protein, high carbohydrate diet
  Nutritional supplements (orally, or via nasogastric tube or gastrostomy tube)
  Extra table salt or salty snacks
Distal intestinal obstructive syndrome
Acute therapy
  Polyethylene-glycol-electrolyte solution (orally, or via nasogastric tube or gastrostomy tube)
  Gastrograffin enema
  Surgical repair
Maintenance therapy
  Correct dosage and administration of enzymes
  Fiber laxatives
  Regular administration of polyethylene-glycol-electrolyte solutions
Hepatobiliary disease
  Ursodiol (Actigall)

containing lipase, protease and amylase. Titration of enzyme dosage is determined by quality and frequency of bowel movements, by weight gain, and by measures of adequate fat absorption such as normal vitamin A, D, and E levels. In some cases, enzymes are ineffective despite higher than expected dosing. This may be due to inadequate bicarbonate secretion into the duodenum; such patients often benefit from a trial of H_2-blockers or proton pump inhibitors to reduce the acidity of the intestine and permit optimal enzyme activity. In addition to enzyme supplementation, patients require supplementation with the fat-soluble vitamins, A, D, E, and K.

Patients with CF have high resting energy requirements[37]. These caloric requirements increase dramatically during exacerbations of bronchitis. Furthermore, pulmonary function directly correlates with nutritional status[22]. For these reasons, patients are encouraged to eat a high calorie, high protein diet. As pulmonary disease progresses, if the caloric needs outpace the patient's ability to achieve daily calorie requirements, alternative modes of nutritional therapy are implemented including nasogastric or gastrostomy tube nighttime feedings. With a supplemental high calorie formula delivered at night, patients can increase daily calorie intake by 1000–2000 calories per day.

Salt Replacement

Because of increased electrolyte loss, especially during the summer and with exercise, CF patients are encouraged to increase their intake of table salt. Infant formulas are supplemented with one-quarter teaspoon of salt per day.

Treatment of DIOS

DIOS is often a recurrent acute problem; therefore management is targeted to both the acute events and long-term prevention. For acute management, if the obstruction is partial with no abdominal distension, then a hyperosmolar agent such as polyethylene-glycol-electrolyte solution delivered orally or via nasogastric tube, is useful to dislodge the fecal mass. If obstruction is severe, or the patient is unable to tolerate the hyperosmolar agent via the stomach, then a gastrograffin enema should be performed to clear the obstructed stool. Finally, if the obstruction is complete and unresponsive to gastrograffin enema, or the patient is toxic, surgery may be required to clear the obstruction. Recurrent obstructions can result from failure to take enzymes, insufficient enzyme dosing, low duodenal pH so that enzyme therapy is relatively ineffective, or colonic abnormalities such as fibrosing colonopathy[38]. Risk of fibrosing colonopathy is associated with very high enzyme supplementation; patients with recurrent DIOS should be evaluated by gastrograffin enema to rule out fibrosing colonopathy (Figure 7-7). If fibrosing colonopathy or incorrect enzyme supplementation are ruled out, then preventive therapy can be initiated including fiber supplements or regular therapy with a polyethylene-glycol-electrolyte solution.

Ursodeoxycholic Acid

The findings of hepatosplenomegaly or elevated liver enzymes suggest that further evaluation for biliary cirrhosis is indicated. As part of a complete evaluation, infectious etiologies of hepatitis are investigated. An ultrasound examination is extremely useful to evaluate for cirrhosis and to evaluate the biliary tract including the gall bladder. Once cholestasis, fibrosis, or cirrhosis is diagnosed, then therapy with ursodeoxycholic acid is initiated. This therapy may improve bile flow and reduce hepatic inflammation[39], but its effectiveness in reducing the risk of cirrhosis is not known. When cirrhosis becomes symptomatic with hyperammonemia, encephalopathy and poor synthetic function, then medical treatment includes salt restriction, protein restriction, and diuretics. Lactulose increases gut motility, and neomycin reduces the load of enteric bacteria; both therapies help to control hyperammonemia.

Liver Transplantation

This therapy is reserved for patients with complications of cirrhosis that are recalcitrant to medical therapy. Outcomes are similar to those for patients undergoing liver transplantation for other etiologies[40].

SUMMARY

CF is a complex disorder affecting many organ systems with remarkable heterogeneity in presentation and clinical course. Current therapies have significantly improved quality of life and long-term outcomes. Yet, this disease still causes early mortality. Further significant improvements in outcome await therapeutic breakthroughs based on new information about the cellular and molecular pathogenesis of the disease.

MAJOR POINTS

1. CF is an autosomal recessive disease caused by mutations in the cystic fibrosis transmembrane conductance regulator gene on chromosome 7.
2. CF can be diagnosed by a quantitative pilocarpine iontophoresis sweat test or by genetic testing.
3. CF-associated pulmonary disease is characterized by chronic bronchitis with pathogenic organisms including *S. aureus* and *P. aeruginosa*, leading to bronchiectasis and respiratory failure.
4. CF associated gastrointestinal disease is characterized by pancreatic exocrine insufficiency leading to failure to thrive, and distal intestinal obstruction syndrome. Other gastrointestinal complications include cholestatic liver disease, pancreatitis, and diabetes.
5. Therapy is palliative and targeted to optimize mucociliary clearance, treat chronic bronchitis, replace pancreatic enzymes, and optimize nutrition.

Barium Radiogram   Histologic Slide

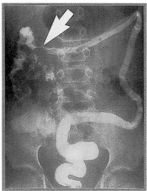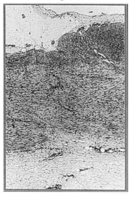

Figure 7-7 Gastrograffin enema of a CF patient with fibrosing colonopathy reveals narrowing of the transverse colon (arrow).

REFERENCES

1. Welsh MJ, Ramsey BW, Accurso F, Cutting GR. Cystic fibrosis. In Scriver CR, Beaudet AL, Sly WS, Valle D, editors: The metabolic and molecular bases of inherited disease, 8th edition, pp. 5121–5188. New York: McGraw-Hill, 2001.

2. Robinson C, Scanlin TF. Cystic fibrosis. In Fishman AP, editor: Pulmonary diseases and disorders, pp. 803-824. New York: McGraw-Hill, 1997.

3. Kerem BS, Rommens JM, Buchanan JA, Markeiwicz D, Cox TK, Chakravarti A, et al. Identification of the cystic fibrosis gene: genetic analysis. Science 245:1073-1080, 1989.

4. Rich DP, Anderson MP, Gregory RJ, Cheng SH, Paul S, Jefferson DM, et al. Expression of cystic fibrosis transmembrane conductance regulator corrects defective chloride channel regulation in cystic fibrosis airway epithelial cells. Nature 347:358-363, 1990.

5. Welsh MJ, Smith AE. Molecular mechanisms of CFTR chloride channel dysfunction in cystic fibrosis. Cell 73:1251-1254, 1993.

6. Chillon M, Casals T, Mercier B, Bassas L, Lissens W, Silber S, et al. Mutations in the cystic fibrosis gene in patients with congenital absence of the vas deferens. N Engl J Med 332:1475-1480, 1995.

7. Cohn JA, Friedman KJ, Noone PG, Knowles MR, Silverman LM, Jowell PS. Relation between mutations of the cystic fibrosis gene and idiopathic pancreatitis. N Engl J Med 339:653-658, 1998.

8. Zielenski I, Corey M, Rozmahel R, Markeiwicz D, Aznarez I, Casals T, et al. Detection of a cystic fibrosis modifier locus for meconium ileus on human chromosome 19q13. Nat Genet 22:128-129, 1999.

9. Garred P, Pressler T, Madsen HO, Frederiksen B, Svejgaard A, Hoiby N, et al. Association of mannose-binding lectin gene heterogeneity with severity of lung disease and survival in cystic fibrosis. J Clin Invest 104:431-437, 1999.

10. Rhim AD, Stoykova L, Glick MC, Scanlin TF. Terminal glycosylation in cystic fibrosis (CF): a review emphasizing the airway epithelial cells. Glycoconj J 18:649-659, 2001.

11. Voynow JA, Rosenthal Young L, Wang Y, Horger T, Rose MC, Fischer BM. Neutrophil elastase increases *MUC5AC* expression in A549 lung carcinoma cells. Am J Physiol 276:L835-L843, 1999.

12. Lundgren JD, Rieves RD, Mullol J, Logun C, Shelhamer JH. The effect of neutrophil proteinase enzymes on the release of mucus from feline and human airway cultures, Respir Med 88:511-518, 1994.

13. Fuchs HJ, Borowitz DS, Christiansen DH, Morris EM, Nash ML, Ramsey BW. Effect of aerosolized recombinant human DNase on exacerbations of respiratory symptoms and on pulmonary function in patients with cystic fibrosis. N Engl J Med 331:637-642, 1994.

14. Vasconcellos CA, Allen PG, Wohl ME, Drazen JM, Janmey PA, Stossel TP. Reduction in viscosity of cystic fibrosis sputum in vitro by gelsolin. Science 263:969-971, 1994.

15. Ziegler M. Meconium ileus. Curr Probl Surg 3:731-777, 1994.

16. Palmer J, Dillon-Baker C, Tecklin JS, Wolfson B, Rosenberg B, Burroughs B, et al. Pregnancy in patients with cystic fibrosis. Ann Intern Med 99:596-600, 1993.

17. Stern RC. The diagnosis of cystic fibrosis. N Engl J Med 336:487-491, 1997.

18. Rosenstein BJ, Cutting GR. The diagnosis of cystic fibrosis: a consensus statement. J Pediatr 132:589-595, 1998.

19. Castile R, Filbrun D, Flucke R, Franklin W, McCoy K. Adult-type pulmonary function tests in infants without respiratory disease. Pediatr Pulmonol 30:215-227, 2000.

20. Lang BJ, Aaron SD, Ferris W, Hebert PC, MacDonald NE. Multiple combination bactericidal antibiotic testing for patients with cystic fibrosis infected with multiresistant strains of *Pseudomonas aeruginosa*. Am J Respir Crit Care Med 162:2241-2245, 2000.

21. Brody AS. Cystic fibrosis: when should high-resolution computed tomography of the chest be obtained? Pediatrics 101:1071, 1998.

22. Zemel BS, Jawad AF, FitzSimmons S, Stallings VA. Longitudinal relationship among growth, nutritional status, and pulmonary function in children with cystic fibrosis: analysis of the Cystic Fibrosis Foundation National CF patient registry. J Pediatr 137:374-380, 2000.

23. Moran A, Hardin D, Rodman D, Allen HF, Beall RJ, Dorowitz D, et al. Diagnosis, screening and management of cystic fibrosis related diabetes mellitus: a consensus conference report. Diabetes Res Clin Prac 45:61-73, 1999.

24. Cystic Fibrosis Foundation. Patient registry 2001 annual report. Bethesda, MD: CFF.

25. Ramsey BW. Management of pulmonary disease in patients with cystic fibrosis. N Engl J Med 335:179-188, 1996.

26. Duijvestijn YCM, Brand PLP. Systematic review of *N*-acetylcysteine in cystic fibrosis. Acta Paediatr 88:38-41, 1999.

27. Reisman JJ, Rivington-Saw B, Corey M, Marcotte J, Wannamaker E, Harcourt D, et al. Role of conventional physiotherapy in cystic fibrosis. J Pediatr 113:632-636, 1988.

28. Prasad SA, Main E. Finding evidence to support airway clearance techniques in cystic fibrosis. Dis Rehab 20:235-246, 1998.

29. Ramsey BW, Pepe MS, Quan JM, Otto KL, Montgomery AB, Williams-Warren J, et al. Intermittent administration of inhaled tobramycin in patients with cystic fibrosis. N Engl J Med 340:23-30, 1999.

30. Wolter J, Seeney S, Bell S, Bowler S, Masel P, McCormack J. Effect of long term treatment with azithromycin on disease parameters in cystic fibrosis: a randomised trial. Thorax 57:212-216, 2002.

31. Nepomuceno IB, Esrig S, Moss RB Allergic bronchopulmonary aspergillosis in cystic fibrosis: role of atopy and response to itraconazole. Chest 115:364-370, 1999.

32. Hjelte L, Petrini B, Kallenius G, Strandvik B. Prospective study of mycobacterial infections in patients with cystic fibrosis. Thorax 45:397-400, 1990.

33. Eigen H, Rosenstein BJ, FitzSimons S, Schidlow DV. A multicenter study of alternate-day prednisone therapy in patients with cystic fibrosis. J Pediatr 126:515-523, 1995.

34. Konstan MW, Byard PJ, Hoppel CL, Davis PB. Effect of high-dose ibuprofen in patients with cystic fibrosis. N Engl J Med 332:848-854, 1995.

35. Kerem E, Reisman J, Corey M, Canny GJ, Levison H. Prediction of mortality in patient with cystic fibrosis. N Engl J Med 326:1187–1191, 1992.

36. Yankaskas JR, Mallory GB Jr. Lung transplantation in cystic fibrosis: consensus conference statement. Chest 113: 217–226, 1998.

37. Zemel BS, Kawchak DA, Cnaan A, Zhao H, Scanlin TF, Stallings VA. Prospective evaluation of resting energy expenditure, nutritional status, pulmonary function, and genotype in children with cystic fibrosis. Pediatr Res 40:578–586, 1996.

38. Smyth RL, vanVelzen D, Smyth AR, Lloyd DA, Heaf DP. Strictures of ascending colon in cystic fibrosis and high-strength pancreatic enzymes. Lancet 343:85–86, 1994.

39. Lindblad A, Glaumann H, Stsrandvik B. A two-year prospective study of the effect of ursodeoxycholic acid on urinary bile acid excretion and liver morphology in cystic fibrosis-associated liver disease. Hepatology 27:166–174, 1998.

40. Milkiewicz P, Skiba G, Kely D, Weller P, Bonser R, Gur U, et al. Transplantation for cystic fibrosis: outcome following early liver transplantation. J Gastroenterol Hepatol 17:208–213, 2002.

CHAPTER 8

Primary Ciliary Dyskinesia (Immotile Cilia Syndrome–Kartagener Syndrome)

DANIEL V. SCHIDLOW, M.D.

JONATHAN STEINFELD, M.D.

DEFINITION

Primary ciliary dyskinesia (PCD) is an autosomal recessive genetic disease, characterized by dysfunction of the synchronous beating and propulsive function of ciliated epithelia and spermatozoa. Clinical features include early onset of persistent nasal and paranasal sinus disease, bronchial infection and obstruction. A subtype of this condition called Kartagener syndrome is characterized by mirror-image reversal of thoracic and abdominal organs (situs inversus) and occurs in 50% of affected individuals. Infertility occurs in almost 100% of affected males due to abnormal or absent movement of spermatozoa. The incidence of this condition is approximately 1:30,000 to 1:35,000 live births. The incidence of Kartagener syndrome is estimated to be roughly half that of PCD. The incidence of isolated situs inversus, without ciliary abnormalities is about 1:11,000 in the United States.[1]

PCD was first described in the beginning of the 20th century. The ultrastructural and functional defects of cilia associated with PCD were described in the 1970s and 1980s, and the terms "immotile cilia syndrome" and "primary ciliary dyskinesia" were coined. Recent research has been focused on determining the site for the gene(s) and mutations responsible for this condition. Conditions similar to PCD have also been described in animals[2].

GENETICS

The pattern of inheritance of PCD appears to be autosomal recessive, with some rare exceptions[3]. Higher incidence of this disease has been observed in consanguineous marriages and certain isolated population groups than in the general population. The exact location of the affected gene and its mutations has not yet been determined. Candidate genes have been reported in both chromosomes 6 and 7[2,4]. There are at least 10 different genes that encode dynein and others that encode tubulin, both constituent proteins of cilia. Further, it appears that the presence of situs inversus may be governed by mutations in separate genes that lie close to the PCD gene and interact in some form with it. Genes causing reversal of normal organ asymmetry have been reported in mice and other animals. In some cases random orientation occurs; some investigators have reported a gene mutation in chromosome 4 in mice which in its homozygote state results in 100% of affected animals having situs inversus[5].

Thus, it appears that the interaction of several genes and mutations and not the product of a single gene mutation determines the occurrence of PCD. Further work is necessary to better understand the relationship between ciliary defects, situs abnormalities and identification of genes and mutations associated with this disease in humans.

ANATOMY

Normal Anatomy and Function of Cilia

Ciliated epithelium lines the human respiratory tract from the posterior third of the nose to the bronchioles. In humans, cilia are present in the paranasal sinuses, the Eustachian tubes, the ependymal lining of the central nervous system, in the male vasa efferentia, and the female oviducts, among other structures. Each cilium measures 6 μm in length and 250 nm in diameter. The respiratory tree has 10 cilia per square centimeter. The surface of the respiratory tract is "carpeted" with beating cilia that expel extraneous substances and propel mucus from distal areas towards the oropharynx. It is, then, easy to understand how a malfunction of this system will result in mucus stasis and secondary infection.

The structure of a cilium is complex and consists of an axoneme, anchored by a basal body and a rootlet to the cell, and it possesses some smaller claw-like formations on its tip (Figure 8-1). The direction in which the basal body points defines the orientation of the cilium and the direction of the effective beat. The axoneme contains nine pairs of microtubules which surround a central pair of microtubules, as well as radial spokes and peripheral nexin links, which to a great extent maintain the wheel-like arrangement of the cilium[6]. Inner and outer arms attach to the microtubules (Figure 8-2). The main structural protein of the doublets is tubulin. The arms (inner and outer) contain dynein, which is a protein classified as an ATPase. Dynein generates the force that results in a sliding movement of the microtubules, responsible for ciliary movement. It is generally accepted that the outer dynein arms are mostly responsible for beating frequency whereas the inner dynein arms together with the radial spokes and nexin links have a role in the waveform of the beating[7]. Changes in the structural integrity of the axoneme can result in abnormal movement that ranges from stillness to aberrant patterns of hyperactivity.

Normal cilia beat synchronously in a characteristic whip-like fashion propelling mucus from the distal airways to the nasopharynx. The tips of the cilia will only touch the viscous mucus layer when fully extended (effective stroke) and return to the much less viscous

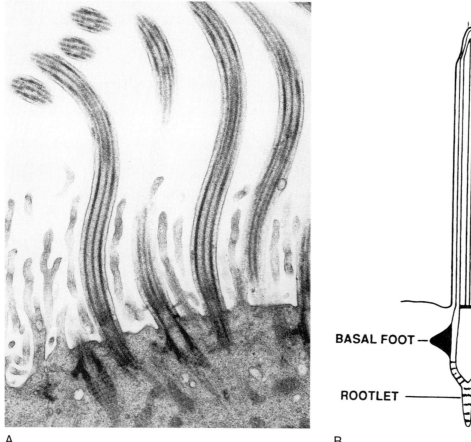
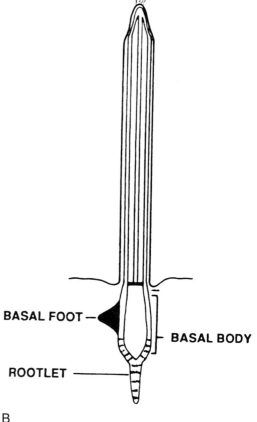

A   B

Figure 8-1   (**A**) Electron microscopic view of a longitudinal cut of cilia appearing to be beating synchronously. Note that the basal foot processes are aligned in the same direction. (**B**) Diagram of a cilium showing the axoneme and the anchoring structures.

BASAL FOOT —

BASAL BODY

ROOTLET —

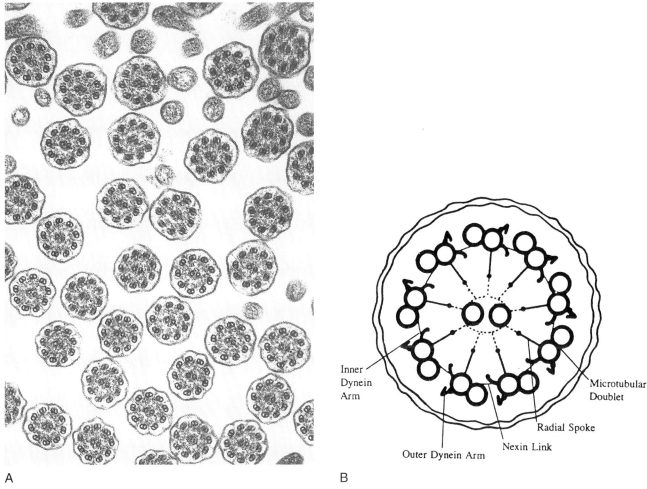

A   B

Figure 8-2   (**A**) Electron microscopic view of a transverse cut across ciliated epithelium, showing the axonemal structure. All cilia are properly oriented within normal relative angles (see text).
(**B**) Diagram of a cross-section of a cilium showing the wheel-like arrangement of the axonemal
structures.

periciliary fluid that lies underneath (recovery stroke)
before the next beat (Figure 8-3)[6]. Neural and chemical
mechanisms, and cell-to-cell signaling control this action.
The net effect is the so-called metachronal wave, a constant movement similar to the movement of sea or lake
waters casting their particles onto a beach. Effective ciliary beating requires proper hydration to preserve the
integrity of the layer of fluid in which the organelles are
immersed (periciliary fluid). Both dehydration and overhydration result in less effective movement of mucus.

Ciliary Defects

In PCD all defects are genetically determined, irreversible and constant in each affected family. A wide
range of abnormalities of ciliary structure has been
described, including absence of cilia, excessively long
axonemes, cilia with normal structure but abnormal
function and orientation, as well as a variety of axonemal
defects (Table 8-1)[2,8,9]. Because of their genetic origin,

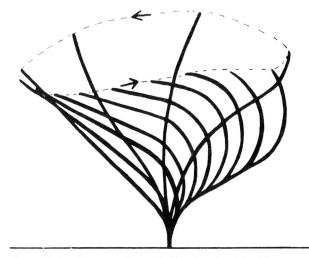

Figure 8-3   Diagram of normal ciliary beating. The cilium moves
from the resting position in a whip-like fashion until fully extended,
subsequently recoiling into the recovery stroke (Reproduced with
permission from Sleigh MA. The nature and action of respiratory
tract cilia. In Brain JD, Proctor DF, Reid LM, editors. Respiratory
defense mechanisms. New York: Marcel Dekker, 1977.)

Table 8-1	Primary and Secondary Ciliary Abnormalities in PCD

Ciliary Abnormalities in PCD	
Dynein arms	Total or partial absence of inner, outer, or both types of arms
Nexin links	Absence of nexin links and inner dynein arms with axonemal disorganization
Tubular defects	Transposition
	Absence of central micro-tubular pair
Radial spoke	Absence of the head of the spoke
	Total absence of spokes
Normal structure with random orientation (disorientation)	
Elongated cilia	
Absence of cilia (ciliary aplasia due to defective ciliogenesis)	
Secondary (acquired) ciliary abnormalities	
Compound cilia (fusion of two or more cilia)	
Rupture of ciliary membrane	
Ciliary fragmentation	
Missing tubules	
Extra tubules	

affected individuals within a family unit share the identical ultrastructural defect. Ciliary movement abnormalities range from total absence to movement resembling a windshield wiper or an eggbeater. Cilia with these defects are rendered "dyskinetic," insofar as their action is ineffective in propelling mucus adequately, although movement is present.

Widespread ciliary disorientation (or random orientation) even in the absence of structural defects is a sign of dyskinesia[10]. Drawing a line through the central tubule pair of adjacent cilia and measuring the relative angle can determine the orientation of cilia. The line across the central tubule is perpendicular to the direction of beating. Angles beyond 25° or 30° are indicative of ciliary disorientation and disorganized beating.

Smokers, patients with asthma and cystic fibrosis, and individuals afflicted by viral respiratory infections can exhibit reversible ciliary lesions[11,12]. In these instances, however, the percentage of cells with ciliary abnormalities is much lower than in patients with PCD. Further, many of the defects seen in these conditions (referred to as "secondary," as opposed to genetically determined) involve the cell membrane and peripheral doublets. Typical secondary defects are compound cilia, where two or more cilia coalesce into one larger structure, and breaks in the cell membrane with injury to doublets. In some instances dynein arm defects have been described, but, as was stated above, the number of affected cells is much lower than in PCD and the defects are reversible.

PATHOPHYSIOLOGY

Patients with PCD have poor mucociliary clearance and therefore have ineffective bacterial removal. The respiratory tract of these individuals is chronically colonized with bacteria. Bacteria multiply locally and virulence factors accumulate. Bacterial toxins may further slow ciliary movement, disrupt their beat, and even lead to further ciliary disorganization[13].

Many bacteria, such as *Pseudomonas aeruginosa* and *Haemophilus influenzae*, prefer to bind to mucus rather than to normal epithelium. When bacteria colonize mucus they release toxins that damage the underlying epithelium, further enhancing bacterial adhesion and causing damage. Activated neutrophils are attracted to the damaged area in an attempt to clear bacteria. Proteases, reactive oxygen species, and elastases attack the bacteria and the lung itself, leading to even more lung inflammation and damage[13]. Chronic infection and obstruction leads to the development of bronchiectasis, lung scarring and loss of function. In the sinuses, faulty clearance of mucus and subsequent infection causes chronic inflammation and recurrent exacerbations. Thickening of the mucosa, chronic bacterial infection, and meatal obstruction are the rule.

CLINICAL MANIFESTATIONS

Lower Respiratory Tract

Pulmonary manifestations can be present as early as in the neonatal period. Recurrent pneumonia and atelectasis, often multifocal, have been reported in babies in the nursery. Later in life, recurrences of "chest congestion," and signs of airways obstruction such as wheezing not totally responsive to bronchodilator therapy, are common complaints. PCD should be suspected in patients with asthma and severe upper respiratory complaints that do not respond to standard therapy. Chronic respiratory infections are the hallmark of PCD. The presence of chronic mucopurulent expectoration from which bacteria are consistently recovered (including *Pseudomonas aeruginosa*) and bronchiectasis in imaging studies should alert clinicians to the diagnosis as well.

Chest radiographs may show areas of atelectasis, infiltrates, hyperinflation, and other changes associated with chronic infections. Peribronchial thickening and nodular cystic lesions with evidence of bronchial dilatation heighten the suspicion of bronchiectatic changes (Figure 8-4). These must be confirmed by computed tomography (CT). Pulmonary function testing may show a wide range of severity of obstruction including decreased forced vital capacity and forced expiratory flows through large and small airways (FEV_1 and $FEF_{25-75\%}$). Bronchodilator responsiveness is very variable.

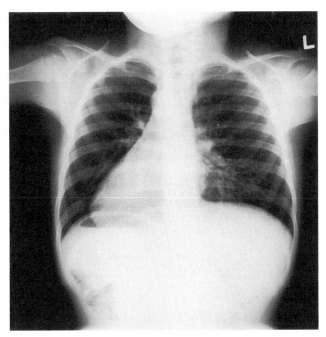

Figure 8-4 Complete situs inversus in a patient with Kartagener's syndrome. Dextrocardia in addition to finding the liver on the left side and the stomach on the right. There is an infiltration with an air bronchogram in the left lung as well as peribronchial thickening bilaterally (especially in the left upper and left lower lobes). Some nodular-cystic lesions are seen in the lower left lung field, suggestive of bronchiectasis.

The development of bronchiectasis is a late event in the disease, which results from untreated infection and airways obstruction. In an era of increased recognition of this condition due to awareness by pediatric caregivers, finding widespread or severe bronchiectatic changes in the lungs of these patients is uncommon. Likewise, the onset of restrictive disease due to destruction of lung tissue and scarring is very unusual in the pediatric population nowadays.

Upper Respiratory Tract

Otitis media and sinusitis are very common and occur early in life. Most children have protracted or recurrent otitis media with effusion, and conductive hearing loss necessitating tympanostomy. Mucopurulent nasal secretions are a hallmark of this condition, due to persistent nasal and paranasal sinus inflammation and infection.

Frequent exacerbations of sinus disease are common, especially in the ethmoid and maxillary sinuses. Patients frequently complain of chronic nasal congestion, purulent rhinorrhea, sinus pressure and headaches. Drainage from the maxillary sinuses is frequently ineffective, as cilia must be able to move mucus against gravity in order to drain adequately. Poor mucus clearance, as in the lungs, leads to chronic infection and further inflammatory response by the surrounding tissues[14]. Twenty percent of

children develop nasal polyps[15]; many develop chronic nasal obstruction, snoring, postnasal drip, hyponasal speech, halitosis and a poor sense of smell.

Radiographs of the sinuses frequently show opacities with mucosal thickening of the maxillary sinuses. The preferred imaging technique is CT of the sinuses which often reveals meatal obstruction, air–fluid levels, mucosal thickening, and bone erosion in severe cases. The frontal sinuses are often hypoplastic[16].

One conspicuous feature of respiratory disease in PCD is the almost universal need for antimicrobial therapy to curb the symptoms, and their common recurrence upon discontinuation of such therapy. Thus, many individuals affected with PCD require ongoing "suppressive" antibiotics to avert recurrences.

Reproductive System

Male patients almost universally have immotile spermatozoa and are, therefore, sterile. Spermatozoa have normal structure but are completely immotile. Intracytoplasmic injection of sperm from men with PCD has been used successfully to fertilize eggs[17]. Typically, sperm flagella and respiratory cilia share the same ultrastructural defect in affected individuals. Very rare cases of PCD with motile sperm have been reported, pointing to the very heterogeneous nature of this condition[1]. Women with immotile cilia may have abnormal ciliary movement in the oviducts and the fimbriae, however there is no evidence to date to indicate that female fertility is reduced or that affected women have a higher risk for ectopic pregnancy[18].

Situs inversus

Kartagener syndrome refers to the association of chronic sinusitis, bronchiectasis and situs inversus, as described by a Swiss physician about 70 years ago. Situs inversus is defined as a complete mirror image of normal organ placement. Situs inversus as an isolated finding (not associated with ciliary dysfunction) in some people is widely known to occur[19]. Because these individuals are essentially healthy, it is very likely that the true incidence of complete situs inversus without underlying conditions is underreported.

Fifty percent of patients with immotile cilia syndrome have complete situs inversus. What leads to this randomization of laterality is unclear. It is unknown whether the mechanics of abnormal ciliary movement leads to situs inversus. It is possible that a gene that controls left–right determination is related to one of the genes responsible for ciliary development. Another hypothesis is that ciliary movement is necessary for normal organ lateralization in utero. Absence of dynein arms could lead to lack of direction and random visceral situs determination.

DIAGNOSIS

Clinicians must consider the diagnosis of PCD in every child with complete situs inversus. Clear definition of organ position is necessary, because individuals with other situs abnormalities are not afflicted by PCD (see below). It must also be remembered that not every child with situs inversus has PCD; the constellation of situs abnormalities and chronic, severe respiratory disease is indicative.

The diagnosis of PCD in children without situs abnormalities is difficult, given the similarities between this and other conditions. PCD becomes almost a diagnosis of exclusion because it is much less common than respiratory allergy or cystic fibrosis. A very suggestive feature is the presence of persistent respiratory symptoms—particularly upper airway congestion with otitis, purulent rhinitis and sinusitis that abate with antibiotics, but suffer almost immediate recrudescence after antibiotic discontinuation.

In the neonate, the diagnosis must be suspected if respiratory distress is accompanied by unexplained abnormal findings on chest radiograph[8]. Lobar or subsegmental opacifications are suspicious, especially if they are recurrent, multifocal and resolve with administration of antimicrobial drugs and physiotherapy. Purulent rhinitis in a newborn, especially in the absence of other epidemiologic history, is also suggestive of PCD.

In adult males, infertility associated with chronic respiratory symptoms should make clinicians suspect the diagnosis. Sperm immotility on analysis of seminal fluid followed by ultrastructural examination can be used to confirm the diagnosis[20]. Absent spermatozoa alert clinicians to the diagnosis of cystic fibrosis or Young syndrome (a disease characterized by chronic sinusitis and lung disease with azoospermia).

The first phase of the diagnosis is the establishment of the anatomic abnormalities or lack thereof. This can be accomplished by a variety of imaging studies listed in Table 8-2. The examination of the paranasal sinuses is, in the opinion of the authors, a very important element in the diagnostic constellation, in that chronic sinusitis with frontal sinus aplasia or hypoplasia is almost universal. CT is the best imaging modality in defining this problem.

The first phase of diagnosis also requires the elimination of a more common diagnosis such as cystic fibrosis (sweat test and gene mutation analysis), immune deficiency (quantitative immunoglobulin levels) and allergy. The latter, of course, is non-specific, in that it can (and frequently does) coexist with PCD.

The next phase of diagnosis is the specific diagnosis of PCD and involves tests of ciliary motility and structure. The sequence of tests varies from center to center and is based in the proficiency with which tests of ciliary function are performed.

Table 8-2 Diagnosis of PCD

Clinical
Chronic upper and/or lower respiratory infections
Early (neonatal) onset
Purulent rhinorrhea
Chronic otitis
Persistent or refractory sinusitis
Chronic airways obstruction/mucopurulent expectoration
Situs inversus
Male infertility (adults)

Laboratory: Phase I
Chest radiograph (recurrent atelectasis/pneumonia, right middle lobe syndrome, situs inversus, nodular-cystic lesions)
Computed tomogram of the sinuses (pansinusitis, hypoplasia of frontal sinuses)
Computed tomogram of the chest (bronchiectasis)
Echocardiogram
Biopsy of nasal and tracheal mucosa
Analysis of semen (motility: electron microscopy)
Saccharin test
Studies of ciliary movement/ciliary cultures

Laboratory: Phase IIa
Direct examination of ciliary beating
Saccharin test
Radioactively tagged particle test

Laboratory: Phase IIb
Analysis of semen (adolescent/adults)
Biopsy of respiratory mucosa/electron microscopy
Ciliary culture

The direct microscopic observation of ciliary beating or the use of phase-contrast videomicroscopy requires the brushing or scraping of epithelium from the nose[8]. Such tests have traditionally been used in combination with studies of ciliary ultrastructure from biopsies to confirm a diagnosis of PCD.

The saccharin test involves the placement of a particle of saccharin on the inferior turbinate and measurement of the amount of time before the patients feels a sweet taste (normally 20–30 minutes)[21]. An alternative is the bronchoscopic placement of radioactively tagged particles in the lower central airway to follow their trajectory.

Another approach is the inhalation of radioactive aerosols and measurement of clearance of radioactivity from the lung over time. All these methods require that individuals remain still for a prolonged period of time with the head tilted, without evidence of sniffing, sneezing, or other maneuvers that would normally accelerate the movement of particles[8]. Likewise, cough can greatly speed clearance of particles from the lung. These exacting conditions make such functional tests of ciliary movement notoriously inaccurate in younger individuals who are unable to keep still for prolonged periods of time. They are very rough qualitative estimates of ciliary function.

We tend to prefer to secure an anatomic diagnosis over all other methods. Samples of mucosa must be obtained from at least two sites, often the posterior third of the nose and the carina. It is essential that one sample at least be obtained deep enough in the respiratory tree (i.e., trachea) to assure a minimum effect of inflammation and a maximum recovery of ciliated cells. Samples must be delicately and proficiently handled, and placed in glutaraldehyde—NOT in saline solution or formaldehyde. Properly handled samples should be examined by electron microscopy with transverse and longitudinal cuts to determine axonemal structure as well as orientation. The diagnosis can thus be confirmed. Viral infections or chronic inflammation can result in the denudation of nasal mucosa, or secondary changes in ciliary function and structure that can interfere with the diagnosis[21]. Thus, biopsies should ideally be obtained after a course of antibiotics and while the patient is not experiencing an intercurrent illness or an exacerbation.

A more recently described approach is the in vitro culture of ciliated epithelium[22]. The cilia thus generated express the primary genetically induced abnormalities, without the secondary defects caused by inflammation. This approach is especially useful in patients with defects other than dynein-arm deficiency (especially outer) in whom the nature of the ciliary defects visualized is unclear[23].

DIFFERENTIAL DIAGNOSIS

Asplenia and polysplenia are conditions associated with abnormalities of visceral position that can occasionally be easily confused with Kartagener syndrome. Characteristically, these patients can have complex congenital heart disease, random positioning of abdominal organs with livers that occupy the entire mid-abdomen (situs ambiguus), absent inferior vena cava, and intestinal malrotation, among other defects. Asplenic patients are prone to sepsis caused by encapsulated organisms and have Howell–Jolly bodies on the peripheral smear.

In the absence of situs inversus, the differential diagnosis must include cystic fibrosis, B-cell immune deficiency, and severe respiratory allergies. Table 8-3 summarizes the salient characteristics of the most important conditions included in the differential diagnosis of PCD.

TREATMENT

Regular care and periodic evaluations by subspecialists are helpful to maintain health in these patients. It is important to remember these individuals have a normal immune system and should, therefore, receive all childhood immunizations. Influenza vaccination on a yearly

Table 8-3   Differential Diagnosis of PCD

Condition	Differentiating feature
Other situs abnormalities Asplenia–polysplenia	Severe cardiac disease Sepsis (capsulated organisms) Howell–Jolly bodies (asplenia) Discordant situs
Cystic fibrosis	Intestinal malabsorption Mucoid strains of *P. aeruginosa* in sputum Positive sweat test Positive mutation analysis Semen analysis: aspermia (adults)
B-cell immune deficiency	Severe respiratory and systemic infections with unusual organisms Abnormal immunoglobulin levels
Respiratory allergies	Positive allergy tests Increased IgE levels Seasonality Normal oropharyngeal flora
Primary ciliary dyskinesia	Situs inversus (50% of patients) Abnormal ciliary biopsy Prominent upper airway disease Semen analysis: absent or abnormal movement of spermatozoa (adults)

basis should be added to their regimen. Patients should have access to physiotherapists, otolaryngologists, audiologists, and, when necessary, urologists and gynecologists[2]. When the patient is old enough to cooperate, periodic pulmonary function testing, radiographs and sputum cultures should be done to monitor the patient's course and adjust therapy.

The two most important therapies for PCD are the aggressive use of antibiotics and the clearance of mucus. The goal of medical treatment is to avoid complications of sinusitis, bronchial obstruction and bronchiectasis due to infection and mucus stasis.

Lower Airway Treatment

Daily chest physiotherapy allows for improved mucus clearance. This includes chest clapping, breathing techniques, and postural drainage twice a day[8]. Newer mechanical devices include mechanical vests, flutter devices, Thera PEP masks and other newly developed techniques.

Bacteria often colonize the damaged respiratory tract of patients with PCD. The aggressive use of antibiotics may help to decrease bacterial colonization. Antibiotics may be given orally, via nebulizer, and intravenously. Sputum cultures, while imperfect, may provide the identification and antibiotic sensitivities of specific bacteria. While bronchoalveolar lavage has a superior diagnostic yield, its routine performance may subject patients to unnecessary risk.

Upper Airway Treatment

There is no standard of care for treatment of otitis media with effusion in patients with PCD[16]. Some physicians advocate bilateral myringotomy tube insertion when patients have impaired speech, language, or educational development. However, these patients often continue to have chronic discharge from their tubes. Patients may also be treated with unilateral myringotomy tube insertion. Hearing aids are helpful and less invasive. They may be used in conjunction with myringotomy tubes or on their own. As many patients experience a spontaneous resolution of hearing abnormalities, hearing aids may not be necessary after childhood[8].

Chronic sinusitis may need to be treated surgically. An inferior meatus antrostomy is helpful because it allows gravitational sinus drainage. Other procedures, such as ethmoidectomy and frontal sinus recess surgery, may also be beneficial[14]. Functional endoscopic sinus surgery also creates a pathway for drainage, aeration, and medical therapy[24]. Even after surgery, patients will clinically benefit from nasal washes, topical corticosteroids, and systemic antibiotics (Table 8-4)[8].

Prognosis

PCD is a chronic and potentially debilitating disease, but it is *not* a lethal condition. Early diagnosis and aggressive therapy are aimed at avoiding complications, especially bronchiectasis and lung scarring. Proper care can assure reasonable well-being and ability to participate fully in all aspects of life.

MAJOR POINTS

1. Primary ciliary dyskinesia (PCD) leads to recurrent upper and lower airway infections due to ineffective mucus clearance.
2. One half of all patients with PCD also have complete situs inversus (known as Kartagener syndrome).
3. Aside from very rare case reports, men with PCD have immotile sperm.
4. There are in vitro fertility methods that allow men with PCD to have children.
5. Infections, asthma, and other airway diseases can lead to temporary ciliary dysfunction.
6. The electron microscopic diagnosis of PCD is difficult to accomplish and must be attempted several weeks after resolution of infection.
7. The treatment of PCD centers around aggressive treatment of infection with antibiotics and mucus clearance.
8. Patients with PCD benefit from a multidisciplinary team approach, regular care and periodic health care visits.

SUGGESTED READING

1. Schidlow DV. Primary ciliary dyskinesia (the immotile cilia syndrome). Ann Allergy 73:457–468, 1994.
2. Sleigh MA. Ciliary function in mucus transport. Chest 80: 791–795, 1981.
3. Knowles MR, Boucher RC. Mucus clearance as a primary innate defense mechanism for mammalian airways. J Clin Invest 109:571–577, 2002.

REFERENCES

1. Afzelius BA. Immotile cilia syndrome: past, present, and prospects for the future. Thorax 53: 894–897, 1998.
2. Meeks M, Bush A. Primary ciliary dyskinesia. Pediatr Pulmonol 29:307–316, 2000.
3. Narayan D, Krishnan SN, Upender M, Ravikumar TS, et al. Unusual Inheritance of primary ciliary dyskinesia (Kartagener's syndrome). J Med Genet 31:493–496, 1994.
4. Pan Y, McCaskill CD, Thompson KH, Hicks J, et al. Paternal isodisomy of chromosome 7 associated with complete situs inversus and immotile cilia. Am J Hum Genet 62:1551–1555, 1998.
5. Yokohoma T, Copeland N, Jenkins NA, Montgomery CA, et al. Reversal of left–right asymmetry: a situs inversus mutation. Science 260:679–682, 1993.
6. Sleigh MA, Blake JR, Liron N. The propulsion of mucus by cilia. Am Rev Respir Dis 137:726–741, 1988.

Table 8-4 Treatment of Respiratory Problems of PCD
Lower airway
Mucus clearance techniques
Continuous or intermittent antibiotics
Treatment of reversible airways obstruction
Therapy similar to asthma
Alpha-dornase[a]
Upper airway
Continuous or intermittent antibiotics
Sinus lavages
Nasal corticosteroids
Endoscopic sinus surgery
Alpha dornase[a]

[a]Off-label use. Some clinicians use inhalation via mask to enhance thinning and clearance of purulent respiratory secretions.

7. de Iongh RU, Rutland J. Ciliary defects in healthy subjects, bronchiectasis, and primary ciliary dyskinesia. Am J Respir Crit Care Med 151:1559-1567, 1995.

8. Bush A, Cole P, Hariri M, Mackay I, et al. Primary ciliary dyskinesia: diagnosis and standards of care. Eur Respir J 12:982-988, 1998.

9. DeBoeck K, Jorissen M, Wouters K, et al. Aplasia of respiratory tract cilia. Pediatr Pulmonol 13:259-265, 1992.

10. Rutland J, de Iongh RU. Random ciliary orientation: a cause of respiratory tract disease. N Engl J Med 323:1681-1684, 1990.

11. Rayner CFJ, et al. Ciliary disorientation in patients with chronic upper respiratory tract inflammation. Am J Respir Crit Care Med 151:800-804, 1995.

12. Rossman CM, et al. Nasal ciliary ultrastructure and function in patients with primary ciliary dyskinesia compared with that in normal subjects and in subjects with various respiratory diseases. Am Rev Respir Dis 129:161-167, 1984.

13. Dowling RB, Wilson R. Bacterial toxins which perturb ciliary function and respiratory epithelium. Soc Appl Bacteriol Symp Ser 84(27S):138-148S, 1998.

14. Hulka GF. Head and neck manifestations of cystic fibrosis and ciliary dyskinesia. Otolaryngol Clin North Am 33:1333-1341, 2000.

15. Levison H, et al. Pathophysiology of the ciliary motility syndromes. Eur J Respir Dis 64(127S):102-116, 1983.

16. El-Sayed Y, Al-Sarhai A, Al-Essa AR. Otological manifestations of primary ciliary dyskinesia. Clin Otolaryngol 22:266-270, 1997.

17. von Zumbusch A, Fiedler K, Mayerhofer A, et al. Birth of healthy children after intracytoplasmic sperm injection in two couples with male Kartagener's syndrome. Fertil Steril 70:643-646, 1998.

18. Afzelius BA, Eliasson R. Male and female infertility problems in the immotile-cilia syndrome. Eur J Respir Dis 64(127S):144-147, 1983.

19. Splitt MP, Burn J, Goodship J. Defects in the determination of left-right asymmetry. J Med Genet 33:498-503, 1966.

20. Munro NC, Currie DC, Lindsay KS, Ryder TA, et al. Fertility in men with primary ciliary dyskinesia presenting with respiratory infection. Thorax 49:684-687, 1994.

21. Canciani M, et al. The saccharin method for testing mucociliary function in patients suspected of having primary ciliary dyskinesia. Pediatr Pulmonol 5:210-214, 1988.

22. Jorissen M, Van Der Schveren B, Van Der Berghe, Cassiman JJ. The preservation and regeneration of cilia on human epithelial cells cultured in vitro. Arch Otorhinolaryngol 246:308-315, 1989.

23. Jorissen M, Van Der Schveren B, Van Der Berghe, Cassiman JJ. Ciliogenesis in cultured human nasal epithelium. ORL J Otorhinolaryngol Relat Spec 52:368-374, 1990.

24. Parsons DS, Green BA. A treatment of primary ciliary dyskinesia: efficacy of functional endoscopic sinus surgery. Laryngoscope 103:1269-1272, 1993.

CHAPTER 9

Pulmonary Complications of Immunologic Disorders

ANAND C. PATEL, M.D.

CLEMENT L. REN, M.D.

The average 4-year-old child inhales approximately 600 liters of air a day, exposing the lung to large quantities of potential pathogens. To protect against potential infection, the respiratory tract has a wide variety of defense mechanisms, including a mucociliary barrier, the innate immune system, and the adaptive immune system. Although abnormalities in the mucociliary system and innate immunity have been described and can lead to pulmonary complications, these conditions are quite rare and not well characterized. In contrast, defects in the adaptive immune system and its effector cells have been extensively studied on a molecular and cellular level, and there is considerable information concerning the acquisition of lung disease and its treatment. For this reason, this chapter will focus on pulmonary complications arising from defects in adaptive immunity.

INFECTIOUS PULMONARY COMPLICATIONS OF IMMUNODEFICIENCY

Each component of the immune system serves a specific role in host defense. A deficiency in any one element of the immune system renders individuals susceptible to specific groups of pathogens. Table 9-1 summarizes the pattern of infections seen in the different immunodeficiency syndromes.

Complications of Neutrophil Defects

Polymorphonuclear neutrophils (PMNs) are the primary phagocytic cells of the immune system. They play a key role in eliminating opsonized bacterial and fungal pathogens through release of proteolytic enzymes and reactive oxidant species (ROS). This function may be impaired through abnormalities in cell adhesion, cell signaling, cell number, granule function or formation, and intracellular killing [1].

The most common PMN disorder is chronic granulomatous disease (CGD), with an estimated incidence of 1 in 200,000 in the United States[1,2]. The primary defect in CGD is a loss of NADPH oxidase function. CGD exists in X-linked and autosomal recessive forms, depending on which gene coding for the NADPH oxidase complex is mutated; the X-linked form is more common. Loss of NADPH oxidase activity leads to a markedly reduced oxidative burst following phagocytosis. PMNs from patients with CGD can phagocytose bacteria but cannot kill them, leading to the development of multiple large granulomas. Organisms that express catalase are particularly resistant to killing by PMNs from CGD patients, because catalase neutralizes any residual ROS produced by these patients by hydrolyzing superoxide to hydrogen peroxide. The most

Table 9-1 Typical Pathogens Associated with Specific Immunodeficiencies

Element of the Immune System Affected	Example Diseases	Typical Pulmonary Pathogens
Neutrophils	CGD	*S. aureus, A. fumigatus*
B lymphocytes	XLA, CVID	*S. pneumoniae, H. influenzae*
T lymphocytes	Severe: SCID Less severe: A-T, WAS	PCP, viruses, fungi Bacterial pneumonia

common catalase-positive organisms that cause pulmonary infections in CGD are *Staphylococcus aureus* and *Aspergillus* species. *Burkholderia cepacia*, *Nocardia* species, and *Serratia marcescens* can also cause pulmonary infections in this group of patients[1].

Patients with CGD present with atypical or unusually severe lymphadenitis, skin abscesses, pneumonia, and/or hepatomegaly secondary to infections with the aforementioned agents. Less common initial presentations include intestinal lymphadenitis that can cause a diarrhea and colitis picture that can be mistaken for Crohn's disease. Data from a national registry of 368 CGD patients in the United States provide considerable insight into the pulmonary complications of CGD[3]. Eighty percent of the patients in the registry had had pneumonia at least once. *Aspergillus* was the most common causative organism, responsible for 41% of pneumonias. *Aspergillus* pneumonia with or without dissemination was also the most common cause of death in patients with CGD, causing 35% of deaths in the series. *Staphylococcus* species caused 12% of pneumonias. *B. cepacia* was the third most common cause of pneumonia (8% of all cases), but the second most common cause of death (18%). Other pathogens reported to cause pneumonia in these patients include *Nocardia*, *Mycobacteria*, and Gram-negative bacteria.

A recent trend in the epidemiology of pulmonary infections in CGD is the growing incidence of *Aspergillus* as the primary pulmonary pathogen. This trend probably reflects advances in the treatment of CGD. Trimethoprim/sulfamethoxazole (TMP/SMX) prophylaxis was introduced in 1990, and has been effective in reducing the frequency of serious bacterial infections[1]. The other therapy that has had a major impact on the clinical course of CGD has been interferon-gamma (IFN-γ). The precise mechanism by which IFN-γ acts in CGD is unclear, although there is some evidence that it augments the oxidative burst in CGD patients[4]. A large multicenter trial of IFN-γ therapy in CGD patients showed

a significant reduction in both bacterial and fungal infections[5]. The combination of these two therapies has significantly reduced bacterial infections, but has had a less dramatic effect on serious fungal infections (Figure 9-1).

Pulmonary abscesses also occur frequently in patients with CGD. Sixteen percent of patients in the registry had a lung abscess at some point in their course. Of those, the most common organism isolated was *Aspergillus* (23%), although *Nocardia* species, *B. cepacia*, and *Staphylococcus* species can also cause abscesses[3].

Other PMN disorders include leukocyte adhesion molecule (LAM) deficiency, hyper-IgE syndrome, and Chediak–Higashi syndrome[1]. LAM deficiency results from defects in expression of either integrin or selectin adhesion molecules on the surface of leukocytes. Without these adhesion molecules, PMNs cannot migrate to sites of infection. Delayed umbilical cord separation, marked leukocytosis, and chronic severe skin infections are common presenting signs. Hyper-IgE syndrome is a rare disorder of unknown etiology associated with impaired PMN function. Patients typically present with coarse facial features, recurrent skin infections, and extremely high serum IgE levels (Figure 9-2). Chediak–Higashi syndrome (CHS) is an autosomal recessive disorder resulting from mutations in a lysosomal protein transport gene. Patients with CHS have multiple abnormalities, including reduced PMN phagocytosis and chemotaxis. In general, pulmonary complications in these disorders are very similar to those of CGD.

Complications Associated with B Lymphocyte Disorders

B lymphocytes are the only source of immunoglobulin (Ig), or antibody[6]. There are five different Ig isotypes: IgM, IgG, IgA, IgD, and IgE. B cells initially can make only IgM and IgD, but with appropriate T lymphocyte help they will switch to making other isotypes. Immunoglobulins play a key role in the opsonization and clearance of encapsulated bacterial organisms. Thus patients with B cell deficiencies are prone to infection with these organisms, primarily *S. pneumoniae* (Pneumococcus) and *H. influenzae*. In contrast, because T cell function is intact, patients tend to have normal defenses against viruses, fungi, and mycobacteria. Because maternal IgG crosses the placental barrier, infants with B cell disorders receive passive protection from infection for the first 6 to 9 months of life. After this age, patients will present with recurrent bacterial infections of the middle ear, sinuses, and lungs. Complications such as mastitis are common. Sepsis and osteomyelitis may also be seen[6].

The most severe forms of B cell disorders arise from defects in B cell development, leading to near total absence of circulating B cells. Of this group, X-linked

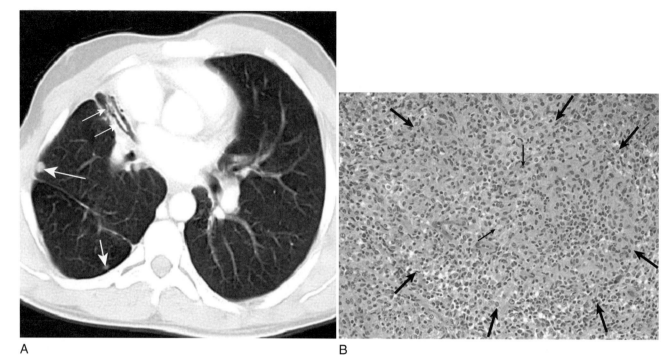

A   B

Figure 9-1 **(A)** Chest CT scan of a 22-year-old man with CGD who had a 2 kg weight loss over 2 weeks and complained of chest pain for 1 month. The study demonstrates several nodules in the right lung (arrows). There is also a patchy density in the right upper lobe and right middle lobe adjacent to the heart (small arrows). The patient had been receiving ciprofloxacin and itraconazole prophylaxis. (CT image courtesy of Avrum N. Pollock, M.D., FRCPC and Kathleen Sullivan, M.D., Ph.D.) **(B)** Thoracoscopic biopsy of one of the nodules demonstrates poorly formed suppurative granulomata (wide arrows) with central necrosis (thin arrows) and surrounding organizing pneumonia. Culture of the lesion grew a fungus, *Paecilomyces lilicanus*. Hematoxylin and eosin stain, magnification ×20. (Photomicrograph courtesy of Bruce Pawel, M.D.)

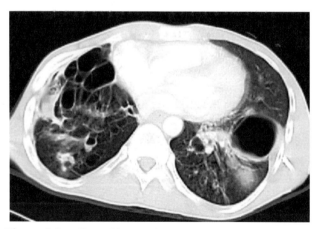

Figure 9-2   Chest CT scan of a 20-year-old man with hyper-IgE syndrome. There are numerous bullae in the right lung along with cystic bronchiectasis. The large cystic lesion in the left lung was a multiloculated abscess arising from the major fissure, which had been percutaneously drained of 500 cc of purulent fluid. In culture, the fluid grew methicillin-resistant *Staphylococcus aureus* and nontypeable *Haemophilus influenzae*. (CT image courtesy of Avrum N. Pollock, M.D., FRCPC and Kathleen Sullivan, M.D., Ph.D.)

agammaglobulinemia (XLA), or Bruton's disease, is the most common. The molecular defect in XLA is due to mutations in the Bruton's tyrosine kinase (BTK) gene[6]. Absence of BTK results in a block in B cell maturation at the pre-B cell stage. Thus patients with XLA have no circulating B cells and make no antibody of any kind. Pulmonary infections are very common in XLA, mainly due to *S. pneumoniae* and *H. influenzae*[7]. In contrast to other B cell disorders, patients with XLA can develop *Pneumocystis carinii* pneumonia (PCP)[6]. The reason for this is unclear, although it may be related to the role of B cells as antigen-presenting cells. Alternatively, it may be that loss of BTK function leads to subtle defects in cellular immunity.

Common variable immunodeficiency (CVID) is the name given to a heterogeneous group of disorders characterized by varying degrees of hypogammaglobulinemia with or without other abnormalities of T cell function[6]. Patients with CVID usually have normal numbers of B cells, but the function of these cells is impaired. Other immunologic abnormalities that can be seen in CVID include impaired lymphocyte proliferative response to antigens, deficiency of antigen-primed T cells, increased macrophage activation, and reduced production and/or expression of cytokines. CVID can frequently occur in older children or adults following a viral infection, and it is sometimes referred to as acquired hypogammaglobulinemia. Although CVID patients may have subtle defects in T cell function, they rarely develop opportunistic infections. More commonly, patients with CVID are prone to recurrent bacterial infections, generally of the sinopulmonary tract. Because the condition may present in later childhood and the diagnosis may be delayed, many of these

patients have bronchiectasis at the time of presentation[8] (Figure 9-3).

IgG subclass deficiency is a subset of CVID characterized by low normal or mildly reduced total IgG and selective decreases in one or more of the four IgG subclasses[6]. Although symptomatic disease has been described in association with all four IgG subclasses, IgG2 subclass deficiency is the syndrome that has been best described. Patients with IgG2 subclass deficiency present with recurrent sinopulmonary infections; most patients also

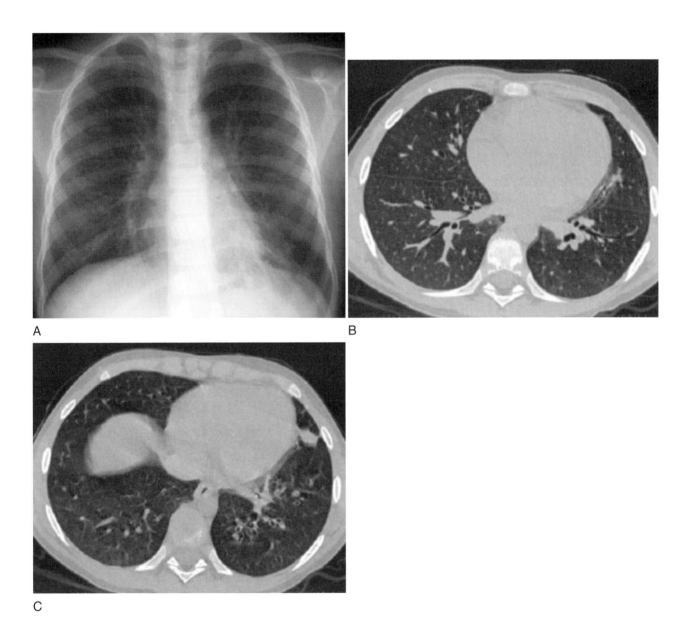

A

B

C

Figure 9-3 (**A**) Posterior-anterior chest radiograph of a 10-year-old male with CVID, demonstrating persistent densities in the left lower lobe and lingula. He had been treated for asthma from infancy until age 8 years, when he presented with severe bilateral pneumonia and staphylococcal sepsis. A sputum culture at the time of this radiograph grew non-typeable *H. influenzae*. (Image courtesy of Avrum N. Pollock, M.D., FRCPC, and Howard B. Panitch, M.D.) **B**, **C**. Chest CT scans of the same patient, demonstrating mild, diffuse bronchiectasis of the right middle lobe and lingula (**B**) and of the left lower lobe (**C**). (Images courtesy of Avrum N. Pollock, M.D., FRCPC and Howard B. Panitch, M.D.)

carry the diagnosis of asthma[9]. Although their total IgG may be normal, they fail to make high titers of antibody against encapsulated organisms, such as *S. pneumoniae* and *H. influenzae*.

IgA deficiency is one of the most common antibody deficiencies, with an approximate incidence of 1 in 400 to 3000 individuals in the general population[6]. Most patients with IgA deficiency are asymptomatic, perhaps because of compensatory protection by IgG. Those who are symptomatic are at increased risk of gastrointestinal and sinopulmonary infections. Symptomatic IgA deficiency is often seen in association with IgG subclass deficiency (Figure 9-4).

The introduction of intravenous immunoglobulin (IVIG) replacement therapy has had a significant impact on the morbidity and mortality of B cell immunodeficiencies[6,10]. IVIG is prepared from pooled plasma collected from a large number of donors. As a blood product, IVIG does carry a potential risk for pathogen transmission. However, improved purification protocols have rendered this risk extremely small. IVIG therapy significantly reduces the incidence and severity of pneumonia and other respiratory tract infections in patients with XLA, CVID, and other antibody deficiency syndromes[10]. However, bronchiectasis can still develop in some patients in spite of IVIG therapy[8,11].

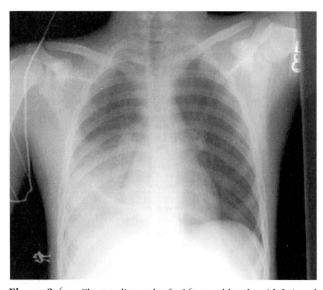

Figure 9-4   Chest radiograph of a 16-year-old male with IgA and IgG$_3$ subclass deficiencies, and possible deficient antibody response to polysaccharide antigens. He presented with a 2 day history of upper respiratory symptoms, fever, diarrhea and vomiting. The study shows consolidation of the right lower lobe along with a right-sided pleural effusion. The sputum grew only normal oropharyngeal flora and a blood culture was sterile. He had a 2 year history of recurrent episodes of pharyngitis and sinusitis, and was treated approximately monthly with antibiotics for recurrent upper respiratory illnesses before the diagnosis of his immunodeficiency was made. (Image courtesy of Avrum N. Pollock, M.D., FRCPC and Kathleen Sullivan, M.D., Ph.D.)

Pulmonary Infections Associated with T Lymphocyte Disorders

Overview of T Cell Disorders

T lymphocytes play important roles in both coordinating the adaptive immune system as well as actively eliminating foreign pathogens[11]. T cells can be roughly divided into two major subsets. Helper T (TH) cells usually express the cell surface receptor CD4, whereas cytotoxic T lymphocytes (CTLs) usually express CD8 and are responsible for cell-mediated immune responses. TH cells are critical for B cell activation and optimal antibody production. Helper T cells also coordinate the activity of CTLs. Because of the multiple roles that T cells play in the immune system, impairment of their function may have profound consequences for immunity.

Severe Combined Immunodeficiency

Severe combined immunodeficiency (SCID) is the term used to identify the most severe forms of T cell disorders. SCID can result from a diverse array of genetic mutations that affect lymphocyte production, development, metabolism, or cell signaling[12]. Regardless of the underlying genetic defect, the immunologic consequence is that there is near total loss of T cell number or function. Because B and T lymphocytes develop from a single lymphoid lineage, many cases of SCID are also associated with absent B cells. In those cases with residual circulating B cells, the lack of T cell help renders them non-functional.

The loss of T cell function in SCID patients leads to their being susceptible to opportunistic infections such as *Pneumocystis carinii*, fungi, and viruses. Patients with SCID tend to present early in infancy because of the severe loss of immune function. Pulmonary infections are a common initial presenting sign in SCID, and up to 67% of SCID patients present with pulmonary disease at diagnosis[13] (Figure 9-5). In patients with pulmonary complaints at presentation, 60% present with a persistent pulmonary infiltrate and chronic cough, while the other 40% present with more acute symptoms of respiratory distress secondary to pneumonia. *P. carinii* is the most common cause of pneumonia and is associated with significant mortality (43%) (Figure 9-6). Bacterial pneumonia can also occur, with *K. pneumoniae*, *S. pneumoniae*, and *S. aureus* being the most common pathogens isolated. Viral infections, though not common at presentation, also contribute to morbidity and mortality in these patients. In patients not treated with immunoreconstitution, pulmonary disease remains a significant cause of morbidity and mortality. Subsequent pulmonary infection can occur in 80–100% of patients after initial diagnosis[13].

Other T Cell Defects

Besides SCID, immunodeficiency can also arise from other, less severe, defects in T cell function. Because some

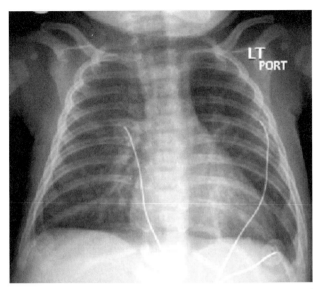

Figure 9-5   Chest radiograph of a 2½-month-old infant with SCID and parainfluenza 3 infection. Note the narrowed mediastinum, resulting from absence of a thymus. The lungs demonstrate diffusely increased interstitial markings and subsegmental atelectasis in the left lower lobe. This infant had seborrheic dermatitis and chronic cough and congestion. (Image courtesy of Avrum N. Pollock, M.D., FRCPC and Kathleen Sullivan, M.D., Ph.D.)

degree of residual T cell function persists in these other conditions, the severity of disease tends to be less than that of SCID. Pulmonary complications, however, continue to be common in this group of patients.

DiGeorge syndrome results from errors in the formation of the third and fourth pharyngeal pouches during embryogenesis, resulting in hypoplasia or complete

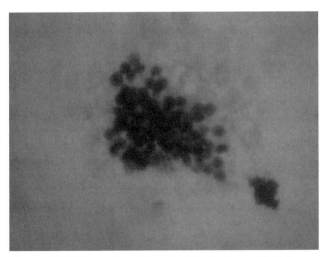

Figure 9-6   Silver stain of bronchoalveolar lavage fluid from a patient with *Pneumocystis carinii* pneumonia. The protozoan appears as cysts, each containing anywhere from one to eight oval bodies called sporozoites. (Courtesy of Howard B. Panitch, M.D.)

absence of the thymus, and parathyroid glands[12]. Other midline structures may also be affected, such as the heart and great vessels, craniofacial bones and tissues, and upper limbs. The immunologic defect is due to thymic dysplasia and ranges from a severe depression of T cell function in patients with no thymus, to near normal function in patients with mild thymic hypoplasia. In contrast to SCID, DiGeorge syndrome patients are not commonly infected with *P. carinii*. Bacterial pneumonia with Gram-negative organisms is more commonly seen. Severe respiratory syncytial virus (RSV) infections have also been reported.

Wiskot–Aldrich syndrome (WAS) is an X-linked recessive syndrome caused by mutations in the Wiskott–Aldrich Syndrome Protein (WASP) gene[12]. The classic clinical triad of WAS is thrombocytopenia, eczema, and recurrent bacterial infection. Although the exact function of WASP is still undetermined, loss of WASP function results in an inability to generate antibody to polysaccharide antigens. WAS patients are therefore susceptible to recurrent infections with bacteria that form polysaccharide capsules, such as *S. pneumoniae* and *H. influenzae*. Although the sites of infection tend to be the middle ear and sinuses, pneumonia can also be seen in this group of patients. Later in life, there is also an increased incidence of PCP.

Ataxia-telangiectasia (A-T) is a complex multisystem autosomal recessive syndrome, with abnormalities of the nervous system, endocrine system, skin, liver, and immune system[12]. Immune dysfunction in A-T is variable and affects both T and B cells. Although A-T is classified as a T cell immunodeficiency, B cell dysfunction due to loss of T cell help is the primary immune problem. IgA and IgG subclass deficiencies are commonly seen in patients with A-T. Pulmonary infections are a common complication in A-T, and a significant cause of mortality. Pneumonia in patients with A-T tends to be caused by bacteria, such as *S. pneumoniae, S. aureus, H. influenzae, Mycoplasma pneumoniae*, and *P. aeruginosa*. RSV and cytomegalovirus (CMV) can also cause lower respiratory tract infection in these patients, but fungi, mycobacteria, and *P. carinii* rarely are pathogens in this disease[12]. The underlying defect in A-T involves a defect in DNA repair, and patients with A-T are at high risk for the development of malignancy. In some patients with A-T, pulmonary lymphoma has led to cavitary lesions on chest radiographs that were mistaken for pneumonia[14]. It is therefore important to consider the possibility of malignancy when evaluating patients with A-T and pulmonary symptoms and to pursue an appropriate investigation.

Hyper-IgM (HIgM) syndrome is characterized by normal or elevated serum IgM levels with decreased or absent levels of IgG, IgA, and IgE[12]. HIgM syndrome exists in both an X-linked and autosomal recessive form. About 55–65% of the patients have the X-linked form, which is due to mutations in the gene for CD40 ligand (CD154), a T cell surface molecule critical for induction of B cell isotype switch. Because of the absence of CD154, B cells from X-linked HIgM patients can only make IgM, with little or no production of other Ig isotypes. An autosomal recessive form also exists, where the defect appears to be due to mutations in a cytidine deaminase gene. Bacterial pneumonia is the most common pulmonary complication in HIgM syndrome (Figure 9-7), but PCP also occurs in the X-linked form, indicating that CD154 also plays a role in T cell function.

NON-INFECTIOUS PULMONARY COMPLICATIONS OF IMMUNODEFICIENCY

In addition to impaired host defense, patients with immunodeficiency can also develop dysregulated immune responses[15]. Non-infectious pulmonary diseases that have been reported in association with immunodeficiency include interstitial lung disease, bronchiolitis obliterans, and hypersensitivity pneumonitis. CVID and A-T are the most common conditions associated with the above disorders[8,12], although they have been reported in other immunodeficiencies[16]. Allergic bronchopulmonary aspergillosis has also been seen in patients with CGD[17].

PULMONARY COMPLICATIONS ASSOCIATED WITH HUMAN IMMUNODEFICIENCY VIRUS INFECTION

Human immunodeficiency virus (HIV) infection is the most common cause of acquired immunodeficiency[18]. HIV infects CD4 positive helper T cells, leading to their loss. As HIV infection progresses, patients have a near total depletion of CD4 T cells. The loss of helper T cells impairs both CTL function as well as B cell function.

Infectious Complications of HIV Infection

PCP is one of the most common complications of HIV[18,19]. PCP infections in HIV infected patients carry a high degree of morbidity and mortality[18]. Prophylaxis against PCP is an important part of HIV treatment and can be accomplished with either TMP/SMX or inhaled pentamidine.

In endemic areas of developing nations, *Mycobacterium tuberculosis* (TB) has emerged as a major pulmonary complication in HIV-infected patients[18]. TB infections tend to be more severe and difficult to treat in HIV-infected patients. Non-tuberculous mycobacteria, such as *Mycobacterium avium* complex (MAC) can also cause significant pulmonary disease in adults with HIV. In contrast,

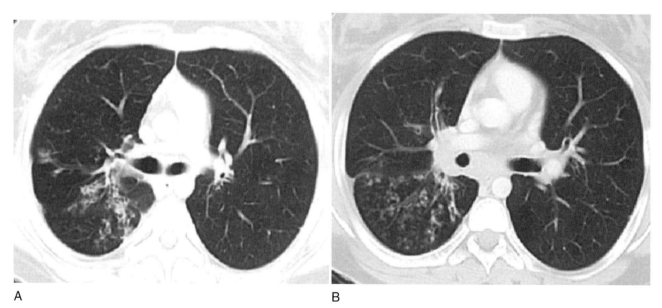

A   B

Figure 9-7 Chest CT scan of a 13-year-old female with hyper-IgM syndrome and a 4 day history of fever, fatigue, and shortness of breath. The images demonstrate bronchiectasis with a "tree-in-bud" pattern in the posterior segment of the right upper lobe (**A**), as well as bronchiectasis of the right middle lobe (**B**). The patient presented at age 6 years with a history of recurrent pneumonia, sinusitis, and otitis media, for which ventilation tubes were placed on three different occasions. She was treated with monthly infusions of IVIG. Quantitative culture by bronchoalveolar lavage yielded >10^5 colonies of α-hemolytic streptococci. (Images courtesy of Avrum N. Pollock, M.D., FRCPC and Howard B. Panitch, M.D.)

the incidence of severe pulmonary MAC disease is less in HIV infected children[20].

Respiratory viral infections are another common complication in HIV infection. RSV, influenza A and B, and parainfluenza viruses can all cause severe lung disease in HIV-infected infants[21]. CMV can also cause pulmonary disease. However, because CMV is often shed asymptomatically, the diagnosis of true pneumonitis should rest upon evidence of systemic dissemination (e.g., retinitis or hepatitis) or demonstration of viral inclusion bodies in lung biopsy specimens.

The other major group of respiratory pathogens in HIV-infected individuals is fungi. *Histoplasmosis* infection is rare, but when present it occurs as disseminated disease that often includes reticulonodular, miliary, and/or lobar infiltrates. It can often progress to septic shock and death if untreated. *Cryptococcus* and *Coccidiomycosis* can also cause pulmonary disease. Pulmonary aspergillosis presents as invasive pulmonary disease rather than as aspergilloma, and can be life-threatening, with poor prognosis despite antifungal therapy[20].

Although patients with HIV primarily suffer from opportunistic infections as a consequence of their loss of cellular immunity, bacterial infections are also common, especially in children[19,20,22]. These occur despite normal or even elevated immunoglobulin levels in patients with HIV, because the loss of CD4 positive helper T cells results in a failure to generate effective specific antibody titers. *S. pneumoniae* is the most common cause of bacterial pneumonia in this patient population. Other common organisms include *S. aureus*, Group A *Streptococcus*, *E. coli*, *P. aeruginosa*, *H. influenzae*, and *Salmonella*.

Non-infectious Complications of HIV Infection

Dysregulation of the immune system is another consequence of HIV infection, leading to an increased incidence of non-infectious disorders of the lung[18,19]. In children, the most common non-infectious pulmonary complication is lymphocytic interstitial pneumonitis (LIP). The precise pathogenesis of LIP is unknown; it is thought to represent a dysregulated immunologic response to Epstein–Barr virus infection. Between 30% and 40% of perinatally infected children will have LIP, with an average age of 2.3 years at presentation. Typically, patients with LIP present with gradual onset of cough and dyspnea. Generalized lymphadenopathy and clubbing are associated clinical findings. The chest radiograph demonstrates diffuse reticulo-nodular densities, frequently with hilar adenopathy. LIP is usually quite responsive to systemic corticosteroid therapy, which is the first line of treatment for this condition. The condition may recur, requiring repetitive courses of oral corticosteroids.

In addition to LIP, a non-specific interstitial pneumonitis (NIP) can also occur in HIV-infected patients, although this is less common in children. NIP is thought to result from localized CTL activity against HIV-infected cells in the lung parenchyma. Therefore it is more commonly seen early in HIV infection, when there is still some residual CD4-positive T cell activity present. However, it can occur at any stage of the disease.

Pulmonary Complications Related to HIV Therapy

Highly active anti-retroviral therapy (HAART) against HIV infection was introduced in the mid-1990s. HAART has had a dramatic effect on the prognosis and clinical course of HIV infection[18]. One result of increased survival has been the increased incidence of chronic lung diseases, such as bronchiectasis[23]. The restoration of immune function in patients with previously longstanding immunodeficiency has also led to unexpected complications resulting from either exuberant inflammatory responses or unmasking of latent opportunistic infections[24]. These complications are summarized in Box 9-1. As immune function is restored, there is an increased inflammatory response against underlying latent mycobacterial infections, both TB as well as MAC. HAART may also be associated with reactivation of latent PCP, leading to acute respiratory failure. Non-infectious complications that have been reported with HAART include a sarcoid-like syndrome, hypersensitivity pneumonitis, and pulmonary hypertension[24]. Although most published reports have focused on adult patients, it is likely that this same phenomenon will be seen in children as HAART increasingly becomes the standard of care in HIV treatment.

PULMONARY EVALUATION OF THE PATIENT WITH IMMUNODEFICIENCY

The approach to evaluating a patient with immunodeficiency is summarized in Box 9-2. The evaluation begins with a thorough history and physical examination. The history should focus on symptoms of chronic infection or bronchiectasis. The patient or patient's parents

---

Box 9-1   Pulmonary Complications of HAART

Increased inflammatory responses to:
  MAC
  TB
  PCP
Sarcoid-like syndrome
Hypersensitivity pneumonitis
Pulmonary hypertension

Box 9-2   Evaluation of the Patient with Immunodeficiency

History
    Delayed umbilical cord separation?
    History of infections?
    Sites and etiologies of infections?
Physical examination
    HEENT
        Presence of tonsils
    Chest
        Crackles
        Wheezes
    Extremities
        Lymphadenopathy
        Clubbing
Radiographic imaging
    Chest radiograph
    High-resolution computed tomography
    Evidence of bronchiectasis?
Pulmonary function testing
    Restrictive versus obstructive pattern
Bronchoscopy

should be questioned about the presence of cough and sputum production. Symptoms of wheezing may suggest an asthma or reactive airways disease component. Elements of the physical examination of particular importance include the patient's height and weight, chest examination, and extremity examination. The height and weight provide important information about the patient's nutritional status, which may be compromised in the setting of chronic pulmonary disease. Auscultation of the chest is important to identify areas of localized crackles or wheezes. The presence of digital clubbing on extremity examination is an indication of underlying bronchiectasis. Other important aspects of the physical examination include evidence of skin infections, absence of lymphoid tissue (e.g., tonsils and lymph nodes), and evidence of chronic or frequently recurring otitis media.

Radiography is an important tool in the evaluation of pulmonary disease in immunodeficient patients. Plain chest radiographs can reveal areas of atelectasis or infiltrate. Although large areas of bronchiectasis can be seen by plain radiographs, high-resolution computed tomography (CT) is a more sensitive tool for the detection of early or mild bronchiectasis[11,25]. CT is also helpful for delineating lesions such as pulmonary abscesses or lymph node pathology.

The results of pulmonary function tests (PFTs) in immunodeficient patients depends on the underlying pulmonary pathology. Patients with bronchiectasis demonstrate an obstructive pattern. Patients with interstitial lung processes will have a restrictive pattern, and the diffusion capacity may also be decreased. PFTs can be helpful in establishing the severity of disease and in tracking disease progression. PFTs can also provide objective assessment of response to medications, such as bronchodilators.

Bronchoscopy can be important both for acute complications as well as for chronic conditions. For patients presenting with acute pulmonary symptoms, bronchoscopy with bronchoalveolar lavage (BAL) can help in the diagnosis of infections such as PCP. For patients with bronchiectasis who cannot expectorate sputum, BAL can provide information about the organisms colonizing the lower respiratory tract. Bronchoscopy can also be helpful in studying the airway anatomy, especially in patients in whom there is concern for compression of the bronchi by enlarged reactive lymph nodes. In most cases, flexible fiberoptic bronchoscopy can be safely performed under conscious or deep sedation on this group of patients.

TREATMENT OF PULMONARY COMPLICATIONS

Treatment of the underlying immune defect is the best way to prevent pulmonary complications. IFN-γ has been shown to improve phagocytic cell function in patients with CGD, leading to a reduced incidence of infections[5]. For patients with SCID or other T cell disorders, bone marrow transplantation can result in complete correction of the immune defect[12]. Antibody deficiency syndromes can be treated with IVIG replacement therapy[6]. HAART has had a dramatic impact on survival and the rates of infection in patients with HIV[18]. It is likely that as our understanding of the molecular and cellular basis of congenital and acquired immunodeficiency increases, more therapies aimed at correcting the underlying defect will become available.

Although specific therapy for immunodeficiencies is available, not all patients are candidates for bone marrow transplantation, and other therapies may not lead to complete absence of pulmonary complications. In this situation, antibiotic prophylaxis can be used to reduce the incidence of pulmonary infections. The choice of antibiotic depends on the pathogens most likely to be involved in the underlying disease process. For CGD, prophylaxis against *S. aureus* is indicated, whereas for T cell immunodeficiencies and HIV infection prophylaxis against *P. carinii* is the major concern. Itraconazole prophylaxis for *Aspergillus* in CGD has been used at some centers[26], but the potential benefits of prophylaxis must be weighed against the known risks of increased drug resistance[27,28].

Many patients with immunodeficiency still develop bronchiectasis, as a result of either delayed diagnosis or continued infection despite treatment. This is especially common in patients with B cell disorders such as XLA and CVID. Treatment of bronchiectasis due to immunodeficiency is similar to that seen in other conditions[25].

Airway clearance in the form of chest physiotherapy or other techniques is important to prevent accumulation of purulent secretions in the respiratory tract. Antibiotics are used to treat acute exacerbations of lung disease as well as to maintain control of chronic infection. For this latter goal, intermittent administration of inhaled tobramycin has been shown to improve lung function without an increase in bacterial resistance in patients with bronchiectasis due to cystic fibrosis[29]. Although there are no published reports of its use in bronchiectasis due to immunodeficiency, it has been used anecdotally for this purpose and a large multicenter trial of this medication in bronchiectasis is currently under way.

For patients with irreversible or progressive respiratory failure, lung transplantation is an option. In general, the 5 year survival rate following lung transplantation is around 55%[30]. Lung transplantation has been performed on patients with immunodeficiency, but there are limited data on their clinical outcomes[8,31]. There are no data that focus specifically on immunodeficient recipients. Any decision for lung transplantation in this patient population requires a careful consideration of the risks and benefits of this procedure.

SUMMARY

Pulmonary complications are common in patients with immunodeficiency, and pulmonary infections are frequently the initial presenting sign in this patient population. Pneumonia and other respiratory tract infections continue to occur in these patients, despite treatment for the underlying disorder and supportive measures, such as antibiotic prophylaxis. In addition to infectious complications, non-infectious pulmonary disorders also can occur in this group of patients. The patient with HIV infection presents an entirely different set of pulmonary complications, and the advent of HAART has led to the emergence of new pulmonary manifestations in patients with HIV infection. The clinician dealing with immunodeficient patients must remain vigilant for these complications.

MAJOR POINTS

1. Pulmonary complications are common in children with immunodeficiency, and are often the presenting illness.
2. The type of pulmonary infections will depend on the specific area of the immune system affected.
3. Early diagnosis and treatment of immunodeficiencies can prevent pulmonary complications.
4. Chest CT, bronchoscopy, and pulmonary function testing can be helpful in evaluating pulmonary disease in patients with immunodeficiency.

REFERENCES

1. Lekstrom-Himes JA, Gallin JI. Immunodeficiency diseases caused by defects in phagocytes. N Engl J Med 343: 1703–1714, 2000.
2. Goldblatt D, Thrasher AJ. Chronic granulomatous disease. Clin Exp Immunol 122:1–9, 2000.
3. Winkelstein JA, Marino MC, Johnston RB Jr., et al. Chronic granulomatous disease. Report on a national registry of 368 patients. Medicine (Baltimore) 79:155–169, 2000.
4. Ezekowitz RA, Dinauer MC, Jaffe HS, et al. Partial correction of the phagocyte defect in patients with X-linked chronic granulomatous disease by subcutaneous interferon gamma. N Engl J Med 319:146–151, 1988.
5. Gallin JI. Interferon-gamma in the management of chronic granulomatous disease. Rev Infect Dis 13:973–978, 1991.
6. Ballow M. Primary immunodeficiency disorders: antibody deficiency. J Allergy Clin Immunol 109:581–591, 2002.
7. Lederman HM, Winkelstein JA. X-linked agammaglobulinemia: an analysis of 96 patients. Medicine 64:145–156, 1985.
8. Cunningham-Rundles C, Bodian C. Common variable immunodeficiency: clinical and immunological features of 248 patients. Clin Immunol 92:34–48, 1999.
9. Umetsu DT, Ambrosino DM, Quinti I, et al. Recurrent sinopulmonary infection and impaired antibody response to bacterial capsular polysaccharide antigen in children with selective IgG-subclass deficiency. N Engl J Med 313: 1247–1251, 1985.
10. Busse PJ, Razvi S, Cunningham-Rundles C. Efficacy of intravenous immunoglobulin in the prevention of pneumonia in patients with common variable immunodeficiency. J Allergy Clin Immunol 109:1001–1004, 2002.
11. Kainulainen L, Varpula M, Liippo K, et al. Pulmonary abnormalities in patients with primary hypogammaglobulinemia. J Allergy Clin Immunol 104:1031–1036, 1999.
12. Buckley RH. Primary cellular immunodeficiencies. J Allergy Clin Immunol 109:747–757, 2002.
13. Deerojanawong J, Chang AB, Eng PA, et al. Pulmonary diseases in children with severe combined immune deficiency and DiGeorge syndrome. Pediatr Pulmonol 24:324–330, 1997.
14. Yalcin B, Kutluk MT, Sanal O, et al. Hodgkin's disease and ataxia telangiectasia with pulmonary cavities. Pediatr Pulmonol 33:399–403, 2002.
15. Conces DJ Jr. Noninfectious lung disease in immunocompromised patients. J Thorac Imaging 14:9–24, 1999.
16. Levy J, Espanol-Boren T, Thomas C, et al. Clinical spectrum of X-linked hyper-IgM syndrome. J Pediatr 131:47–54, 1997.
17. Eppinger TM, Greenberger PA, White DA, et al. Sensitization to *Aspergillus* species in the congenital neutrophil disorders, chronic granulomatous disease and hyper-IgE syndrome. J Allergy Clin Immunol 104:1265–1272, 1999.
18. Moylett EH, Shearer WT. HIV: clinical manifestations. J Allergy Clin Immunol 110:3–16, 2002.

19. Bye MR. Human immunodeficiency virus infections and the respiratory system in children. Pediatr Pulmonol 19:231–242, 1995.

20. Perez MS, Van Dyke RB. Pulmonary infections in children with HIV infection. Semin Respir Infect 17:33–46, 2002.

21. Madhi SA, Schoub B, Simmank K, et al. Increased burden of respiratory viral associated severe lower respiratory tract infections in children infected with human immunodeficiency virus type-1. J Pediatr 137:78–84, 2000.

22. Mofenson LM, Yogev R, Korelitz J, et al. Characteristics of acute pneumonia in human immunodeficiency virus-infected children and association with long term mortality risk. National Institute of Child Health and Human Development Intravenous Immunoglobulin Clinical Trial Study Group. Pediatr Infect Dis J 17:872–880, 1998.

23. Sheikh S, Madiraju K, Steiner P, et al. Bronchiectasis in pediatric AIDS. Chest 112:1202–1207, 1997.

24. Robles AM. HAART and evolving pulmonary manifestations of HIV. Pulmon Perspect 19:9–11, 2002.

25. Barker AF. Bronchiectasis. N Engl J Med 346:1383–1393, 2002.

26. Mouy R, Veber F, Blanche S, et al. Long-term itraconazole prophylaxis against *Aspergillus* infections in thirty-two patients with chronic granulomatous disease. J Pediatr 125:998–1003, 1994.

27. Dannaoui E, Borel E, Monier MF, et al. Acquired itraconazole resistance in *Aspergillus fumigatus*. J Antimicrob Chemother 47:333–340, 2001.

28. Warris A, Weemaes CM, Verweij PE. Multidrug resistance in *Aspergillus fumigatus*. N Engl J Med 347:2173–2174, 2002.

29. Ramsey BW, Pepe MS, Quan JM, et al. Intermittent administration of inhaled tobramycin in patients with cystic fibrosis. Cystic Fibrosis Inhaled Tobramycin Study Group. N Engl J Med 340:23–30, 1999.

30. Huddleston CB, Bloch JB, Sweet SC, et al. Lung transplantation in children. Ann Surg 236:270–276, 2002.

31. Hill AT, Thompson RA, Wallwork J, et al: Heart lung transplantation in a patient with end stage lung disease due to common variable immunodeficiency. Thorax 53:622–663, 1998.

CHAPTER 10

Pneumonia and Bacterial Pulmonary Infections

CHARLES W. CALLAHAN, D.O.

The ancient Greeks knew that the lungs were essential in bringing life from the air into the body. They called the breath, "pneuma" a word they also used for "spirit" and "wind." The organs responsible for moving the "pneuma" into the body from the air were the "pneumon." And when these organs were ill or inflamed, the process was called "pneumonia." With no knowledge of oxygen or gas exchange, they recognized the lungs' crucial role for life.

But the same life-giving contact with the air also poses one of the body's greatest dangers.

The lungs have far greater contact with the surrounding environment and its microbial threats than any other part of the body. An average newborn baby has a body surface area of 0.2 m². The surface area of the infant's lungs is 3–4 m², as much as 20 times greater. As the infant matures, the disparity increases. An adult with a body surface of 2 m² has a pulmonary surface area of 70 m². This huge pulmonary surface area contacts the outside world with every tidal breath, drawing in potential contagion dozens of times each minute. It is no surprise that respiratory illnesses are the most common cause of death for children in the developing world. Two million children die across the globe every year from pneumonia.

The term "lower respiratory tract infection (LRI)" encompasses not only infections of the airspaces and pulmonary parenchyma (i.e., pneumonia), but also infections of the airways below the glottis (e.g., tracheitis, bronchitis). Although deaths from LRIs have declined in the United States by more than 90% since the 1930s, respiratory-associated mortality still remains a common problem for children in developed nations. Twenty-five to forty infants and young children out of 1000 can be expected to contract an LRI per year in the United States. The number in school-age children is half that, and in adolescents one third. In their study of children with LRI in an ambulatory setting in North Carolina, Denny and Clyde diagnosed nearly 6000 cases of LRI over an 11-year period[1]. The diagnosis in 15% of the cases was croup, characterized by hoarseness and inspiratory stridor. In 34% it was tracheobronchitis (rhonchi), in 29% bronchiolitis (airway obstruction and/or wheezing), and in 23% pneumonia (crackles on auscultation or consolidation on radiograph) (Table 10-1). Viruses were the cause of nearly all the infections they reported; 35% from parainfluenza and 22% from respiratory syncytial

Table 10-1	Syndromes of Lower Respiratory Tract Infection
Croup:	Cough with hoarseness and inspiratory stridor
Bronchitis:	Cough with rhonchi, no wheezing or stridor
Bronchiolitis:	Cough with expiratory wheezing and evidence of airway obstruction (hyperinflation on chest radiograph or subcostal retractions)
Pneumonia:	Cough with pulmonary consolidation (crackles on auscultation or consolidation on chest radiograph)

(Adapted from Denny FW, Clyde WA. Acute lower respiratory tract infections in nonhospitalized children. J Pediatr 108:635–646, 1986.)

virus (RSV), for example. In only 15% of cases was a type of bacterium implicated, the atypical *Mycoplasma pneumoniae*. Significantly, all the agents isolated were responsible for each of the four clinical syndromes of LRI identified by the authors in different children[1].

ETIOLOGY OF PNEUMONIA

A variety of factors affect the infectivity of a particular infectious agent in a given child, and influence the conditions that lead to the development of pneumonia or another LRI. Host-specific factors, such as nutritional status and age, contribute to the development as well as the severity of an infection after exposure to an agent. Mortality from measles pneumonia is markedly higher in children with vitamin A deficiency, for example. The child's age is directly related to the size of his or her respiratory tree, and the relative effect that an infection can have on the airways or lung parenchyma. A millimeter of circumferential narrowing in the central airway of a 4-month-old infant can decrease the diameter of the airway by 64%, whereas the same millimeter of swelling narrows an adolescent's airway by only a third. Thus, the clinical syndrome caused by the same agent in each of these two children will be markedly different. The month of the child's birth also influences the infections to which he or she is prone. Children born in the late summer are more susceptible to the viral respiratory infections of winter, when the advantages of maternal antibody may abate, breastfeeding stops as the mother returns to work, and cold, wet conditions favor the spread of infections such as RSV. There is also evidence that preceding viral infection predisposes a child to developing bacterial pneumonia, as the normal pulmonary defense mechanisms may be impaired by the effect of the virus.

There are a number of additional "host-specific" factors that influence the development of a LRI in a given child. In general, pneumonia occurs when the normal pulmonary defense mechanisms are deficient or overwhelmed. Children with bypassed upper respiratory tracts, such as those with tracheostomies, will be more prone to LRI. The plastic of the tracheostomy tube in the upper respiratory tract also disrupts the mucociliary blanket, increasing the risk for infection. In other children, recurrent aspiration from gastroesophageal reflux or dysfunctional swallowing will also impair mucociliary clearance of the airways. Cystic fibrosis is another example of a disease leading to disrupted mucociliary clearance and increased proclivity to infection. Children with musculoskeletal disease have impaired cough and airway clearance. Congenital lung anomalies such as bronchogenic cysts and sequestrations can also become infected because of poor airway clearance. Additionally, there are a number of specific conditions that impair the child's immune response including defects in cellular and humoral immunity and changes in the biochemical airway milieu.

In addition to host factors, physical and biochemical characteristics of the infecting organism have an effect on the type and severity of the LRI. The magnitude of the infective load of a microbial agent, as well as the agent's size relative to the child's airway, influence the agent's infectivity. Infants with smaller airways have a higher deposition rate for the same-sized microbials than do older children and adults. Specific strains of viruses and bacteria are more infectious than others. In one study, *Pneumococcus* serotype 1 caused 24.4% of cases of complicated pneumonia, and only 3.6% of the uncomplicated cases. In at least one study, the majority of severe RSV infections were caused by serotype A[2].

Infections of the airspaces and parenchyma present with different clinical and laboratory findings compared with infections of the airways. The following are typical signs of pneumonia; presentation and laboratory findings of airway infections will be discussed with the particular type of infection below.

PULMONARY PATHOPHYSIOLOGY AND CLINICAL SIGNS AND SYMPTOMS OF PNEUMONIA

Viruses cause the majority of cases of LRI in children. While these infections can be severe and life-threatening, they are usually self-limited. Viral respiratory tract infections are the subject of Chapter 15. However, they share with bacterial infections a common range of pathophysiologic effects on the lungs and airways, and a number of clinical signs and symptoms. Table 10-2 summarizes the clinical signs and symptoms of pneumonia in children.

Table 10-2   Signs and Symptoms Suggestive of Pneumonia

Fever
Cough
Tachypnea
   Infants 2 months   >60 bpm
   Infants 2-12 months >50 bpm
   >12 months   >40 bpm
Retractions
Thoracoabdominal asynchrony
   ("see-saw breathing")
Auscultation
   Heterophonous wheezing   small airway obstruction
   Homophonous wheezing   large airway obstruction
   Coarse crackles/rhonchi   mucus in large airways
   Fine crackles/rales   airspace consolidation
Chest pain
Grunting
Cyanosis

Fever

Infectious agents reach the airways and parenchyma of the lung through the bloodstream or through the inspired air. The majority of agents that cause pneumonia in children are air-borne pathogens, and gain entry to the body through the respiratory tract. The inhaled or aspirated particles impact at some level of the respiratory tree, multiply and stimulate an inflammatory response and the migration of neutrophils to the affected area. Lobar pneumonia develops in one of two ways: either the infection expands and affects surrounding airspaces, or the patient becomes bacteremic and seeds other areas of the lung. The initial stage of infection involves vascular engorgement and infiltration with inflammatory cells, and the inflammation leads to fever. The "red hepatization" phase of lobar pneumonia refers to the color of the lung on gross section, and is characterized microscopically by fibrin deposition and red blood cells in the airspaces. In the "gray hepatization" phase the fibrin strands and inflammatory cells degenerate. In the final "yellow hepatization" phase the inflammatory cells and macrophages predominate and, in uncomplicated cases, resolution begins. The nature and intensity of the leukocytic infiltration determines the degree of fever. In cases of pneumococcal pneumonia, the fever may precede other symptoms, is often associated with an abrupt onset and shaking chills, and may exceed 104°F (40°C).

Cough

Cough can be both a symptom (the reason the parent brings the child to the office) and a sign (observed by the provider during the visit). Myelinated fibers of the vagus nerve innervate receptors in the larynx, upper thoracic airway to the carina and the proximal regions of the major bronchi. Nonmyelinated "C-fibers" innervate receptors in the interstitium and interalveolar spaces. Chemical, osmotic, inflammatory and mechanical irritants stimulate cough receptors in the larynx and airway. Primarily, chemical and inflammatory mediators stimulate the interstitial receptors. Pulmonary infection increases mucus production and inflammation, affecting receptors in the interstitium and airways, leading to cough. Cough is an important presenting symptom of LRI in children. In a survey conducted in our clinic in January 2000, cough was the complaint in 8% of 2725 patients. Eleven percent of the children with cough were diagnosed with an LRI. For many, cough was both a sign and a symptom. Children with cough during the visit were significantly more likely to be diagnosed with lower respiratory disease (including asthma) than those without cough during the visit. Sixty-one percent of children diagnosed with LRI had cough during the office visit, in contrast with less than a third of the children diagnosed with upper respiratory tract infection (Roberts S, Sheets S, Callahan C, unpublished data, January 2000).

Tachypnea

The inflammatory cascade that results from a bacterial infection of the lung parenchyma increases endovascular leakage in the interstitium and airspaces of the lung, altering the viscoelastic forces and surface tension of the affected lung units. In addition, edema and increased secretions in the airway increase airway resistance. If a sufficient number of lung units and associated airways are affected, the dynamic compliance of the lung (the combination of static and dynamic forces to be overcome, described as movement of volume per pressure change) will decrease, so that a greater negative intrapleural pressure will have to be generated to sustain the same tidal volume. Thus, the child will have to work harder to maintain oxygenation and ventilation. In order to preserve the same minute ventilation (respiratory rate times tidal volume) most efficiently in the face of decreased compliance, the child will respire with smaller tidal volumes at a higher rate. Tachypnea is a sensitive sign of pneumonia in children. It is best measured by auscultation over a period of 60 seconds. Rates measured at shorter time intervals (15 or 30 seconds) and multiplied, tend to overestimate the respiratory rate by 3-4 breaths a minute. Tachypnea is defined as a respiratory rate greater than 60 breaths per minute in an infant younger than 2 months of age, greater than 50 in infants 2-12 months and greater than 40 in children over 1 year old.

Retractions ("Chest-Indrawing")

Decreased dynamic respiratory compliance, as discussed above, reflects changes in the tissue properties of the lung as well as increased airway resistance. Either of these conditions can be the result of pneumonia in infants and children. Because the chest wall of the infant or young child is more compliant than that of an adult, it is more pliable and deforms inward more easily when the child decreases intrathoracic pressure in an attempt to move air into stiffer lungs. Examination of the child will reveal retraction of the soft tissue above the clavicles or between the ribs. Depression of the sternum can also reflect greater work of breathing in infants and children with pneumonia. When inflammation of peripheral airways causes enough obstruction to result in air trapping, the diaphragm will become depressed or flattened. Subsequently, contraction of the flattened diaphragm draws in the soft tissues below the ribcage. Thus, subcostal retractions are the clinical sign of hyperinflation.

Thoracoabdominal Asynchrony ("See-Saw Breathing")

Depression of the diaphragm during inspiration displaces the abdominal contents. Normally, the outward movement of the abdomen occurs at the same time as the rise of the thorax from inspiration. This symmetric movement is referred to as thoracoabdominal synchrony. Observed from the side, the infant's chest and belly appear to rise and fall at the same time in healthy infants. Children with pulmonary infection very often have diminished respiratory compliance and increased airway resistance. The movement of air into the lungs, and the rise of the chest, is delayed after the diaphragm contracts, so the abdominal contents are displaced slightly before the chest rise occurs. The resulting asymmetry is called thoracoabdominal asynchrony, which can be measured objectively experimentally but, even better, noted easily by the careful observer. The extreme of thoracoabdominal asynchrony occurs when the chest wall sinks inward as the abdomen moves outward. This paradoxical motion is referred to as "see-saw breathing" and reflects severe respiratory distress.

Auscultatory Changes

Auscultation of the chest of an infant or young child is difficult because the child is often frightened and uncooperative. Experienced providers learn that it is helpful to listen to the child while he or she is still on the mother's lap, before examining ears, eyes or throat, and ideally before the child is placed on the examination table. It is often helpful to talk to and touch the child before placing the stethoscope on the chest, and occasionally the child will remain quiet during auscultation if he or she is allowed to lie against the parent while the provider listens to the posterior lung fields. Generally speaking, percussion for consolidation is not helpful for the same reasons. Breath sounds over the consolidated area, however, will sound coarse or "vesicular," like listening over the trachea, because sound is transmitted better in the fluid-filled consolidated lung than in air-filled areas. Airway inflammation associated with LRIs can result in airway narrowing and wheezing. As discussed in Chapter 2, small airway obstruction causes "heterophonous" or "polyphonic" wheezing, while central airway obstruction causes "homophonous" or "monophonic" wheezing that often can be heard at the mouth without the use of a stethoscope. Crackles are caused by the sudden, explosive opening of tiny narrowed or collapsed airways on inspiration. Tachypnea and crackles are the most sensitive predictors of LRI in infants and children.

Chest Pain

There are no pain sensors in the pulmonary parenchyma. Pulmonary pain comes from significant inflammation of large airways, or more commonly from pleural involvement. Infection that occurs close to the surface of the lung causes changes in the pleural surface. The visceral pleura will become inflamed and disrupted, so that the smooth interface with the parietal pleura is lost. Thus with breathing, the raw surface of the visceral pleural membrane rubs against that of the parietal pleura causing pain. Of course, an inflammatory or infectious process in the pleural space, such as empyema, can also lead to inspiratory or "pleuritic" chest pain.

Grunting

Small children and infants with pneumonia may present with a "grunting" expiratory sound. These children often have loss of pulmonary volume due to their infectious process. The grunting noise is caused by approximation of the vocal cords during expiration. This airway narrowing elevates the intraluminal airway pressure and results in a concomitant increase in distending pressure for the airspaces.

Cyanosis

Loss of functional airspaces due to infection and inflammation leads to mismatching of ventilation and pulmonary perfusion. If unventilated lung units continue to be perfused in sufficient number, the mean oxygen saturation will decrease. Subtle decreases in oxygenation can be detected by pulse oximetry before they are evident to the provider. Although it may not be immediately dangerous, a hemoglobin saturation less than 95%

in a child is abnormal. A rough rule to estimate the partial pressure of oxygen in the blood based on the saturation is "40-50-60, 70-80-90": at 90% saturation, the oxygen tension is approximately 60 mmHg, at 80% it is 50 mmHg and at 70% it is 40 mmHg. Local cyanosis can result from venous stasis and vascular instability in young infants and children, often associated with decreases in ambient temperature. It does not represent decreased oxygen saturation, and in fact pulse oximetry will be normal. Generalized cyanosis is noted in the oral mucosa and lips, nailbeds, ears and malar regions, and occurs when the concentration of reduced hemoglobin exceeds 5-6 g/100 ml blood. For a child with a hemoglobin concentration of 12 g/100 ml, this requires that the saturation be as low as 50–60% before cyanosis becomes visible[3].

DIAGNOSTIC EVALUATION OF THE CHILD WITH PNEUMONIA

Pneumonia is a clinical diagnosis. It should be suspected in the febrile child with cough, tachypnea (especially out of proportion to the degree of fever) and crackles. Studies conducted to determine the sensitivity of clinical signs and symptoms of pneumonia generally use a positive radiograph as the "gold standard" for the presence of pneumonia. However, a normal chest radiograph in a febrile, ill-appearing child with cough, tachypnea and crackles should not deter the clinician from initiating treatment for pneumonia, as the radiograph can lag behind the clinical findings by several days.

There are three radiographic patterns used to describe pneumonia. Alveolar or airspace disease with consolidation and air-bronchograms characterizes lobar pneumonia. In the vast majority of cases, bacterial organisms gain access to the distal airways and airspaces by inhalation or aspiration of oropharyngeal secretions in the presence of inadequate or impaired pulmonary defenses. The infection may be limited initially to a lobe or segment of the lung, and in fact may initially appear radiographically as a subsegmental consolidation or "round" pneumonia. The infection can spread to adjacent segments along airways or through the intra-alveolar connections: the pores of Kohn, and canals of Lambert and Martin. Lobar pneumonia is most often caused by *Streptococcus pneumoniae* in the United States. Type B *Haemophilus influenzae* was another cause of this clinical syndrome before widespread vaccination against the organism began in the 1980s.

The second type of radiographic finding results from infection of the airways with a bacterial agent, with subsequent airway obstruction and spread to airspaces. This pattern, called bronchopneumonia, may not be distinguishable from airspace disease if the radiograph is obtained later in the course. Pathologically, the airways become infected and ulcerated. On the chest radiograph there will be prominence of the bronchovascular markings and later, multiple ill-defined nodular opacifications develop with coalescence to airspace disease. The mechanism of this infectious process is thought to be aspiration of oropharyngeal or gastric contents. *Staphylococcus aureus* is a frequently implicated source, as are the Gram-negative organisms, anaerobes and *Legionella pneumoniae*.

Interstitial pneumonias cause the third radiographic pattern. They primarily affect the tissue spaces between alveoli and vasculature, rather than the airspaces. These infections begin with aspiration of infectious agents leading to a bronchopneumonia with spread of the infection distally along the interstitial spaces. Radiographically, thickened linear (interlobular septa) markings can be seen early in the course of the disease. Reticular densities on a chest radiograph result from "summation" of linear interstitial lines. Here, the two-dimensional view of a three-dimensional object (the lung) causes linear opacifications that occur at a wide range of angles to intersect one another when projected onto the radiographic film. A nodular pattern may result from a combination of both linear and reticular opacities overlaying one another and causing larger opacities. The reticulonodular radiographic pattern represents the range of different sized opacities. Infections with a number of organisms cause this radiographic pattern, including viruses. In children, the atypical bacteria *Mycoplasma pneumoniae*, *Chlamydia trachomatis*, and *Chlamydia pneumoniae* are common causes. Indeed, it is worth noting that there is no single pathognomonic radiographic pattern for *Mycoplasma* pneumonia in children[4]. Table 10-3 summarizes radiographic patterns and includes an agent that may (but does not always) present with the corresponding radiographic picture. Radiographic evidence of pneumonia generally resolves within 4–6 weeks, and persistent opacifications beyond that suggest inadequate pulmonary drainage, a chronic, persistent problem or

---

Table 10-3 Radiographic Patterns of Pneumonia

Alveolar/Airspace (e.g., *Streptococcus pneumoniae*)
  Consolidation
  Air bronchograms
Bronchopneumonia (e.g., *Staphylococcus aureus*)
  Bronchovesicular markings
  Nodular opacification
  Consolidation
Interstitial (e.g., *Mycoplasma pneumoniae*)
  Linear
  Reticular
  Nodular
  Reticulonodular
  Ground-glass

the possibility of an anatomic lung anomaly. Children whose radiographic infiltrates persist beyond this point warrant referral to a pediatric pulmonologist.

The laboratory evaluation of children with pneumonia usually adds little to the diagnosis. If a child is able to produce a sputum sample for analysis, however, Gram stain and culture can direct therapy towards the causative organism. Blood cultures are routinely obtained on ill, hospitalized children with pneumonia, although they will not usually be positive. While earlier literature suggested that as many as 25% of children with pneumococcal pneumonia will have a positive blood culture, in a more recent review of 580 children aged 2–34 months with a diagnosis of pneumonia, only 1.6% of the children had positive blood culture. In all nine cases, *Pneumococcus* was the agent isolated[5]. Latex agglutination tests for bacterial antigens in collected urine are more sensitive than blood cultures and may provide additional information. A leukocyte count greater than 15,000 cells per high-power field (hpf) predicts those children who will respond to antibiotics within 48 hours (and who are likely to have pneumococcal disease). Erythrocyte sedimentation rate and C-reactive protein levels will both be elevated in bacterial diseases, although neither is completely sensitive nor specific for pulmonary infection. Serum sodium may be decreased in children with bacterial pneumonia and a component of the syndrome of inappropriate antidiuretic hormone secretion. Additionally, a low serum phosphorus level may be a predictor of illness severity in patients with pneumonia admitted to the hospital. No single symptom, sign or laboratory test is adequately sensitive and specific to predict the presence of pneumonia in a child[6,7]. In fact, the best predictor for the presence of pneumonia (compared with the radiograph) is the "overall clinical impression" of the provider prior to obtaining the radiographic study.

CLINICAL SYNDROMES OF BACTERIAL PULMONARY INFECTION

Bacterial diseases of the respiratory tract in children occur as recognizable clinical syndromes. Pneumonia in most children will follow a predictable clinical course, and the specific etiology of the infection can often be inferred based upon the child's presentation, symptoms and signs. Viruses cause the overwhelming majority of LRIs in children and infants, including all of the clinical syndromes described by Denny and Clyde[1] in addition to pneumonia. Thus, antibiotics are not necessary for most children with respiratory tract infection. The provider, however, must recognize the clinical syndromes that can be the result of bacterial infection, remember that these infections can be life-threatening and cause rapid clinical deterioration, and take aggressive steps toward intervening in affected children. The following scenarios illustrate important points about various clinical syndromes, which will lead the clinician to consider a diagnosis of bacterial infection of the lower respiratory tract.

Tracheitis

Case

The pediatrician was called to the emergency room to evaluate a 14-month-old child of a close friend with fever, cough, and stridor in the winter months. Her presentation was very typical for viral laryngotracheobronchitis (LTB) although she had shown improvement in her initial symptoms over the previous 2 days. Now, however, the child seemed somewhat sicker than the usual child with croup, and was considerably fussier. In addition, her temperature exceeded 103°F (39.5°C) on presentation. She was stridulous at rest and tachypneic, though not hypoxemic. During the physical examination of her oropharynx, a normal epiglottis was visualized, but there were copious purulent secretions in her hypopharynx. A repeat of the same examination revealed the same copious secretions when her stridor became worse sometime later, and she remained febrile. As her clinical condition deteriorated, the decision was made for elective, rapid sequence intubation, and when the endotracheal tube was introduced through her vocal cords, a large amount of pus was noted. Suctioning of her endotracheal tube revealed secretions containing many neutrophils. The sputum sample grew pure colonies of *Staphylococcus aureus*. Bronchoscopy several days later confirmed the diagnosis of bacterial tracheitis.

This bacterial infection of the central airway usually begins with a viral respiratory tract infection in a child less than 3 years of age. A clue to the diagnosis is that the child begins to recover from the initial illness but the clinical course subsequently worsens. Presumably, the virus disrupts the normal airway defenses and *Staphylococcus* aspirated from the nasopharynx into the airway infects the mucosal epithelium. Neutrophils migrate into the area and the combination of necrotic mucosa, bacteria, white blood cells and fibrin strands form a membrane along the tracheal wall that can extend into the bronchi. The condition is sometimes referred to as "pseudomembranous croup" for this reason.

Conservative management of the child with bacterial tracheitis in a pediatric intensive care unit with early intubation is the most important part of treatment. While death can result from sepsis, most deaths in this disease occur from airway obstruction and hypoxemia. Antibiotic coverage should target *Staphylococcus aureus*, and a third-generation cephalosporin (ceftriaxone) is sufficient to treat the infection until therapy can be tailored to sputum culture results. Patients often remain intubated for up to a week, and are a challenge to keep adequately sedated. Little is known about the likelihood of long-term sequelae, although it is not difficult to imagine that patients could develop tracheal stenosis or tracheomalacia following a severe infection.

Acute Bronchitis

Case

A nine-year-old was evaluated for protracted cough and fever of 101°F (38.5°C). He complained of chest pain, especially with coughing spells. He was treated in the emergency room a week ago with guaifenesin and amoxicillin for "bronchitis," but there had been no improvement. He also complained of headache and abdominal pain. He was not ill-appearing on examination, but he coughed during the examination. Auscultation of his chest revealed coarse rhonchi. A chest radiograph showed no evidence of pneumonia, but some mild, bilateral peribronchial thickening was present. A serum *Mycoplasma* enzyme-linked immunoassay for IgM was positive.

In more than 80% of cases, acute bronchitis in children is caused by viruses. Rhinovirus, parainfluenza, influenza, and RSV are frequently implicated in this clinical syndrome. As a primarily viral illness, acute bronchitis is self-limited and requires no specific antimicrobial therapy. Few bacteria have been implicated as causes of acute bronchitis in childhood, aside from the atypical bacterium *Mycoplasma pneumoniae*. *Mycoplasma* was also the most frequently identified agent in a study of young American soldiers with protracted cough (>21 days) who probably had bronchitis. Eighty-five percent had an agent isolated, and in 61% of cases the agent was *Mycoplasma*. *Bordetella* species and *Chlamydia pneumoniae* were the other two agents most commonly identified[8]. Pertussis is a common cause of protracted cough and bronchitis in older children and adults. In a review of 442 adolescents (older than 12 years of age) and adults with prolonged cough syndrome (1–8 weeks) 19.9% had laboratory evidence of *Bordetella pertussis*[9]. Importantly, there are no bacterial causes of acute bronchitis in childhood for which amoxicillin is an appropriate treatment, despite the frequency of its use for this syndrome in a variety of clinical settings.

Acute bronchitis is caused by inhalation of infectious agents, which bind to receptors on airway epithelium, multiply and induce an inflammatory response. Cough receptors are stimulated directly by inflammatory mediators, and by the increased mucus production that accompanies the inflammatory response. The clinical syndrome is characterized by cough, and rhonchi or coarse wheezing on auscultation, without evidence of inspiratory stridor (thereby excluding extrathoracic airway obstruction) or small airway wheezing. Cough usually follows 3–4 days of nasal congestion and increased mucus production, and represents spread of the infection to the large, subglottic

airways where the highest density of cough receptors can be found. The cough is frequently productive, and the presence of neutrophils in the sputum is common.

Treatment of acute viral bronchitis is supportive, and there is little indication for cough suppressants. Guaifenesin derivatives and over-the-counter cough suppressants are generally of little or no value, despite the frequency with which they are prescribed. Cough generally resolves within 3 weeks, and most clinicians will begin to consider other etiologies for cough, including chronic bacterial bronchitis or sinusitis, when it persists beyond 21 days. However, one placebo-controlled trial of antibiotics for children with suspected sinusitis showed little benefit. Children were randomized after 2 weeks of symptoms to treatment with amoxicillin/clavulanate, amoxicillin or placebo. Fourteen days after treatment, there was no difference between any of the three groups in sinus symptom score[10]. Thus, the specific etiology of protracted cough in these children is not clear, and may represent dysfunction or persistent inflammatory effects of the infection on the cough receptor.

Chronic Bronchitis

Case

A mother brought her 9-month old infant to the pediatric pulmonologist for persistent cough, congestion, wheezing and "noisy breathing." The child developed a severe cough during an episode of RSV bronchiolitis at 3 months of age. The cough had never resolved. The child's cough was present both day and night, was often associated with paroxysms, and sounded "loose" to the mother. The mother also mentioned that she often felt "rattling" in the baby's chest. The child was drinking 12 ounces of formula four or five times a day in addition to bottles of juice, and had frequent regurgitation. In fact the baby had always been "spitty." On examination, the child was not tachypneic, had wheezing audible without a stethoscope, and homophonous ("central") wheezing and coarse rhonchi on auscultation. Fiberoptic bronchoscopy was notable for erythematous, edematous, friable airways. A bronchoalveolar lavage revealed numerous neutrophils (normally macrophages predominate) and lipid-laden macrophages (suggestive of aspiration from her clinically diagnosed gastroesophageal reflux). The lavage culture grew >10^5 cfu of non-typeable *Haemophilus influenzae*. She was treated with 21 days of amoxicillin/clavulanate. Her mother was counseled to decrease the volumes of liquid consumption, and the child experienced complete resolution of her symptoms.

The diagnosis of chronic bacterial bronchitis in pediatrics is controversial. Many infectious disease and pulmonary experts do not believe that it exists. However, there is clearly a subset of children who develop persistent cough and bronchorrhea following a viral infection or accompanying persistent insult to the airways such as microaspiration of stomach contents or exposure to environmental tobacco smoke. The etiology of the chronic symptoms is suspected to be similar to that of chronic bronchitis in adults: disruption of the normal epithelial barriers of the airway by an acute or chronic insult followed by bacterial colonization, infection and associated inflammatory response.

A series of 30 children evaluated at St. Christopher's Hospital for Children over a 4-year period is representative. Average age (+/− SD) was 14 +/− 18 months (range 1 month to 8 years). Respiratory symptoms had been present for an average (+/− SD) of 8 +/− 8 months (range 1 month to 3 years), either on a continuous or frequently recurrent basis. Thirteen of 30 (43%) of subjects had been prescribed 10-day courses of oral antibiotics as treatment for otitis media, possible sinusitis, or "bronchitis"; amoxicillin was most commonly prescribed. In most cases, antibiotics had been ineffective in reducing respiratory symptoms. In 6 cases, parents reported that antibiotics had been associated with transient improvement, but symptoms returned shortly after antibiotics were discontinued.

The children presented with chronic cough (77%) or recurrent wheezing that did not resolve completely with bronchodilators and corticosteroids (83%). Physical examination revealed homophonous ("central") wheezing in 57% of the children. Many of the children also had asthma (97%) or gastroesophageal reflux (40%). In 63% of the bronchoscopies, *Moraxella catarrhalis* was recovered and in 29% non-typeable *Haemophilus influenzae* was found in significant numbers by quantitative culture. The children were treated with a beta-lactamase resistant antibiotic and 87% of the children experienced resolution or improvement of the symptoms (C. Papastamelos, C. Callahan, B. Alpert, H. Panitch, J. Allen, D. Schidlow, unpublished data 1992–1996.)

Additional agents may cause chronic bacterial bronchitis in children. Vaccine-induced immunity to *Bordetella pertussis* is not life-long, and this agent can cause tracheobronchitis. It should be suspected in adolescents and young adults who have protracted episodes of cough that is often paroxysmal and may lead to post-tussive vomiting. Mycobacterium tuberculosis can also cause endobronchial disease in children and adolescents, often as a recurrence of a previous infection. Children will have productive cough that does not respond to the usual antibiotic therapy. The chest radiograph may demonstrate calcifications, and induced sputum or gastric lavage may reveal acid-fast bacilli.

The primary care provider should suspect chronic bronchitis in infants and children with persistent symptoms of cough and an abnormal physical examination suggestive of bronchorrhea associated with a history or suspected ongoing airway insult. Asthma should be considered and, if the history is suggestive, these children should be treated aggressively with corticosteroids and bronchodilators. If the cough persists greater that 14 days, despite an adequate course of corticosteroids (5–10 days) and bronchodilator therapy, a course of beta-lactamase-resistant antibiotics is a reasonable next step in treating these children. If the symptoms persist despite 3 weeks of appropriate treatment, the child should be referred to a pediatric pulmonologist and considered for diagnostic bronchoscopy with bronchoalveolar lavage[11].

Bronchiectasis

Case

A 2-year-old child experienced an episode of choking and coughing after eating a small tree-seed in August. His initial radiograph showed mild hyperinflation, but no bronchoscopy was performed. His radiograph was normal a week later. He continued to have cough, however, and was treated with two courses of antibiotics for presumed pneumonia by a different clinician. His coarse cough persisted, and several providers noted coarse crackles on auscultation. He had no digital clubbing. In late September, a chest radiograph showed abnormalities of his left lower lobe (Figure 10-1), and a CT scan demonstrated a small segment of bronchiectasis (Figure 10-2).

Bronchiectasis is a condition of dilated, damaged airways usually due to chronic inflammation, infection and obstruction. It has been considered an "orphan" disease but it is common in the developing world, and is likely more common in the developed world than is currently recognized.

The pathology of bronchiectasis has been recognized for more than a century yet the reasons why some children develop bronchiectasis and others do not remains unclear. Airway obstruction and mucus stasis, coupled with chronic infection and inflammation of the bronchial wall, leads to bronchiectasis in animal models of the disease. Inflammation usually results from bacterial infection or "colonization" of the airways, either as a primary process (e.g., aspiration syndromes), or secondary following airway injury (e.g., viral respiratory tract infection). Airway injury can occur as a result of mechanical obstruction (e.g., prolonged foreign body aspiration) or as a result of injury from a single potent pathogen, such as adenovirus or *Mycoplasma pneumoniae*. Pertussis, measles, and tuberculosis remain childhood diseases that predispose children at risk to subsequent bronchiectasis[12].

Children develop bronchiectasis after an insult to the respiratory tree. They present with symptoms of chronic, productive cough and crackles on auscultation. Half of children have clubbing at presentation. The plain film will often be normal, but may reveal bronchial dilation, volume loss or bronchial wall thickening. The "tram-track"

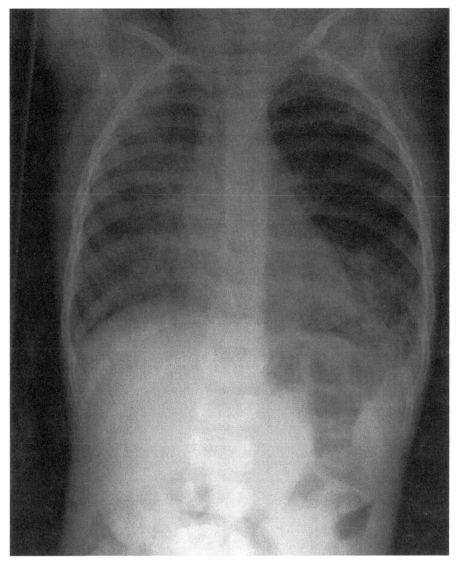

Figure 10-1   Chest radiograph of a child with bronchiectasis.

sign that can be present on a chest radiograph of a patient with bronchiectasis refers to parallel linear densities reflecting thickened bronchial walls seen in longitudinal section. The "signet ring" sign on CT examination is a dilated airway in cross-section that is larger than its associated artery. Definitive diagnosis is made with thin-section, high-resolution computed axial tomography of the chest demonstrating dilated peripheral bronchi with thickened bronchial walls.

Children with bronchiectasis suffer from inadequate pulmonary drainage, and therapy of affected lobes generally involves vigorous chest physiotherapy with postural drainage often several times a day. Short-term courses of antibiotics are often given to decrease bacterial colonization or infection, and sputum cultures can be used to guide therapy. The outcome of these children cannot be predicted, as in some cases clinical and radiographic evidence of bronchiectasis can disappear when underlying conditions (e.g., chronic aspiration) are addressed. Surgical resection of the affected lobe is indicated in cases where children develop repeated episodes of pulmonary sepsis in the bronchiectatic lobe. Table 10-4 summarizes the clinical syndromes and microbiology of bacterial airway infections.

Newborn with Pneumonia

Case

A pediatric intern was called to the delivery room to assess a term newborn infant with respiratory difficulty. The infant was less than 2 hours old. His respiratory effort remained labored and he grunted with each exhalation.

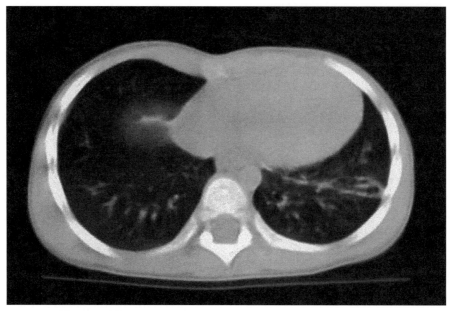

Figure 10-2   High-resolution CT scan of a child with bronchiectasis.

His mother's prenatal history was unknown, and her labor was too rapid for her to have had any prenatal antimicrobial screening or antibiotics. She reported having had a baby die in the first days of life from an infection. This infant was tachypneic with a respiratory rate of 75 breaths per minute. He had decreased breath sounds bilaterally with rare fine crackles. His airway was intubated for severe respiratory distress and his radiograph demonstrated bilateral "ground-glass" alveolar filling (Figure 10-3). His white blood cell count was 2200 cells/hpf and his platelet count was 66,000/ml. His clinical condition deteriorated despite antibiotic therapy. Both initial blood cultures grew group B beta-hemolytic streptococcus (GBBS) within 6 hours. He died before he was 12 hours old.

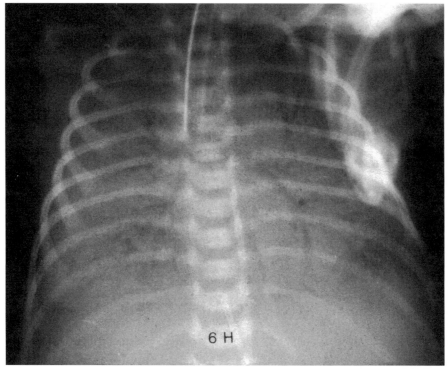

Figure 10-3   Chest radiograph of an infant with GBBS pneumonia.

Clinical Syndrome	Typical Age	Symptoms	Signs	Etiology	Treatment
Tracheitis	1 month–6 years	Fever Croupy cough	Stridor	*Staphylococcus*	Nafcillin/oxacillin
Acute bronchitis	6 months–2 years 9–15 years	Cough Fever	Rhonchi	*Mycoplasma* Viruses	Macrolide Symptomatic
Chronic bronchitis	5 months–15 years	Cough Wheezing Noisy breathing Rattling in chest	Homophonous wheeze Rhonchi	*Moraxella catarrhalis* Non-typeable *Haemophilus*	Amoxicillin/clavulanate
Bronchiectasis	2–6 years	Productive cough Recurrent pneumonia Chest pain	Crackles Rhonchi	Viruses (adenovirus) Pertussis Tuberculosis Aspiration	Chest physiotherapy Postural drainage Beta-agonists Periodic antibiotics

Table 10-4 Bacterial Infections of the Airway

The pretreatment and screening of mothers for GBBS has made a significant impact on the prevalence of "early" GBBS disease in the newborn, so that residents training today are much less likely to see a child with this condition than those who trained 15 years ago. Prenatal and perinatal pneumonia can also be caused by coliforms such as *Escherichia coli*, anerobes, and *Listeria monocytogenes*. Babies can present with very subtle initial symptoms including the full spectrum of respiratory distress from mild to life-threatening, temperature instability, feeding intolerance, and metabolic derangements including hypoglycemia. Often, there is little that can be done once they are delivered, so that maternal prenatal screening and treatment become the most important factors in infant survival.

Since newborns are immunocompromised by definition, a number of different opportunists including *Pseudomonas aeruginosa* can cause infection in infants hospitalized for extended periods. Viruses including cytomegalovirus and fungi such as *Candida albicans* can also cause pneumonia in infants. These agents should be suspected in babies who do not respond to standard therapy. Initial therapy should include aggressive evaluation for sepsis including blood and urine cultures, and antibiotics targeting the most common causes. Typically, an aminoglycoside or third-generation cephalosporin and ampicillin are chosen as initial therapy. Newborns with pneumonia should be cared for in neonatal intensive care units where expertise in mechanical ventilation is available if needed.

Well-Appearing Infant with Pneumonia

Case

A 7-week-old infant was admitted to the pediatric ward with hypoxemia and cough. The child was still eating fairly well and there was no history of fever. On examination, the child was not ill-appearing but his respiratory rate was 70–80 breaths per minute when awake. He had some scattered crackles on examination, and mild subcostal retractions. The chest radiograph showed patchy opacifications and hyperinflation (Figure 10-4). Evaluation for bacterial infection was negative; however, a urine culture grew cytomegalovirus (CMV) and the serum CMV IgM was positive. The child recovered from this illness, but had recurrent episodes of wheezing and dyspnea with variable responsiveness to bronchodilators and oral corticosteroids.

Stagno and his colleagues described the "afebrile pneumonia syndrome of infancy" more than two decades ago[13].

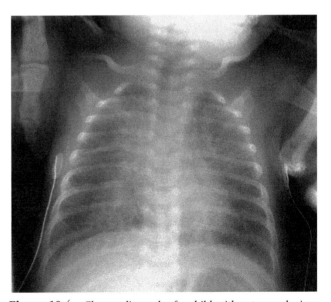

Figure 10-4 Chest radiograph of a child with cytomegalovirus pneumonia.

They reported a group of 104 infants (age 1–3 months) who were not consistently ill-appearing and who had a syndrome of cough, tachypnea and radiographic findings of pneumonia. Eighty-three percent of the infants they reported were afebrile, and 77% had rales (crackles). Paroxysmal cough was uniformly noted. Fifty percent of these hospitalized infants required supplemental oxygen, and 15% required mechanical ventilation. They stayed in the hospital an average of 17 days.

The investigators isolated four agents from these infants with pneumonia: *Chlamydia trachomatis* (25%), *Ureaplasma urealyticum* (21%), cytomegalovirus (20%), and *Pneumocystis carinii* (18%). This last organism, long felt to be a protozoan, has recently been identified to be a phylogenetic fungal species and reclassified as *Pneumocystis jiroveci*. Pneumonia from this organism is still referred to as "PCP": Pneumocystis pneumonia. In many cases, multiple organisms were recovered from the same infant with this clinical syndrome. Organisms were identified by culture and in the case of Pneumocystis, by counter immunoelectrophoresis and indirect immunofluorescence of serum. These studies are not available in every clinical setting today, so aside from culture for CMV, the other organisms are seldom isolated. Thus the diagnosis is often made clinically[13].

Infants with this clinical syndrome will often require hospitalization because of hypoxemia or decreased feeding due to respiratory difficulty. If the child is to be managed as an outpatient, he or she should be followed daily until the clinical symptoms begin to improve significantly. Additionally, the parents should be given specific, concrete signs and symptoms to watch for that might herald deterioration. Treatment is usually empiric, and includes oral erythromycin for 3 weeks primarily to treat chlamydial infection. In a follow-up study, 46% of the children had recurrent episodes of wheezing and airway obstruction, requiring medical therapy[14].

Ill-Appearing Infant with Pneumonia

Case

An 11-month old girl presented to the emergency room with a fever of 102°F (39°C), congestion, cough and a history of "grunting" respirations. The infant was not eating well. On examination the child was ill, but not septic-appearing. The chest was clear to auscultation and a chest radiograph was normal. The child was discharged with a diagnosis of viral respiratory tract infection and instructions to follow-up in a pediatric clinic in the morning. The parents did not return to the doctor the next morning, but instead returned a day later, after the child developed progressive respiratory distress. A chest radiograph showed a large left-sided pneumonia. The child's blood culture grew *Staphylococcus aureus*, and despite heroic measures the child succumbed to overwhelming sepsis 48 hours later.

It is easy to forget that pneumonia in children is potentially a life-threatening illness. Most bacterial infections in this age group are preceded by a viral respiratory tract infection. Historically, influenza virus has been identified as a frequent preceding infection. Many of the near 25 million deaths worldwide during the 1918–1919 influenza epidemic are thought to have been from secondary bacterial pneumonia. It is likely that the viral infection alters the ability of the respiratory tract to resist infection from inhaled or aspirated bacterial pathogens.

Infants with pneumonia will often be tachypneic and may have grunting respirations. They can also have other signs associated with sepsis: fever, poor feeding, and lethargy. Initial radiographs may be normal despite findings on physical examination. The diagnosis of a respiratory tract infection will often be made on the basis of clinical findings, and the decision to attempt to diagnose or treat for bacterial disease may be a subjective one. Children with fever should be evaluated according to established protocols. Under 1 month of age, all children with fever and no identifiable source should undergo a sepsis evaluation, and receive inpatient intravenous antibiotic therapy. In older infants and children, a high index of suspicion for pneumonia should be maintained. Any infant or young child with pneumonia should be followed closely. The child with a lower respiratory tract infection should be seen again within 24 hours of the initial visit for a reassessment, regardless of whether bacterial disease is suspected on the initial presentation. Serious, even life-threatening bacterial illness may not be apparent at first.

Pneumonia in an ill-appearing infant is most often due to *Streptococcus pneumoniae*. *Haemophilus influenzae*, Type B (HIB) was seen previously but has diminished with the successful vaccination programs for this organism. Pockets of invasive HIB disease still occur in the developed world, and an immunization history is an important part of the evaluation of a child with pneumonia. *Staphylococcus aureus* may also cause severe pneumonia in infants and young children. Fortunately, it is not a common cause in the developed world. It should be suspected in a child who develops a rapid "white-out" pattern of consolidation radiographically. Children with staphylococcal pneumonia develop pleural disease in up to 90% of cases, and pneumatoceles develop in half of children. This agent should be suspected especially in children with pneumonia and pulmonary abscess or empyema.

When bacterial pneumonia is suspected and the child appears only mildly or moderately ill, ampicillin is an acceptable initial intravenous agent to use pending culture results. Penicillin-resistant *Pneumococcus*, however, has been recognized with increasing frequency since 1978. Organisms produce one or more proteins with variable affinity for penicillin. Approximately 10% of

Pneumococcus isolates are penicillin resistant. Resistance to ceftriaxone is uncommon, and occurs in less than 2.5% of isolates. Therefore, when the child appears ill, initial treatment should be with a second- or third-generation cephalosporin (cefuroxime or ceftriaxone) for *Pneumococcus* or HIB. If the child is septic and *Pneumococcus* is suspected, treatment should begin with vancomycin. If *Staphylococcus* is suspected, treatment with penicillinase resistant penicillin (nafcillin or oxacillin) should be started.

Well-Appearing Toddler or Child with Pneumonia

Case

A 4-year-old preschooler stayed home from his nursery school for 2 days with low-grade fever, rhinitis, and cough. His symptoms became worse and his mother brought him to your office. He had paroxysms of cough, especially at night, but was relatively well between episodes. He did not cough during the visit, and he had no previous history of severe cough with respiratory infections, or with exercise. On examination he was not tachypneic. He had mild rhinitis. Auscultation of his chest revealed diffuse heterophonous wheezing (small airway obstruction) and fine crackles. He had no hepatomegaly and no digital clubbing. A chest radiograph revealed scattered interstitial infiltrates and mild hyperinflation.

Viral pneumonias are not the focus of this chapter, yet deserve mention because they are the most common cause of pneumonia in children of any age. The child in this case was well-appearing, but viruses can certainly cause severe, life-threatening infections. The most commonly isolated viruses in children with LRIs are parainfluenza (35%), RSV (22%), influenza virus (12%), adenovirus (7%) and assorted others (enterovirus, rhinovirus, 9%). *Mycoplasma pneumoniae* is responsible for 15% of infections[1].

The absence of severe episodes of cough with other respiratory tract infections and exercise makes a diagnosis of asthma less likely. Most viral pneumonia begins with inhaled infectious agents, and the airways are commonly involved. Thus wheezing and hyperinflation (subcostal retractions) are frequently noted. A chest radiograph may be normal. It may also show interstitial or airspace disease.

Children with LRI managed in an ambulatory setting should be followed daily until the symptoms of respiratory tract infection begin to resolve. Follow-up is critical because it is difficult to predict the course of pneumonia. In addition, viral pneumonia may become secondarily infected with a bacterial pathogen and parents may not be sophisticated enough to recognize respiratory deterioration in their children.

Child with Pneumonia

Case

A 7-year-old girl with a viral respiratory tract infection awoke one night with shaking chills, worsening of cough, malaise and fever. She also complained of right-sided chest pain. On presentation to her pediatrician in the morning, she was ill-appearing and had a temperature of 104°F (40°C). Her respiratory rate was 42 breaths per minute and auscultation of her chest revealed crackles on her posterior right lung fields. A chest radiograph showed a right-sided opacification. Her white blood cell count was 21,000 WBC/hpf. A course of amoxicillin/clavulanate PO was started, but she returned to her physician 2 days later with persistent fever, worsening cough, and increased difficulty breathing. A repeat radiograph revealed complete opacification of her right lung (Figure 10-5). Room air pulse oximetry was 87%. Blood cultures obtained on her original presentation grew *Streptococcus pneumoniae*.

She was admitted to the hospital for intravenous antibiotics, but her respiratory condition deteriorated. She was transferred to the pediatric intensive care unit where she was intubated and started on mechanical ventilation. Her hypoxemia was unresponsive to increasing levels of positive pressure on conventional ventilation so she was started on a high-frequency oscillator ventilator. She stabilized, but a pleural effusion and eventual pneumothorax on the right side necessitated chest tube placement 2 days later. She remained on high-frequency ventilation for 2 weeks, before returning to conventional ventilation and extubation after a total of more than 3 weeks of ventilator therapy. She recovered but her radiograph remained abnormal, with decreased volume on the right (Figure 10-6).

Pneumococcal pneumonia in childhood usually presents as a distinct, clinical syndrome characterized by an acute onset and fever. It is not rare. Laboratory studies reveal leukocytosis, and sputum Gram stain in older children will demonstrate more than 25 WBC/hpf and Gram-positive diplococci. The spectrum of pneumonia from this organism can vary from a very mild course managed in an ambulatory setting, to the severe case of complicated pneumococcal pneumonia presented here. Complicated pneumonia is characterized by significant pleural effusion often requiring chest tube placement and, in some cases, pulmonary necrosis.

Children with complicated pneumonia are more likely to be older (45 vs. 27 months in one series)[2], are more likely to present with chest pain and to require decortication for pleural disease. In the same series, complicated pneumonia was caused by pneumococcal serotypes 1, 6, 14, and 19 in 24% of cases, as opposed to 3.6% of the children with uncomplicated pneumonia. Serotype 1, which accounted for 24% of complicated

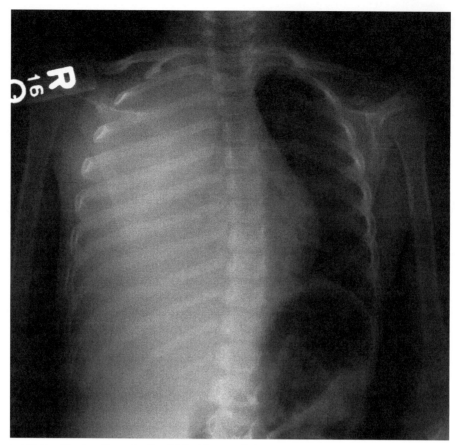

Figure 10-5   Chest radiograph of a child with overwhelming *Streptococcus pneumoniae* pneumonia.

pneumonia, is not included in the currently licensed pneumococcal vaccine.

Children who develop pneumococcal pneumonia are often carriers of this organism. Twenty to forty percent of children are carriers, and risk factors for the development of invasive pneumococcal disease include frequent episodes of otitis or upper respiratory tract infections (>3 in 6 months) and daycare attendance. Organisms are aspirated or inhaled, and escape the lung's extensive defense systems, including the mechanical barriers of the upper airway, the mucociliary blanket and cough, and the macrophages and humoral defenses of the distal airways. Onset of symptoms is usually abrupt with shaking chills and spiking fever. Younger children may present with febrile seizure[2].

Ambulatory children with suspected pneumococcal pneumonia should be treated with high-dose amoxicillin or a cephalosporin. Children ill enough to require hospitalization should receive a second- or third-generation cephalosporin or ampicillin in combination with sulbactam. Vancomycin or clindamycin should be used for severely ill children with suspected complicated pneumococcal disease.

Adolescent with Pneumonia

Case

A previously healthy 16-year-old stayed home from school with headache, abdominal pain, and sore throat. She did not have any nasal congestion, but developed paroxysms of cough. She developed a fever of 101°F (38.5°C) and generalized malaise. After 4 days of symptoms and progressive cough, her mother took her to the physician. She was uncomfortable, but not ill-appearing. She was not hypoxemic or tachypneic. Auscultation of her chest revealed crackles and heterophonous wheezing. She had a mild erythematous maculopapular exanthem. A chest radiograph revealed mild, bilateral increased interstitial infiltrates (Figure 10-7). A complete blood count disclosed a mild anemia and the smear suggested hemolysis. Bedside serum cold agglutinins were positive (Figure 10-8), and serologic testing for *Mycoplasma pneumoniae* IgM was positive >1:32. She was treated with oral doxycycline, and recovered uneventfully within 2 weeks, although episodes of cough persisted for two additional weeks.

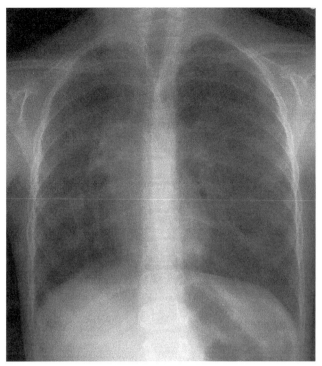

Figure 10-6 Chest radiograph of resolved complicated *Streptococcus pneumoniae* pneumonia.

Pneumonia due to *Mycoplasma pneumoniae* was called "atypical" initially because, in 1935, it did not respond to the typical pneumonia treatment, sulfonamides. It is also sometimes called "walking" pneumonia because it does not render affected children so sick that they are confined to bed. The onset of symptoms, in contrast to *Pneumococcus*, is usually insidious with malaise, low-grade fever and cough. Rhinitis is significant for its absence, and can help the clinician discern *Mycoplasma* from viral pneumonia due to adenovirus, which can have a similar clinical course. Pharyngitis is frequently noted, but may be more prominent in atypical pneumonia due to *Chlamydia pneumoniae*, another of the causes of this clinical syndrome. Headache and abdominal pain are also frequently seen.

The physical examination will often provide no additional clues to help discern the specific cause of pneumonia. Clinical signs of pneumonia will often be present, including crackles, wheezes or coarse breath sounds. However, they may be absent early in the course of the disease. A range of different rashes may be noted from a slight erythematous eruption in mildest cases, to life-threatening Stevens–Johnson syndrome. Cardiac involvement has also been noted in some cases, including myocarditis and pericarditis leading to signs and symptoms of congestive heart failure. Rarely, hepatitis may occur and hepatomegaly will be noted on physical examination.

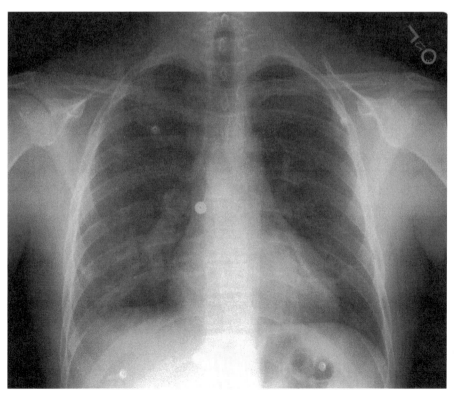

Figure 10-7   Chest radiograph of an adolescent with *Mycoplasma* pneumonia.

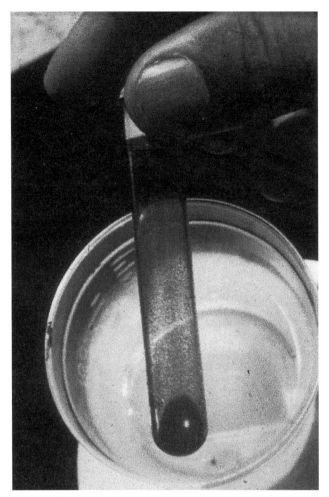

Figure 10-8 Bedside serum cold agglutinins (from the collection of Dr. Jim Bass).

There is no pathognomonic pattern of the chest radiograph for children with *Mycoplasma* pneumonia. The radiograph can be completely normal. Bilateral interstitial infiltrates may be noted, or there may be a unilateral lobar infiltrate. Parapneumonic pleural effusion may occur in up to 20% of children with *Mycoplasma* pneumonia when it is carefully sought. There is usually no reason for pleurocentesis in these children. Serologically, the immunogenicity of *Mycoplasma* leads to production of a host of antibodies, including one to the red blood cell "I/I antigen" that causes cold agglutination of the blood cells. While this antibody may be absent in up to half of children with *Mycoplasma*, its presence in this clinical setting would make the diagnosis of a *Mycoplasma* infection all but assured. If blood is being drawn anyway, the clinician can perform the bedside "cold agglutinin" test for *Mycoplasma*[15].

Two to three milliliters of blood are placed in a small "blue-top" sodium citrate blood tube. The blood is placed in a cup of ice water for several minutes, then removed, held in front of a white piece of paper, tilted and rolled slowly between the fingers. Clumps of red blood cells will be visible lining the surface of the tube, and the clumps dissolve when the tube is warmed by holding it in the closed hand for several minutes. In a true positive test, this process can be repeated multiple times. This predominantly IgM antibody may lead to a mild hemolytic anemia in some children. A positive cold agglutinin test should be confirmed with serologic evaluation for the presence of anti-*Mycoplasma* IgM. This test will diagnose an acute infection, as culture for *Mycoplasma* is costly and not available in every clinical setting.

Chlamydia pneumoniae is the other agent commonly associated with atypical or "walking" pneumonia, although the specific diagnosis is even more difficult to make. Pharyngitis and hoarseness in an adolescent or young adult with interstitial pneumonia who does not have rhinitis should prompt the clinician to consider *Chlamydia* in addition to *Mycoplasma*. While erythromycin is generally considered the first choice for therapy in this syndrome, there is some evidence that *Chlamydia* is more susceptible to tetracycline than to erythromycin[16]. Doxycycline is an excellent agent for the treatment of this syndrome in children 12 years and older. Other macrolides are also effective and the newer agent, azithromycin, shows greatest effectiveness in experimental settings.

OTHER BACTERIAL INFECTIONS OF THE RESPIRATORY SYSTEM

Pulmonary Abscess

Two populations of children develop pulmonary abscess: otherwise healthy children who develop severe pneumonia and abscess are said to have primary pulmonary abscess. In 62% of cases, *Staphylococcus aureus* is the etiology. Children with underlying disorders of swallowing or effectiveness of the cough reflex, such as children with static encephalopathy, comprise the other group and can develop secondary pulmonary abscess. In these children, *Staphylococcus* is the cause of the abscess in only a third of cases, and two thirds of the cases are caused by other agents including anaerobic organisms and coliforms. In either group, the condition is generally first suspected when the abscess is noted on a chest radiograph obtained in an ill child with pneumonia (Figure 10-9).

Children with pulmonary abscess present with high fever, cough, chest pain and sputum production. The radiograph will demonstrate air–fluid levels in most cases. In one series the right lung was more commonly affected, and associated pleural effusion was common[17]. Children with primary abscess generally respond to therapy with antibiotics, usually for 2–3 weeks. It may take 14 days for

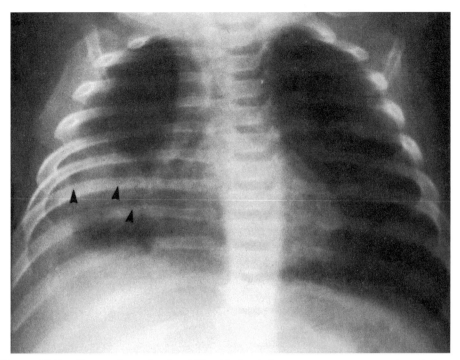

Figure 10-9   Chest radiograph of a child with *Staphylococcus aureus* pneumonia and abscess (from the collection of Dr. Jim Bass).

fever to resolve. Antibiotics to cover *Staphylococcus* and anaerobes should be considered. For this reason, clindamycin or penicillin and metronidazole therapy can be used. Other excellent alternatives are ticarcillin in combination with clavulanate, or ampicillin and sulbactam.

Younger children and children with underlying disorders that impair cough mechanisms often require surgical drainage. Options include the radiographic placement of small bore "pigtail"-type catheters, or open drainage. Children with pulmonary abscess should be managed in a medical center where pediatric specialty and surgical support is available, but children with this condition can be expected to recover completely. In one series of almost a dozen children, three-quarters had normal pulmonary functions when assessed 9 years after the diagnosis[17].

Empyema and Parapneumonic Effusion

Children with bacterial pneumonia near the pleural surface will frequently develop parapneumonic effusions. The concomitant bacterial infection leads to sympathetic inflammation of the pleura, and increased pleural fluid production. Typically, the fluid will have low numbers of white blood cells, and a low LDH concentration. The initial treatment for parapneumonic effusion is to treat the underlying pneumonia. Children with simple effusions will defervesce quickly and no further treatment of the effusion

is required, although radiographic evidence may persist for weeks. The only reasons for pleurocentesis in this setting are clinical deterioration of the patient with need for microbiologic diagnosis, and respiratory compromise due to the mass effect of the pleural fluid.

Empyema occurs when the bacterial infection breaks into the pleural space, and causes infection. Children will often have persistent, elevated temperature and marked pleuritic chest pain. Analysis of fluid obtained by pleurocentesis will demonstrate large numbers of white cells and often organisms on Gram stain, low pH (<7.2) and high levels of LDH (typically above 1000 IU/l).

The chest radiograph demonstrates layering of the effusion on lateral decubitus films if the fluid is free-flowing, or blunted costophrenic angles with smaller volumes of fluid. Air–fluid levels may also be noted in children with pleural infections due to gas-producing organisms. CT of the chest is sensitive and specific for effusion, and the presence of significant pleural thickening on CT scan is relatively specific for empyema (Figure 10-10). Ultrasound is useful in determining whether the fluid is free flowing, and whether there are septations or loculations. The presence of intrapleural septae, echogenicity of the pleural fluid or pleural thickening all are consistent with a complicated empyema and suggest the need for more aggressive surgical drainage of the pleural space.

Like children with pulmonary abscess, children with empyema should be cared for in a center with pediatric

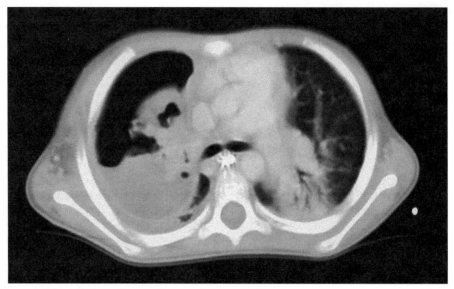

Figure 10-10 High-resolution CT scan of a child with complicated *Streptococcus pneumoniae* pneumonia, empyema, pleural thickening, and free pleural air.

specialists, and thoracic surgeons capable of assisting with drainage of the pleural space when needed. Goals in the treatment of children with empyema include elimination of the infection, re-expansion of the lung, return of respiratory function, elimination of complications and reduced recovery time. Therapy with antibiotics alone is often effective, but may lead to a protracted hospital course. Chest tube placement is most effective when used early in the course of the disease, with antibiotic treatment. This combination is sufficient treatment for many children with uncomplicated effusion. Fibrinolytics can be instilled through the chest tube, and in many studies therapy with streptokinase or urokinase have been demonstrated to be effective in treating loculated pleural effusion. However, there are no pediatric studies comparing the use of fibrinolytics with other forms of treatment.

Thoracotomy with removal of the pleural "peel" (decortication) is a major surgical procedure, but early surgical intervention in children whose empyema will invariably require surgical therapy has been shown to hasten resolution of the infection, and shorten the child's hospital course. The ideal time for intervention seems to be between 2 and 6 weeks after the onset of symptoms. Sooner than 2 weeks into the course, the pleural fibrin "peel" is rarely organized enough to facilitate surgical removal. Beyond 6 weeks, the thickened fibrin is adherent to the pleura, and difficult to remove.

Another new option in the management of some children with empyema is video-assisted thorascopic decortication (VATD). This technique utilizes two surgical trocars: one with a video camera and the other as a port for surgical instruments. In smaller children, the ports may be too small to be effective for the removal of thick secretions and debris. However, in experienced hands, this technique is as effective as open thoracotomy. Thus far small comparative studies between VATD and chest tube placement with fibrinolysis have shown some advantage to the video-assisted technique, but controlled trials have not been conducted[18].

In summary, a child with parapneumonic effusion should be treated for the underlying pneumonia with appropriate antibiotic therapy and drainage of the effusion should not be attempted unless essential for diagnosis or to alleviate respiratory distress. If the child does not respond to appropriate therapy, or has worsening effusion or persistent fever, he or she should be suspected of having empyema. Empyema requires chest tube placement and fibrinolysis is indicated if the tube fails to drain the effusion. If the effusion persists, CT of the chest or ultrasound should be used to determine whether the effusion is organized or septated. Depending on the expertise of the consulting surgeon, thoracotomy or VATD and chest tube drainage will speed resolution of the symptoms and shorten the hospital stay. Table 10-5 summarizes infections of the pulmonary parenchyma and pleural space.

Unusual Pneumonias

There are a host of unusual causes of pneumonia that generally affect children who are "unusual": those who are immunodeficient or have received immunosuppressive therapy. Commonly, these are children who have been treated for malignancy or who have received tissue transplantation, children with inflammatory diseases

Table 10-5   Bacterial Infections of the Parenchyma and Pleura

Clinical Syndrome	Typical Age	Symptoms	Signs	Etiology	Treatment
Pneumonia Newborn	Birth	Respiratory distress Grunting Cyanosis	Tachypnea Retractions Crackles	Group B beta- hemolytic *Streptococcus* *Escherichia coli* *Listeria monocytogenes*	Ampicillin and aminoglyco- side
"Well" Infant	2 weeks–3 months	Crackles Staccato cough Congestion	Afebrile Heterophonous wheeze Tachypnea	*Chlamydia* *pneumoniae* Cytomegalovirus *Ureaplasma urealyticum* *Pneumocystis jiroveci*	Erythromycin
"Ill" Infant	2 weeks–6 months	Fever Cough Respiratory distress	Respiratory distress Tachypnea Crackles	*Streptococcus* *pneumoniae* *Staphylococcus* *aureus* *Haemophilus* *influenzae*, Type B	Ceftriaxone Vancomycin
"Well" child	7 months–5 years	Rhinitis Cough Congestion	Afebrile Rhonchi Heterophonous wheeze	Viruses	Symptomatic
"Ill" child	7 months–5 years	Fever and chills Productive cough Malaise Chest pain	Tachypnea Crackles Percussion dullness	*Streptococcus* *pneumoniae*	Ceftriaxone
Child/adolescent	6 years–adult	Fever Malaise "Hacking" cough	Crackles Rhonchi	*Mycoplasma* *pneumoniae* *Chlamydia* *pneumoniae*	Macrolide Tetracycline
Abscess	2 weeks–adult	Fever Cough	Crackles Percussion dullness	*Staphylococcus* *aureus* Anaerobic organisms	Ceftriaxone Clindamycin Penicillin and metronidazole
Empyema	6 months–adult	Fever Cough Pleuritic pain	Tachypnea Crackles Pleural rub	*Streptococcus* *pneumoniae* *Staphylococcus aureus* *Haemophilus* *influenzae*, Type B	Ceftriaxone Nafcillin/oxacillin Vancomycin

such as connective tissue disorders, and those with primary immunodeficiencies and acquired immunodeficiency (AIDS).

An opportunistic organism should be suspected at the outset in any immunocompromised child with pneumonia. Viruses (herpesviruses, CMV, varicella), fungi (*Aspergillus*, *Mucor*, *Pneumocystis*), bacteria (*Pseudomonas*, nontuberculous mycobacterium), and other organisms (*Toxoplasma*, *Cryptosporidium*) can all cause pneumonia in this population. Therapy should be initiated with broad-spectrum antibiotics, and aggressive measures must be taken to identify the cause of the infection. Sputum examination and culture is the first step, and should proceed when therapy is begun in older children and adolescents along with blood cultures and the appropriate antigen studies. If the child fails to respond to broad-spectrum therapy, invasive procedures must be performed in order to identify the organism. Flexible fiberoptic bronchoscopy with bronchoalveolar lavage or transbronchial biopsy is the first invasive procedure to be considered. If this procedure is unfruitful, transthoracic needle biopsy using ultrasound or CT guidance is the next method of choice. Finally, open lung biopsy or thorascopic biopsy is the standard to

Table 10-6 When to Refer to a Pediatric Pulmonary Specialist

Severe, life-threatening infection
Recurrent pneumonia (> 3 episodes per year)
Recurrent croup or bronchitis (> 3 episodes per year)
Pneumonia unresponsive to therapy
Progressive pneumonia despite therapy
Complicated pneumonia (abscess or empyema)
Unusual organism causing pneumonia
Physical examination findings suggestive of chronic disease
  (i.e., clubbing)
Persistent pulmonary infiltrate > 6 weeks after resolution of
  symptoms

which all other diagnostic procedures are compared. Aggressive effort to obtain tissue diagnosis of an opportunistic pneumonia offers the immunocompromised child the best chance for survival.

The primary care provider in the ambulatory or the community hospital setting can manage most children with uncomplicated pneumonia. An "unusual" pneumonia or any pneumonia in an "unusual child," i.e., one with altered immune competence, requires more specialized care. It is one of a list of different clinical syndromes of lower respiratory tract infection that warrant more in-depth investigation by a pediatric pulmonary specialist (Table 10-6). In every case, it is essential that the provider consider the possible etiologies based on the child's presentation and clinical syndrome. Aggressive recognition and appropriate antimicrobial therapy are the keys to a successful outcome[19,20].

MAJOR POINTS

1. Viruses are the cause of most lower respiratory tract infections in children.
2. Cough in the office may predict the presence of lower respiratory tract disease in children, and at least should prompt a careful examination of the patient's chest.
3. Tachypnea and crackles are the most sensitive predictors of LRI in infants and children.
4. Pneumonia is a clinical diagnosis. A normal chest radiograph in a febrile, ill-appearing child with cough, tachypnea and crackles should not deter the clinician from initiating treatment for pneumonia.
5. The most important component of treatment of a child with tracheitis is conservative management of the child in a pediatric intensive care unit with early intubation.

MAJOR POINTS —Cont'd

6. Guaifenesin derivatives and other over-the-counter cough suppressants are generally of little or no value in the treatment of children with respiratory tract infections, despite the frequency with which they are prescribed.
7. Suspect chronic bacterial bronchitis in infants and children with persistent symptoms of cough and an abnormal physical examination suggestive of bronchorrhea associated with a history of airway insult.
8. *Chlamydia trachomatis, Ureaplasma urealyticum*, cytomegalovirus, and *Pneumocystis* should be suspected in infants who present with afebrile pneumonia.
9. Under a month of age, all children with fever and no identifiable source should have a sepsis evaluation, and receive inpatient intravenous antibiotic therapy.
10. Children with lower respiratory tract infection managed in an ambulatory setting should be followed daily until the symptoms of respiratory tract infection begin to resolve.
11. Younger children and children with underlying disorders that impair cough mechanisms often require surgical drainage of pulmonary abscess.
12. A child with parapneumonic effusion should be treated for the underlying pneumonia with appropriate antibiotic therapy, and drainage of the effusion should not be attempted unless essential for diagnosis or to alleviate respiratory distress.
13. Aggressive efforts to obtain tissue diagnosis of an opportunistic pneumonia offers the immunocompromised child the best chance for survival.
14. The primary care provider in the ambulatory setting or the community hospital can manage most children with uncomplicated pneumonia.

ACKNOWLEDGMENT

"The views and opinions expressed in this manuscript are those of the authors and do not reflect the official policy or position of the Department of the Army, the Department of Defense, or the United States Government."

REFERENCES

1. Denny FW, Clyde WA. Acute lower respiratory tract infections in nonhospitalized children. J Pediatr 108: 635-646,1986.
2. Tan TQ, Mason EO, Wald ER, et al. Clinical characteristics of children with complicated pneumonia caused by *Streptococcus* pneumoniae. Pediatrics 110:1-6, 2002.
3. Polgar G. A functional analysis of symptoms and therapeutic measures in respiratory disorders of newborn infants. Pediatr Clin North Am 20:303-322, 1973.

4. Correa AG, Starke JR. Bacterial pneumonia. In Kendig's disorders of the respiratory tract in children, 6th edition, pp 485-503. Philadelphia: WB Saunders, 1998.

5. Shah SS, Alpern ER, Zwerling L, McGowan KL, Bell LM. Risk of bacteremia in young children with pneumonia treated as outpatients. Arch Pediatr Adolesc Med 157: 389-392, 2003.

6. Sankaran RT, Mattana J, Pollack S, Bhat P, Ahuja T, Patel A, Singhal PC. Laboratory abnormalities in patients with bacterial pneumonia. Chest 111:595-600, 1997.

7. Grossman LK, Caplan SE. Clinical, laboratory and radiological information in the diagnosis of pneumonia in children. Ann Emerg Med 17:43-46, 1988.

8. Vincent JM, Cherry JD, Nauschuetz JD et al. Prolonged afebrile nonproductive cough illness in American soldiers in Korea: a serologic search for causation. Clin Infect Dis 30:534-539, 2000.

9. Senzilet LD, Halperin SA, Spika JS, Alagaratnam M, Morris A, et al. Pertussis is a frequent cause of prolonged cough illness in adults and adolescents. Clin Infect Dis 32: 1691-1697, 2001.

10. Garbutt JM, Golsstein M, Gellman E, Shannon W, Littenberg B. A randomized, placebo-controlled trial of antimicrobial treatment for children with clinically diagnosed acute sinusitis. Pediatrics 107:619-625, 2001.

11. Smith TF, Ireland TA, Zaatari GS, Gay BB, Zwiren GT, Andrews G. Characteristics of children with endoscopically proved chronic bronchitis Am J Dis Child 139:1039-1044, 1985.

12. Callahan C, Redding G. Bronchiectasis in children: An orphan disease that persists. Pediatr Pulmonol 33:492-496, 2002.

13. Stagno S, Brasfield DM, Brown MB et al. Infant pneumonitis associated with cytomegalovirus, *Chlamydia*, *Pneumocystis* and *Ureaplasma*: a prospective study. Pediatrics 68: 322-329, 1981.

14. Brasfield DM, Stagno S, Whitley RJ, et al. Infant pneumonitis associated with cytomegalovirus, *Chlamydia*, *Pneumocystis* and *Ureaplasma*: follow-up. Pediatrics 79:76-83, 1987.

15. Shebab ZM. Mycoplasma infections. In Taussig LM, Landau LI, editors: Pediatric respiratory medicine, pp 737-742. St. Louis: Mosby, 1999.

16. Thom DH, Grayston JT. Infections with *Chlamydia pneumoniae*, strain TWAR. Clin Chest Med 12:245-256, 1991.

17. Asher MI, Spier S, Bland N, et al. Primary lung abscess in childhood. Am J Dis Child 136:491-494, 1982.

18. Lewis RA, Feigin RD. Current issues in the diagnosis and management of pediatric empyema. Semin Pediatr Infect Dis 13:280-288, 2002.

19. Schidlow DV, Callahan C. Pneumonia. Pediatr Rev 17:300-309, 1996.

20. Gaston B. Pneumonia. Pediatr Rev 23:132-140, 2002.

Tuberculosis

GAIL L. RODGERS, M.D.

Tuberculosis (TB) has plagued mankind for millennia. It is estimated that one third of the world's population is infected with *Mycobacterium tuberculosis*. There are an estimated 8 million new cases a year and up to 2 million annual deaths[1]. Children represent approximately 1.3 million new cases and 400,000 deaths annually. The vast majority of cases (95%) occur in the developing world. Public health efforts in the United States were responsible for a steady decrease in the case rate from 100 cases/ 100,000 persons in 1930 to 10 cases/100,000 persons in 1984. An unexpected 20% increase in reported cases occurred in the United States between 1984 and 1992[2]. The increase in pediatric cases was substantial; a 51% increase was seen in children less than 15 years of age from 1988 to 1992[3]. Contributory factors for this increase were a decrease in public health infrastructure, increased immigration from countries with high prevalence of tuberculosis, socioeconomic factors such as poverty, homelessness, illicit drug use and incarceration, and the epidemic of human immunodeficiency virus infection. Since 1992 there has been a yearly decrease in tuberculosis cases in the United States, from 26,673 cases in 1992 to 15,078 cases in 2002[4-6]. The prevalence of tuberculosis in the United States in 2002 was the lowest ever at 5.2 cases/100,000 persons, representing a 68.4% decline in rates since 1992[6]. This decrease has been highly significant in the pediatric population and in US-born persons, with less of a decrease in foreign-born persons[6]. For the first time ever, in 2002, foreign-born persons accounted for the majority (51%) of cases in the United States[6]. The most common native countries for foreign-born persons with TB are Mexico, the Philippines, Vietnam, India, China, Haiti, and South Korea[6]. The overall dramatic decrease in TB in the United States is due primarily to strengthening of public health programs that emphasize prompt identification of cases with education of healthcare workers, contact investigation and aggressive institution of directly observed therapy that ensures both availability of antituberculous medications and patient compliance. Other important contributory measures include improvement in infection-control policies and practices in hospitals, jails, and prisons[7].

THE ORGANISM AND PATHOGENESIS

TB is caused by the pleomorphic, aerobic acid-fast bacillus, *Mycobacterium tuberculosis*. It requires special media to sustain its growth, which is slow. The bacterium replicates once every 24 hours, thus requiring weeks to months for visible growth in the laboratory.

Overall, acquisition of TB, known as infection, is mainly caused by factors extrinsic to the host and related to exposure to a contagious individual. If infection produces no clinical disease it is known as latent TB. Progression to symptomatic disease after infection is caused by factors intrinsic to the host, mainly immunologic mechanisms that can kill, contain, or allow progression of the bacilli.

The pathogenesis of TB starts with the inhalation of infectious droplet nuclei. These are small enough to avoid entrapment by the mucociliary defenses and reach the lung where they are ingested by macrophages. At this point the mycobacteria have one of two fates: they are killed by the macrophage without establishment of infection or they persist within the macrophage where they can replicate. As the mycobacteria replicate they disseminate to all organs of the body via the bloodstream and lymphatics. At this time the infection can become clinical and manifest as primary tuberculous pneumonia or as miliary disease, although in the majority of infected persons the immune system contains the infection and it becomes latent.

The complex immune mechanisms that govern the interaction of the host with the tuberculous bacilli are the key to understanding of TB[8,9]. In response to mycobacteria, lung macrophages elaborate cytokines. These cytokines, tumor necrosis factor-α (TNF-α), interleukin-12 (IL-12), and multiple chemokines, act together to contain the infection. Some bacilli are able to multiply and cause lysis and death of the macrophages. These bacilli migrate to regional lymph nodes within dendritic cells, which function as antigen presenting cells. Antigen-specific response occurs when the dendritic cells elaborate cytokines and present mycobacterial antigens to CD4+ T cells. These cells play an essential role in the host defense against mycobacteria by producing cytokines, particularly interferon-γ (IFN-γ) and IL-2. IFN-γ in turn activates macrophages to inhibit or kill *M. tuberculosis*. The efficiency of the CD4+ T cell response determines whether active infection will ensue or whether latency will be established. This response is responsible for the production of delayed hypersensitivity manifested as a positive skin reaction to purified protein derivative (PPD). The importance of the CD4+ T cell response is seen clinically in a wide variety of hosts who are at increased risk of reactivating latent TB as they become immunocompromised. The most notable example is HIV-infected persons, who are at significantly higher risk of reactivation of latent TB (10% per year) in comparison with healthy individuals, whose risk is 10% over their lifetime[10,11]. The risk of TB in HIV-infected individuals is inversely related to their CD4+ T cell count; Alpert et al.[12] found that 81% of HIV patients with TB had CD4+ T cell counts less than 200/mm[3]. Because of the association between TB and HIV, all patients with tuberculous disease should be tested for HIV infection.

The immune response and hypersensitivity that occur to the tuberculosis antigens are responsible for the pathologic features associated with TB. In efforts to contain the infection, the components of the immune system organize into granulomas and incomplete necrosis occurs, giving the distinctive pathologic appearance of caseous necrosis.

The immune system's response to *M. tuberculosis* also explains the higher risk of disease following exposure and infection in children compared with adults. The risk of young children with untreated infection developing symptomatic TB is up to 43% in those less than 1 year of age and 24% in those aged 1–5 years, compared with 2% for adults >30 years[13]. The age-related immune defects postulated to enhance the risk in children include: impaired alveolar macrophage killing (despite normal numbers) secondary to high concentration of lung surfactant, less efficient antigen presentation, decreased monocyte chemotaxis, and decreased IFN-γ and TNF-α production by natural killer cells and T lymphocytes[9]. In addition, the proximity to an infectious primary caretaker has been postulated as a factor for the increased risk in infants.

Other factors associated with susceptibility to TB disease include genetic variations[14,15], race[16], and environmental factors.

TRANSMISSION

TB is transmitted from person to person via the respiratory route. The infectious bacilli are contained in droplet nuclei that are less than 10 μm in diameter. Droplet nuclei are expelled from the lungs of an infected person usually by coughing, although infection has been associated with talking loudly and singing. The droplet nuclei dry and disperse rapidly but due to their size these airborne particles may remain suspended for hours. The droplet nuclei are highly infectious, since only a few bacilli contained in one droplet nucleus are required for infection and an infected adult can expel approximately 3000 droplet nuclei with one cough.

The degree of contagiousness is influenced by several factors such as the presence of acid-fast bacilli (AFB) on sputum smears, cough, duration and intensity of exposure, environmental ventilation, and host characteristics. The most important factor is the presence of AFB on sputum smear. Studies have shown that among household contacts of smear-positive cases the rates of tuberculin positivity (i.e., infection) are 30–50% above those among age-matched community controls, and in contacts of smear-negative cases the tuberculin positivity is approximately 5%[17]. The likelihood of AFB smear positivity is enhanced by cavitary lung lesions, which are usually full of bacilli.

Since children rarely have cavitary lung lesions, transmission from children is rare. However, if cavitary lesions are present, children may be the infectious source[18,19]. Most outbreaks involving children (daycare, schools, children's hospitals) have been traced to adults with active contagious disease. Coughing is also important, with those with a greater number of coughs at higher risk of transmitting TB.

The effect of duration and intensity of exposure has been detailed in various outbreaks. These have been seen in offices, clinics, hospitals, classrooms, buses and airplanes, among others. In these situations, the distance from the infected person and the duration of contact were significantly associated with infection. In a school bus outbreak where the driver was the infectious source, children who sat in the front of the bus, close to the driver, and for longer periods of time were more likely to be infected[20]. Kenyon described transmission during a long airplane flight in which the index patient had multidrug-resistant TB. Passengers seated within two rows of the index patient were more likely to have positive tuberculin skin tests[21]. In hospital outbreaks, the intensity of exposure may be more important than duration. Fourteen percent of employees exposed for 4 hours in an emergency department to an intubated patient who required frequent suctioning, became positive[22]. Ventilation has become an important factor for TB transmission, highlighted by outbreaks aboard ships, in jails, and hospitals.

To decrease the risk of transmission in hospital settings, strict infection control practices are recommended[23]. For patients with known or suspected TB, these include isolation in a negative-pressure room and respiratory protection with N95 respirators for all who enter. Special attention should be paid to cough-inducing procedures such as nebulization therapy, which has been associated with enhanced transmission[24]. An employee health program that performs routine PPD testing is essential in recognizing conversions and monitoring employees for active disease[25,26].

Host characteristics may be important factors in transmission. Persons with a positive PPD may be somewhat immune to acquisition of a second infection, although reinfection has occurred in immunocompromised patients. Being immunocompromised does not affect the likelihood of infection but greatly influences the risk of disease. Furthermore, immunocompromised patients may transmit more effectively, if the disease has an unusual presentation or extrapulmonary manifestations that delay diagnosis and proper implementation of infection control measures.

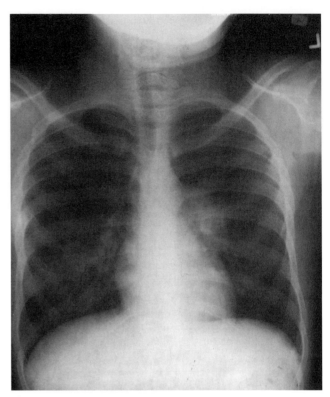

Figure 11-1   Frontal radiograph of the chest demonstrates left hilar adenopathy.

CLINICAL MANIFESTATIONS

Pulmonary Disease

Primary infection in children is usually asymptomatic. Occasionally, patients will have mild fever and cough heralding infection, but these usually resolve without intervention. Symptomatic infection, known as primary pulmonary tuberculosis, occurs more commonly in infants and small children. Forty to fifty percent of infected infants have symptoms or radiographic abnormalities compared with 10% of older children. This syndrome is characterized by fever, respiratory symptoms, failure to thrive, pulmonary infiltrate(s), and enlarged regional lymphadenopathy (Figures 11-1, 11-2). Sometimes the lymphadenopathy causes obstruction followed by segmental atelectasis. In small children this may mimic foreign body aspiration. Although lymphadenopathy and pulmonary infiltrate/atelectasis are the classic findings in pulmonary TB, any radiographic findings can be associated with TB. Thus, it

is of vital importance to inquire about risk factors for TB in any patient with pneumonia. Frequently the symptomatic small infant or child is the first recognized person with TB in a family with a contagious adult contact. Vallejo et al. studied 47 infants under 1 year of age with TB and found that there was an infectious adult contact in 68% of cases[27]. The common symptoms recognized in adults such as night sweats, anorexia, and weight loss are usually absent in infants and children.

Infrequently primary pulmonary disease becomes progressive with an enlarging pulmonary focus that may liquefy in the center resembling a lung abscess. These patients are usually symptomatic with fever, severe cough, anorexia, and night sweats. Although primary pleural and pericardial TB are rare in children a pulmonary cavity can rupture into the pleura and/or pericardium. The pleura may show a hypersensitivity response to bacilli released from a subpleural focus. Pleural fluid characteristically has between 100 and 1000 white blood cells/mm^3, predominantly polymorphonuclear leukocytes, high protein and low glucose. Pleural fluid smears for AFB are typically negative and biopsy of the pleura is usually needed to make the diagnosis. Pericardial involvement can be detected by echocardiography. Pericardial fluid is usually serofibrinous or hemorrhagic and, like the pleura, direct AFB smear is usually negative. Pericardial biopsy is often AFB-smear-positive and culture-positive. Although these

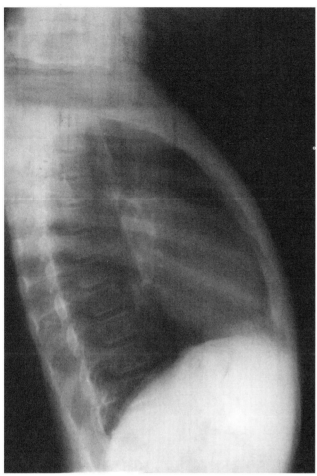

Figure 11-2 Lateral radiograph of the chest demonstrates bilateral hilar adenopathy. Note airway compression by enlarged nodes.

extrapulmonary foci conveyed a high mortality in the pretreatment era, full recovery is the rule with current therapy.

More than half of children with pulmonary TB are completely asymptomatic. Most come to medical attention as a result of contact investigation of an adult case, although infants and small children may be missed in contact evaluations due to the lack of comfort of evaluators with infants. Lobato found many missed opportunities for TB prevention in children younger than 5 years; improvements in contact investigation may have prevented TB in 17 of the 43 children evaluated[28]. Children may also come to attention as part of routine medical care in which a PPD is placed. These asymptomatic children may have moderate or severe pulmonary disease.

Most untreated cases of pulmonary TB in children will resolve. Sequelae that may be seen as a result of pulmonary TB include calcifications and parenchymal scarring that may lead to pulmonary complications.

Older children and adolescents can have reactivation disease. For reasons that are not totally understood adolescence is a high-risk period for reactivation disease. These patients frequently present, as do adults, with symptoms of fever, productive cough, chest pain, night sweats, anorexia, weight loss, and hemoptysis. Radiographically, upper lobe disease is usually evident with infiltrate or cavitary lesions.

Extrapulmonary tuberculosis

Since the tuberculous bacilli disseminate throughout the body after primary infection, any organ can be a site of reactivation and clinical disease. Infants and immunocompromised hosts, especially those with acquired immune deficiency syndrome (AIDS), are most likely to have extrapulmonary TB. Twenty-five percent of children evaluated by Burroughs et al.[29] with TB had extrapulmonary disease. Most had concomitant pulmonary involvement but 13 of 156 had extrapulmonary disease only. Miliary disease is the most common serious, disseminated form of TB and occurs most frequently in infants. It usually occurs as a complication of primary infection in which there is a massive mycobacteremia and clinical disease manifests in more than two organs. Miliary disease commonly presents as an indolent infection with low-grade fevers, malaise, and failure to thrive. Respiratory symptoms are not usually prominent initially but with time pulmonary involvement becomes evident with respiratory distress, and the chest radiograph may show the characteristic miliary pattern (so named because the appearance is similar to millet seeds) (Figure 11-3). Hepatosplenomegaly is usually present as is generalized lymphadenopathy. PPD testing is negative in approximately 30% of patients with miliary disease. Diagnosis of miliary disease requires a high index of suspicion. In one review premortem diagnosis was established in only one-third of children[30]. Often, liver or bone marrow specimens are required for diagnosis. With adequate treatment the prognosis of miliary TB is excellent.

A miliary pattern on the chest radiograph can also be seen in neonates with congenital TB. Congenital TB is exceedingly rare because it requires placental and/or amniotic fluid infection for transmission of bacilli to the fetus[31]. Blackall found three affected patients among 100 infants of mothers with active TB[32]. Patients with congenital TB present in the neonatal period with symptoms compatible with septicemia, commonly respiratory distress, hepatosplenomegaly, and often have a miliary pattern on the chest radiograph. Some may have a more indolent course. A very high index of suspicion is required to make this diagnosis since many infected mothers are asymptomatic and only diagnosed after diagnosis of the infant.

Although most cases of mycobacterial lymphadenitis in children are caused by non-tuberculous mycobacteria (NTM), commonly *M. avium-intracellulare* and *M. kansasii*, lymphadenitis is the most common extrapulmonary manifestation of TB. It occurs most frequently in the lymph nodes of the neck and supraclavicular regions.

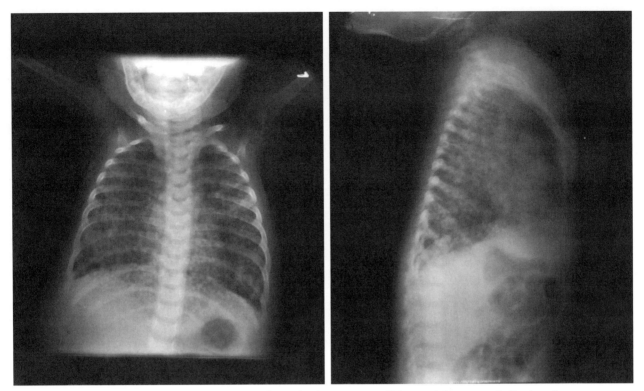

Figure 11-3 Frontal and lateral radiographs demonstrate a diffuse nodular pattern indicative of miliary tuberculosis.

Differentiating lymphadenitis caused by NTM from that caused by *M. tuberculosis* may be difficult. Pulmonary involvement is not seen in normal children with NTM infection and is seen in the majority of children with tuberculous lymphadenitis. The PPD is frequently positive with TB and although it may cause a reaction in NTM infection, it is usually <10 mm. Assessment of risk factors for TB and epidemiologic investigation are essential in making the distinction between TB and NTM lymphadenitis. Often culture of drainage or excisional biopsy is necessary to establish the correct diagnosis.

Other extrapulmonary forms of TB disease include central nervous system infection, with TB meningitis being the most serious complication. Disease can also be seen in bones (typically vertebrae), joints, skin, and the gastrointestinal and genitourinary systems.

DIAGNOSIS

Tuberculin skin tests (TST) such as the PPD, also known as the Mantoux test, are routinely used to evaluate for TB infection. This test is a standardized product composed of *M. tuberculosis* proteins. The multiple puncture test (Tine test) is a non-standardized test that should not be used. Proper application of the PPD is

imperative for an accurate result; 0.1 ml (5TU) is applied intradermally to produce a wheal. In 48–72 hours a cell mediated response will be elicited in patients who have been infected with TB. Induration in those with a positive test may remain for days to weeks. The incubation period for this response to occur after exposure to TB is 2–12 weeks. This response is manifest as an indurated area surrounding the site of application. The diameter of induration transverse to the long axis of the forearm is measured. Studies evaluating skin reaction in patients with TB and those without have yielded interpretative criteria. Interpretation is based on the pretest probability that the patient has TB; populations with low prevalence, at low risk, should not be tested routinely since most reactions will be falsely positive. Thus, to interpret a PPD skin test one must first do a risk assessment for TB (Table 11-1). Reactions that are immediate or accelerated, usually occurring within 24 hours of placement, represent hypersensitivity to polysaccharides or components in the diluent and do not represent positive reactions to TB. Erythema alone does not constitute a positive reaction and only induration should be measured. Unfortunately, antigens present in NTMs may cross-react with TB antigens present in the PPD test. Reactions secondary to NTMs are typically smaller than 10 mm. Vaccination with Bacille Calmette-Guérin (BCG),

Table 11-1   Definitions of Positive Tuberculin Skin Test Results in Infants, Children, and Adolescents

Induration	Interpret as Positive in:
>5 mm	Children in close contact with known or suspected contagious cases of TB
	Children suspected of having TB disease
	Children receiving immunosuppressive therapy or with immunosuppressive conditions, including HIV infection
≥10 mm	Children at increased risk of disseminated disease:
	Younger than 4 years
	With underlying medical conditions such as Hodgkin disease, lymphoma, diabetes, chronic renal failure and/or malnutrition
	Children with increased exposure to tuberculosis disease:
	Children born or whose parents were born in areas of high TB prevalence
	Children frequently exposed to high-risk persons, i.e., HIV-infected, homeless, illicit drug users, nursing home residents, incarcerated or institutionalized, or migrant farmers
	Children who travel to or immigrated from high-prevalence regions of the world
≥15 mm	Children >4 years of age without any risk factors

(Adapted from American Academy of Pediatrics. Tuberculosis. In Pickering LK, editor: Red Book: 2003 Report of the Committee on Infectious Diseases, 26th edition, pp 648-658. Elk Grove Village, IL: American Academy of Pediatrics, 2003.)

which is routinely done in infancy throughout the world, may produce a positive PPD test, but within a year most are less than 10 mm. Thus, the current recommendation is to interpret PPD results in BCG-vaccinated individuals as though they had never been vaccinated. Approximately 10% of children with active pulmonary TB will not respond to skin testing and up to half with miliary disease and/or tuberculous meningitis may have an initial negative test. Frequently these become positive during the course of therapy. Anergy testing is not recommended because a standardized protocol does not exist and many patients who have TB may have global anergy or anergy solely to TB antigens. Thus, a positive anergy test with a negative Mantoux test in a patient with suspected TB would not deter one from further evaluation and treatment[33].

The chest radiograph is the next step in evaluation of a child with a positive PPD. The most common abnormalities include mediastinal lymphadenopathy, consolidation, and interstitial densities, although any abnormality may be compatible with TB (Figures 11-4, 11-5, 11-6). Computed tomography (CT) may be more sensitive for pulmonary involvement in the symptomatic patient with a normal chest radiograph, but there is no role for CT in asymptomatic patients with positive skin tests and negative chest radiographs[34].

Microbiologic investigation is essential in patients who are symptomatic and in those with a positive PPD skin test and a positive chest radiograph. The only exception to this is patients whose known contact has microbiologic proof of *M. tuberculosis* with available susceptibility data. Evaluation of expectorated sputum for AFB is the gold standard for diagnosis of TB. In children, obtaining sputum can be difficult and obtaining first morning gastric aspirates on 3 consecutive days, if done in a standardized

manner, has been shown to have good sensitivity (presumably because of swallowing of pulmonary secretions which pool in the stomach)[35]. Although most are not AFB-smear-positive due to low organism load, culture of gastric aspirates can be positive in up to 70% of infants and 50% of children with pulmonary TB[36]. Abadco and Steiner demonstrated that obtaining gastric aspirates was more sensitive than performing bronchoalveolar lavage for isolation of *M. tuberculosis* in children[37]. For patients with extrapulmonary disease, specimens should be obtained from the affected site, although the positive culture rate is only approximately 50%[34].

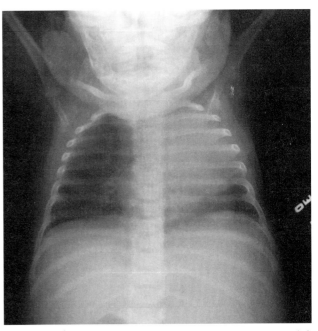

Figure 11-4   Frontal radiograph of the chest demonstrates left upper lobe atelectasis in a patient with pulmonary tuberculosis.

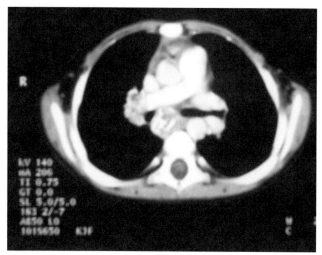

Figure 11-5 Axial contrast-enhanced CT scan demonstrates necrotic right hilar and subcarinal adenopathy.

Conventional culture methods usually take 3–8 weeks for growth to be detected, although newer systems with broth media have decreased that interval to 1–3 weeks.

Recently, nucleic acid amplification assays (polymerase chain reaction [PCR] using the insertion sequence IS*6110* as the target for DNA) have been developed for the diagnosis of TB. In limited pediatric studies PCR had a sensitivity of 40% and a specificity of 80%, which is not significantly better than culture[38]. Use of PCR tests in pediatrics is limited by Food and Drug Administration approval for sputum samples only, poor sensitivity and specificity on gastric aspirates and false positives in pediatric patients with *M. avium-intracellulare*[38-40]. At present, routine use of PCR methodology in pediatrics cannot be recommended.

TREATMENT

Mycobacteria are present in infected tissues in different stages. Some are rapidly dividing, others exhibit spurts of metabolic activity, and some may be dormant. Access to mycobacteria in macrophages can be difficult for some drugs. Since mycobacteria are in these different growing cycles and may exhibit primary drug resistance, a basic principle is to use combination antituberculous therapy. The goal of antituberculous therapy is to make the patient non-contagious rapidly and to cure the disease. In pediatric patients, an immunocompetent host with a susceptible organism and assured compliance has a 100% response rate to therapy with less than 5% risk of relapse. Recent comprehensive guidelines for treatment of TB have been established by the American Thoracic Society, Centers for Disease Control and Prevention and Infectious Diseases Society of America as well as the American Academy of Pediatrics[41,42]. The most common regimen for treatment of susceptible TB strains is shown in Table 11-2. Treatment protocols for patients with multidrug-resistant TB must be individualized and consultation with a specialized treatment center is recommended[41].

Treatment for all pediatric patients with tuberculous disease should be monitored by directly observed therapy (DOT). DOT is performed by the public health department and involves providing the antituberculous drugs directly to the patient and watching as he or she swallows the medications. This is the best way to assure compliance and success of therapy[43,44].

For patients with HIV infection, the American Academy of Pediatrics recommends consultation with a specialist and continuation of therapy for 9 months[42].

Corticosteroids have been used as adjunctive therapy in the treatment of TB. Evidence-based recommendations are present for use of corticosteroids in tuberculous pericarditis and central nervous system disease including meningitis[41,45].

New treatment strategies have emerged from knowledge of the immunobiology of TB. These include administration of aerosolized INF-γ and subcutaneous IL-2[46,47]. Thus far these have been studied in patients with multidrug-resistant TB with good outcomes. This is a new and promising area of TB research.

Although a vaccine for TB exists, BCG vaccine, it is of very limited efficacy; estimates of efficacy have ranged

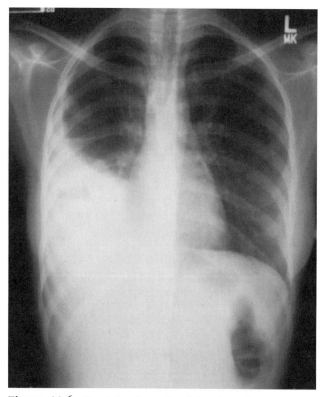

Figure 11-6 Frontal radiograph of the chest demonstrates a large right pleural effusion in a patient with tuberculosis.

Table 11-2   Recommended Treatment Regimens for Drug-Susceptible TB in Infants, Children, and Adolescents

Infection/Disease Category	Treatment
Latent infection (positive Mantoux test, negative chest radiograph)	Isoniazid (INH) daily for 9 months if INH-susceptible Rifampin (RIF) daily for 9 months if INH-resistant Consult specialist if INH- and RIF-resistant
Pulmonary and extrapulmonary TB except TB meningitis	INH, RIF and pyrizinamide (PZA) daily or twice a week[a] for 2 months, followed by INH and RIF for 4 months In areas of high prevalence of resistance add ethambutal (ETH) or aminoglycoside for initial 2 months or until susceptibilities known Consult specialist for multidrug-resistant TB
TB meningitis	INH, RIF PZA, ETH or aminoglycoside daily for 2 months, followed by INH and RIF daily or twice a week[a] for 7-10 months

(Adapted from American Academy of Pediatrics. Tuberculosis. In Pickering LK, editor: Red book: 2003 Report of the Committee on Infectious Diseases, 26th edition, pp 648-658. Elk Grove Village, IL: American Academy of Pediatrics, 2003.)
[a] Drugs can be given twice weekly under directly observed therapy (DOT).

from 0 to 100%, with an average efficacy of 50%[48]. The highest efficacy is in prevention of disseminated disease and death in neonates, thus its continued use worldwide in areas of high TB prevalence. Major limitations of BCG are lack of standardization and side effects that can be severe and life-threatening in immunocompromised infants. Because of the current limitation of BCG and the worldwide burden of TB, one third of the world's population is infected; development of an effective, safe vaccine is an international public health priority. Vaccines under development include whole-cell live, whole-cell inactivated, subunit, DNA and prime-boost vaccines[48,49]. Several vaccines show promise and are undergoing human trials[48].

MAJOR POINTS

1. Diagnosis of tuberculosis (TB) in children requires a high index of suspicion. Since pulmonary TB can manifest in many ways one must inquire about risk factors for TB in patients presenting with pulmonary disease.
2. In view of the close association between TB and HIV, all pediatric patients with TB should be HIV-tested.
3. The Mantoux test or PPD is used for evaluation of TB infection. The multiple puncture test (Tine test) is not standardized and should not be used. The PPD test is read 48-72 hours after placement and induration, not erythema, is measured. To interpret the PPD skin test one must take into account the patient's risk for TB.
4. Treatment of TB is highly effective. To assure adherence with therapy, all patients with TB should be monitored by directly observed therapy, through the public health department.

REFERENCES

1. Dye C, Scheele S, Lolin P, et al. Global burden of tuberculosis: estimated incidence, prevalence and mortality by country. JAMA 282:677-686, 1999.
2. CDC. Reported tuberculosis in the United States, 1993. Atlanta: US Department of Health and Human Services, CDC, 1994.
3. Ussery XT, Valway SE, McKenna M, et al. Epidemiology of tuberculosis among children in the United States: 1985 to 1994. Pediatr Infect Dis J 15:697-704, 1996.
4. CDC Tuberculosis morbidity—United States, 1997. MMWR 47:253-257, 1998.
5. Bloom BR. Tuberculosis: the global view. N Engl J Med 346:1434-1435, 2002.
6. Trends in tuberculosis morbidity—United States, 1992-2002. MMWR 52:217-222, 2003.
7. Frieden TR, Fujiwara PI, Washko RM, et al. Tuberculosis in New York City: turning the tide. N Engl J Med 333:229-233, 1995.
8. Schluger NW, Rom WN. The host immune response to tuberculosis. Am J Respir Crit Care Med 157:679-691, 1998.
9. Smith S, Jacobs RF, Wilson CB. Immunobiology of childhood tuberculosis: a window on the ontogeny of cellular immunity. J Pediatr 131:16-26, 1997.
10. Selwyn PA, Hartel D, Lewis VA, et al. A prospective study of the risk of tuberculosis among intravenous drug users with human immunodeficiency virus infection. N Engl J Med 320:545-550, 1989.
11. Guelar A, Gatell JM, Verdejo J, et al. A prospective study of the risk of tuberculosis among HIV-infected patients. AIDS 7:1345-1349, 1993.
12. Alpert PL, Munsif SS, Gourevitch MN, et al. A prospective study of tuberculosis and human immunodeficiency virus infection: clinical manifestations and factors associated with survival. Clin Infect Dis 24:661-668, 1997.

13. Starke JR, Jacobs RF, Jereb J. Resurgence of tuberculosis in children. J Pediatr 120:839-855, 1992.

14. Bellamy R, Ruwende C, Corrah T, et al. Variations in the *NRAMP1* gene and susceptibility to tuberculosis in West Africans. N Engl J Med 338:640-644, 1998.

15. Goldfeld AE, Delgado JC, Thim S, et al. Association of an HLA-DQ allele with clinical tuberculosis. JAMA 279:226-228, 1998.

16. Stead WW, Senner JW, Reddick WT, et al. Racial differences in susceptibility to infection by *Mycobacterium tuberculosis*. N Engl J Med 322:422-427, 1990.

17. Sepkowitz KA. How contagious is tuberculosis? Clin Infect Dis 23:954-962, 1996.

18. Curtis AB, Ridzon R, Vogel R, et al. Extensive transmission of *Mycobacterium tuberculosis* from a child. N Engl J Med 341:1491-1495, 1999.

19. Ridzon R, Dent JH, Valway S, et al. Outbreak of drug-resistant tuberculosis with second-generation transmission in a high school in California. J Pediatr 131:863-868, 1997.

20. Rogers EFH. Epidemiology of an outbreak of tuberculosis among school children. Public Health Rep 77:401-409, 1962.

21. Kenyon TA, Valway SE, Ihle W, et al. Transmission of multidrug resistant *Mycobacterium tuberculosis* during a long airplane flight. N Engl J Med 334:933-998, 1996.

22. Haley CE, McDonald RC, Rossi L, et al. Tuberculosis epidemic among hospital personnel. Infect Control Hosp Epidemiol 10:204-210, 1989.

23. Guidelines for preventing the transmission of *Mycobacterium tuberculosis* in health-care facilities, 1994. MMWR 43(RR13):1-132, 1994.

24. Nelson JD, McCracken GH. TB in day-care. Pediatr Infect Dis J [Oct]:[Yellow Pages], 1998.

25. Bock NN, Sotir MJ, Parrott PL, et al. Nosocomial tuberculosis exposure in an outpatient setting: evaluation of patients exposed to healthcare providers with tuberculosis. Infect Control Hosp Epidemiol 20:421-425, 1999.

26. Bolyard EA, Tablan OC, Williams WW, et al. Guideline for infection control in healthcare personnel, 1998. Infect Control Hosp Epidemiol 19:407-463, 1998.

27. Vallejo JG, Ong LT, Starke JR. Clinical features, diagnosis, and treatment of tuberculosis in infants. Pediatrics 94:1-7, 1994.

28. Lobato MN, Mohle-Boetani JC, Royce SE. Missed opportunities for preventing tuberculosis among children younger than five years of age. Pediatrics 106:1-6, 2000.

29. Burroughs M, Beitel A, Kawamura A, et al. Clinical presentation of tuberculosis in culture-positive children. Pediatr Infect Dis J 18:440-446, 1999.

30. Hussey G, Chisholm, T. Kibel M. Miliary tuberculosis in children: a review of 94 cases. Pediatr Infect Dis J 10:832, 1991.

31. Cantwell MF, Shehab ZM, Costello AM, et al. Brief report: congenital tuberculosis. N Engl J Med 330:1051-1054, 1994.

32. Blackall PB. Tuberculosis: maternal infection of the newborn. Med J Aust 1:1055-1058, 1969.

33. Slovis BS, Plitman JD, Haas DW. The case against anergy testing as the routine adjunct to tuberculin skin testing. JAMA 283:2003-2007, 2000.

34. Starke JR. Diagnosis of tuberculosis in children. Pediatr Infect Dis J 19:1095-1096, 2000.

35. Pomputius WF, Rost J, Dennehy PH, et al. Standardization of gastric aspirate technique improves yield in the diagnosis of tuberculosis in children. Pediatr Infect Dis J 16:222-226, 1997.

36. Khan EA, Starke JR. Diagnosis of tuberculosis in children. Increased need for better methods. Emerging Infect Dis 1:115-123, 1995.

37. Abadco DL, Steiner P. Gastric lavage is better than bronchoalveolar lavage for isolation of *Mycobacterium tuberculosis* in childhood pulmonary tuberculosis. Pediatr Infect Dis J 11:735-738, 1992.

38. Smith KC, Starke JR, Eisenach K, et al. Detection of *Mycobacterium tuberculosis* in clinical specimens from children using a polymerase chain reaction. Pediatrics 97:155-160, 1996.

39. Delacourt C, Poveda JD, Chureau C, et al. Use of polymerase chain reaction for improved diagnosis of tuberculosis in children. J Pediatr 126:703-709, 1995.

40. Pierre C, Oliver C, Lecossier D, et al. Diagnosis of primary tuberculosis in children by amplification and detection of mycobacterial DNA. Am Rev Respir Dis 147:420-424, 1993.

41. American Thoracic Society, CDC, and Infectious Diseases Society of America. Treatment of tuberculosis. MMWR 52(RR-11):1-77, 2003.

42. American Academy of Pediatrics. Tuberculosis. In Pickering LK, editor: Red book: 2003 Report of the Committee on Infectious Diseases, 26th edition, pp 648-658. Elk Grove Village, IL: American Academy of Pediatrics, 2003.

43. Weis SE, Slocum PC, Blais FX, et al. The effect of directly observed therapy on the rates of drug resistance and relapse in tuberculosis. N Engl J Med 330:1179-1184, 1994.

44. Chaulk CP, Moore-Rice K, Rizzo R, et al. Eleven years of community-based directly observed therapy for tuberculosis. JAMA 274:945-951, 1995.

45. Dooley DP, Carpenter J, Rademacher S. Adjunctive corticosteroid therapy for tuberculosis: a critical reappraisal of the literature. Clin Infect Dis 25:872-887, 1997.

46. Condos R, Rom WN, Schluger NW. Treatment of multidrug-resistant pulmonary tuberculosis with interferon-γ via aerosol. Lancet 349:1513-1515, 1997.

47. Johnson B, Bekker LG, Ross S, et al. Recombinant interleukin-2 adjunctive therapy in multidrug resistant tuberculosis. Novartis Found Symp 217:99-106, 1998.

48. Fordham von Reyn C, Vuola JM. New vaccines for the prevention of tuberculosis. Clin Infect Dis 35:465-474, 2002.

49. Young DB. Current tuberculosis vaccine development. Clin Infect Dis 30:S254-256, 2000.

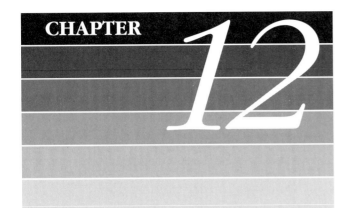

Interstitial Lung Diseases

BRIAN P. O'SULLIVAN, M.D.

The lungs consist of a fine, lacy network of parenchyma and blood vessels surrounding air spaces. The normal alveolar wall is extremely thin, in some places as little as 0.3 µm thick, allowing close approximation of red blood cells in the capillaries to air in the alveolar space (Figure 12-1). The surface area of the gas exchange apparatus in an adult is 50–100 m². The extremely thin, large surface area of the lung is possible due to the fact that 95% of epithelial lining cells are of the type 1 variety—cells which become attenuated and spread very thinly across the blood–air interface. The other 5% of epithelial lining cells are surfactant-producing type 2 cells. Fibroelastic tissue containing fibroblasts, collagen, and elastic fibers in combination with pulmonary capillaries makes up the rest of the alveolar wall (Figure 12-2). Under usual circumstances a red blood cell passing through the lung can become fully saturated with oxygen in just 0.25 seconds, approximately one-third of the time it spends in an alveolar capillary.

Interstitial lung disease (ILD) is the result of an insult to the lung, which leads to inflammation of the alveolar structures (alveolitis). With chronic inflammation there is increased production of fibroblasts and matrix-connective tissue components. The resultant fibrosis and increased cellularity lead to a thickened alveolar-capillary membrane, abnormal gas exchange, and decreased tissue elasticity. Clinically, these changes are expressed as hypoxemia and restrictive lung disease. Although evolution from stimulus to clinically apparent ILD sounds simple, it is likely that the true pattern of development of ILD is much more complex and involves repeated stimuli, environmental exposures in addition to the original insult, host genetic factors (e.g., inflammatory response, immune cell production, wound healing), and chance. Thus, it is impossible to predict who will develop ILD even in the familial forms (where the penetrance of ILD is far below 100%).

The term ILD comprises an amorphous class of pulmonary disease and can mean different things to different physicians. The most all-encompassing definition of ILD is that of a process which leads to thickening of alveolar septa and resultant interference with gas exchange and pulmonary mechanics. Many disease states lead to an end stage consisting of thickened alveolar walls, including rheumatologic disorders, inflammatory bowel disease, vasculitis, hematologic diseases, infection, and reaction to exogenous substances including allergens, medications, and illicit drugs. Most commonly, no inciting agent or disease is identified and the term idiopathic or cryptogenic is applied to the process.

Traditionally, internists think of the entities usual interstitial pneumonia (UIP) and desquamative interstitial pneumonia (DIP) when ILD is discussed. Included in this category is idiopathic pulmonary fibrosis (IPF), the

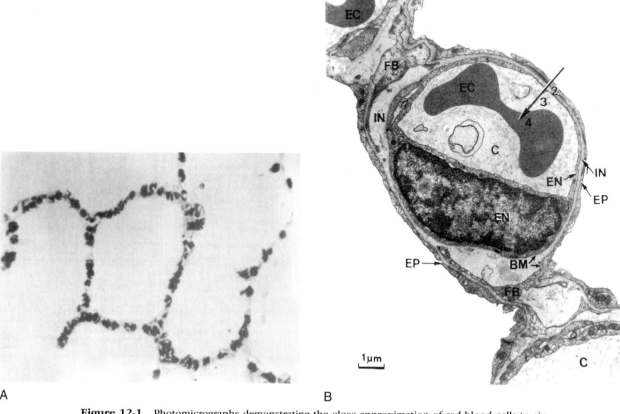

Figure 12-1   Photomicrographs demonstrating the close approximation of red blood cells to air in the lung. (**A**) Section of lung from a dog which was fixed while being perfused. Note that the capillary network forms a sheet of blood in contact with the alveolar air. (**B**) Electron micrograph showing the extremely thin blood–air barrier, as little as 0.3 μm in places. BM, basement membrane; C, capillary; EC, erythrocyte; EP, alveolar epithelium; EN, capillary endothelium; FB, fibroblasts; IN, interstitium. Large arrow shows the diffusion pathway across four layers: surfactant (not shown), cell membranes and interstitium, plasma, and red blood cell membrane. (Reproduced with permission from West JB. Respiratory physiology, the essentials. Philadelphia: Lippincott, Williams & Wilkins, 2000.)

clinical correlate to UIP[1-3]. A glossary of ILD terms appears in Table 12-1. Until recently, the pediatrician has had little information about pathophysiology or prognosis when the term ILD was used for his or her patient. Fortunately, this has changed dramatically over the last decade with multiple reports of myriad forms of ILD in patients under 21 years of age[4-10]. In fact, a field full of confusing and overlapping names with an alphabet-soup of abbreviations with which once only internists had to struggle has become a minefield for pediatricians, too[11].

A recent consensus statement from the American Thoracic Society and the European Thoracic Society has brought a semblance of order if not complete clarity to the confusing array of ILD classifications[1]. There is some overlap in conditions and rare reports of adult-type ILD in children; however, in many ways the idiopathic forms of ILD comprise two distinct entities in children and

Table 12-1 Glossary	
UIP	Usual interstitial pneumonia
DIP	Desquamative interstitial pneumonia
AIP	Acute interstitial pneumonia
NSIP	Non-specific interstitial pneumonia
LIP	Lymphocytic interstitial pneumonia
IPF	Idiopathic pulmonary fibrosis
RBILD	Respiratory bronchiolitis-associated interstitial lung disease
BOOP	Bronchiolitis obliterans with organizing pneumonia
PTI	Persistent tachypnea of infancy
PIG	Pulmonary interstitial glycogenosis
CPI	Chronic pneumonitis of infancy
CIP	Cellular interstitial pneumonia

A

B

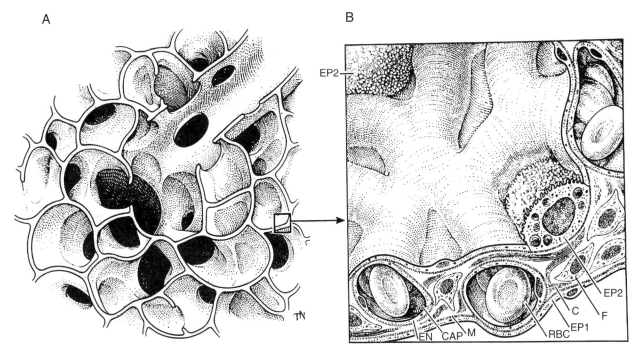

Figure 12-2 Line drawings depicting alveolar architecture. (**A**) Low-power rendering of a terminal bronchiole demonstrating the large surface area and lacy construction of the acinus. (**B**) Cut surface of the alveolar wall. The alveolar wall consists of many cell types, all of which may be involved in ILD. C, connective tissue; CAP, capillary; EP1, epithelial type 1 cell; EP2, epithelial type 2 cell; EN, endothelial cell; F, fibroblast; M, basement membrane; RBC, red blood cell. (Reproduced with permission from Crystal RG, Bitterman P, Rennard SI, Hance AJ, Keough BA. Interstitial lung diseases of unknown cause: disorders characterized by chronic inflammation of the lower respiratory tract. N Engl J Med 310:154–166, 1984.)

adults. Most adult forms of ILD occur later in life (rarely prior to age 50 years) and are associated with tobacco use. In contrast, pediatric ILDs not clearly associated with infection, drug toxicity, or systemic diseases tend to occur in the first months or years of life and are not related to tobacco smoke exposure.

It is important to review the adult entities, both due to their historical importance and because they are used as a basis for describing all ILD, adult and pediatric. This chapter will review the classical internal medicine concept of ILD, the recent revelations specific to pediatric ILD with an emphasis on the idiopathic forms, and a brief overview of secondary causes of ILD.

PRIMARY (IDIOPATHIC) INTERSTITIAL LUNG DISEASE IN ADULTS

Hamman and Rich described patients with an acute form of ILD in 1936, but it was not until the mid-1970s that Liebow offered the various classifications of ILD, a list of varieties of "interstitial pneumonias," which were to become used popularly[12]. Much time and energy has been expended on categorizing these entities in a

reliable and scientifically sound manner. This has proved important for research purposes, for providing prognostic information to patients, and for guiding therapy. Today's categories of adult ILD are very close to those Liebow originally proposed and include: UIP (the pathologic description of the clinical disease known as IPF), DIP, acute interstitial pneumonia (AIP, the disease Hamman and Rich originally described[13]), respiratory bronchiolitis-associated interstitial lung disease (RBILD), non-specific interstitial pneumonia (NSIP), bronchiolitis obliterans with organizing pneumonia (BOOP), and histiocytosis-X (Langerhan cell histiocytosis)[1,2].

Usual Interstitial Pneumonia/Idiopathic Pulmonary Fibrosis

IPF is a disease state typified by shortness of breath, bibasilar crackles, restrictive lung disease, impaired gas exchange with reduced diffusing capacity of carbon monoxide, evidence of diffuse infiltrates on plain radiograph and CT scan of the chest, and biopsy demonstrated inflammation, fibrosis, or both[1,2]. In these clinical, radiographic, and pulmonary function respects it is similar to all the ILDs. IPF is differentiated from the other ILDs by the pathologic changes of UIP seen on light microscopic evaluation of lung biopsy specimens. UIP is defined as consisting of heterogeneous pathologic changes with alternating areas of normal lung, interstitial inflammation, fibrosis, and honeycomb changes. There are scattered fibroelastic foci in fibrotic zones and the subpleural, peripheral parenchyma is most severely involved. Fibrotic areas characteristically vary in age and activity.

What stimulates the chronic inflammation and fibrosis seen in UIP is unclear but that the stimulus is on-going over a long period of time is evident by the chronicity of the disease and the variable stages of the pathologic changes seen on biopsy specimens. As with many disease states, IPF is likely caused by a superimposition of genetic susceptibility and environmental exposure. Up to 75% of patients with IPF have been found to be current or former cigarette smokers in large epidemiologic studies. In addition, latent viral infections have been implicated as causative agents. UIP/IPF is extremely uncommon in childhood, with two-thirds of patients greater than age 60 years and a median age of diagnosis of 66 years.

IPF is a progressive illness with median survival after the biopsy-proven diagnosis of UIP being only 3 years. Although anti-inflammatory and anti-fibrotic therapies have been used extensively there is still no good, proven therapy for IPF. Interferon gamma-1b decreases expression of genes for transforming growth factor beta and connective tissue growth factors in lung tissue and may blunt the chronic fibrosis seen in IPF. A report of immune modulation with interferon gamma-1b and low dose prednisolone showed some promise[14]. At this time IPF remains a poorly understood disease with a dismal prognosis.

Desquamative Interstitial Pneumonia

DIP is an uncommon disease even in the rarefied world of ILDs, accounting for less than 3% of all ILD. This disease is most commonly seen in cigarette smokers in their thirties and forties. The clinical signs and symptoms are similar to those of UIP but occur on a more subacute (weeks to months) rather than chronic scale. Pathologic examination of lung tissue shows a diffuse, uniform alveolar accumulation of macrophages with little fibrosis and only mild or moderate thickening of alveolar walls. DIP lacks the scarring and architectural remodeling seen in UIP[1,2].

The pathologic differences between DIP and UIP are striking, yet over the years many have contended that they are one illness with DIP representing the early, inflammatory stage of a disease process which progresses to the burned-out, fibrotic picture of UIP. Although initially appealing, there is insufficient evidence to support a theory of DIP and UIP lying at different ends of one disease spectrum. There are no biopsy-proven reports of DIP progressing to UIP and several reports of sequential biopsies in DIP patients showing no such progression. Similarly, no patients with early IPF/UIP show pathologic changes consistent with DIP. The differentiation between DIP and UIP is more than academic as DIP has a better response to steroid therapy and an overall survival rate of about 70% after 10 years as compared with the very poor prognosis with IPF/UIP.

Acute Interstitial Pneumonia

Louis Hamman and Arnold Rich described a small series of patients seen at Johns Hopkins University Hospital in reports published in 1935 and 1944[15]. These physicians used the term "acute diffuse interstitial fibrosis" to describe their findings. Today the so-called Hamman–Rich syndrome is more appropriately classified as AIP. Unfortunately, for many years the eponym has been used far too loosely to include many forms of acute and chronic ILD, further confusing the issues surrounding ILD nomenclature. The recent consensus statement report requires the presence of a clinical syndrome of acute respiratory distress syndrome (ARDS) in an idiopathic setting with biopsy confirmation of diffuse alveolar damage with organization in order to make the diagnosis of AIP[1]. As the name implies, this entity is rapid in onset and can be accompanied by fever, cough, and shortness of breath. Chest roentgenograms demonstrate bilateral airspace disease consistent with the underlying diffuse alveolar damage and mimicking ARDS. Mortality is high and there have been reports of survivors having progression to end-stage pulmonary fibrosis. Fortunately, in some cases there is complete healing and return to normal function.

Respiratory Bronchiolitis-Associated Interstitial Lung Disease

This syndrome is generally restricted to current or former cigarette smokers. The presentation of cough, increased work of breathing, and crackles is similar to that of other ILD patients. Patients with RBILD may have mixed obstructive and restrictive defects on pulmonary function testing. Biopsy demonstrates a bronchocentric distribution of luminal pigmented macrophages. Peribronchial fibrosis is seen, as is hyperplasia of type 2 pneumocytes. Cessation of cigarette smoking is the key to therapy for this disease.

Non-specific Interstitial Pneumonia

NSIP is manifested as varying degrees of inflammation and fibrosis that are uniformly distributed within the interstitium of the lung. This entity was first described by Katzenstein and Fiorelli[16] in 1994 in their report of a group of patients with ILD that did not fit readily into the previously described categories. NSIP is known to have a better prognosis than UIP and over the past decade has acquired defined characteristics recognizable on high-resolution CT scanning. The defining pathologic difference between NSIP and UIP is the lack of temporal heterogeneity in NSIP samples. That is, the pathologic changes are uniform in NSIP, all being in the same stage of evolution; whereas in UIP the pathologic changes are in variable stages. The key difference between NSIP and DIP is the paucity of alveolar macrophages seen in the former whereas such airspace debris is the hallmark of the latter (the so-called desquamation of cells into the alveoli). There appears to be a strong correlation between NSIP and connective tissue disorders, especially scleroderma and polymyositis.

Bronchiolitis Obliterans with Organizing Pneumonia

Idiopathic BOOP is seen in the fifth and sixth decades of life and is characterized by a peripheral distribution of opacities on chest X-ray films. Pathologically, BOOP consists of excessive proliferation of granulation tissue within small airways and alveolar ducts. There is chronic inflammation in the surrounding alveoli and buds of granulation tissue may spread from alveolus to alveolus through the pores of Köhn. The fibrosis tends to be of uniform age suggesting a specific, acute insult, in contrast to the heterogeneous changes seen in UIP/IPF. Clinically, BOOP may present similarly to UIP/IPF but some distinguishing features do exist. For example, due to its more acute presentation, clubbing is less common

in BOOP than in UIP/IPF. Unlike many of the ILDs, BOOP is responsive to steroid therapy with recovery in two-thirds of patients. Idiopathic BOOP is rarely seen in children and when it does occur it is in association with another systemic illness. In children, BOOP is most likely to be seen secondary to bone marrow transplant or infection. Figures 12-3 and 12-4 show radiographic studies and biopsy findings from an infant with systemic lupus erythematosus who developed BOOP.

Lymphoid Interstitial Pneumonia

In the adult population LIP is a disease associated with lymphoproliferative disorders, dysproteinemia, Sjögren syndrome, or viral infection (human immunodeficiency virus [HIV], Epstein–Barr virus [EBV]). Idiopathic LIP is felt to be very rare[17]. This disorder is characterized by monotonous polyclonal lymphoid cell infiltrates surrounding airways and expanding the lung interstitium. Viral-induced lymphoid proliferation leading to LIP is seen in some children with HIV or EBV infections. A related condition consisting of more localized follicles of lymphoid hyperplasia known as follicular bronchitis/bronchiolitis has been reported occasionally in adults and children. Pediatric LIP and follicular bronchiolitis are discussed below.

PEDIATRIC INTERSTITIAL LUNG DISEASES

ILD is not a common problem in children. Therefore, collecting data on a large cohort of patients diagnosed

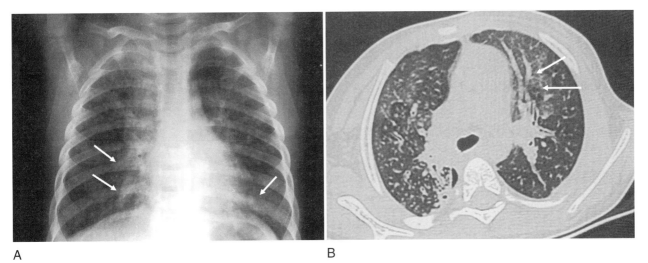

A   B

Figure 12-3   Chest X-ray film (**A**) and CT scan (**B**) from a 15-month-old child who had recurrent respiratory problems. This severe pneumonia was initially thought to be measles pneumonia due to a positive viral titer. This later proved to be a false-positive reaction and the child was found to have systemic lupus erythematosus (SLE) and bronchiolitis obliterans with organizing pneumonia (BOOP). Note the patchy alveolar infiltrates (small arrows) and ground-glass opacities (large arrows).

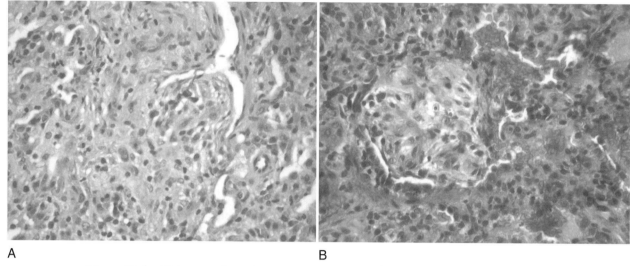

Figure 12-4 (**A**) An area of organizing pneumonia from child with BOOP secondary to SLE. Note the fibroblastic cells forming an airway plug at top center (hematoxylin and eosin, ×200). (**B**) Trichrome stain showing collagen deposition with a fibroblastic plug (Masson trichrome stain, ×200).

and treated in a uniform manner is difficult. The most comprehensive attempts to describe the pattern of primary (idiopathic) ILD in children have been by Fan and Langston in the United States and Nicholson, Bush, and colleagues in the United Kingdom.

The clinical presentation of ILD in childhood is similar to that in adults: shortness of breath, increased work of breathing, hypoxemia, tachypnea, and diffuse, fine, "Velcro-like" crackles. In addition, children with ILD often demonstrate the unique sign of failure to thrive. The age range for presentation of ILD can be from birth through adolescence, although in our experience younger children are more likely to have idiopathic ILD whereas older children tend to have ILD secondary to an underlying systemic disease or drug/toxin. The triad of failure to thrive, fine crackles, and hypoxemia in an infant is highly suggestive of ILD and is grounds for CT scan and lung biopsy once more common causes of chronic lung disease of infancy have been ruled out.

For many years lung biopsies from infants and children with ILD were described in terms of the adult categories listed above. This was unfortunate since the causative factors seen in adults (such as cigarette smoking) do not apply to children and the prognoses of many of the childhood ILDs are clearly different from those of the adult forms. In addition, whatever insult that causes ILD is also superimposed on lung development in children, an issue not relevant to adult pathologies. More recently, a number of separate entities seemingly unique to pediatric patients have been described. These new categories of ILD render the previously used adult classification system obsolete and allow for a more systematic gathering of information regarding ILD in children. Fan and Langston have proposed several variants of the adult

schema[7,9] whereas Nicholson et al.[18] prefer to classify pediatric ILD according to the defined adult histopathologic patterns. The latter investigators ignore the newer designations of pediatric ILD such as cellular interstitial pneumonitis (CIP), persistent tachypnea of infancy (PTI), and pulmonary interstitial glycogenosis, and lump most children into the categories of LIP or NSIP. Placing a majority of the childhood ILDs into a category (NSIP) which even those who use the adult system recognize as a place-holder until more definitive diagnoses come to light does not seem fruitful. It is more beneficial for pediatric pulmonologists and pathologists to modify the category of NSIP by breaking it into component parts.

Pediatric ILDs as defined by Fan and Langston include chronic pneumonitis of infancy (CPI), cellular interstitial pneumonia (CIP), persistent tachypnea of infancy with neuroendocrine cell hyperplasia (PTI), pulmonary interstitial glycogenosis (which may simply be a better histologic description of CIP), and surfactant protein deficiencies[7,9]. Of note is the tremendous overlap between the surfactant protein deficiencies and the other categories of ILD in infancy and childhood. A growing number of studies implicate surfactant protein (SP)-B and C gene mutations in a variety of adult ILDs (UIP, DIP, NSIP) and pediatric ILDs (CIP, CPI)[19-24]. The following sections will focus on the various classes of pediatric ILDs, but it should be kept in mind that despite the histologic differences seen, it is possible that surfactant protein dysfunction plays a role in the pathogenesis of many of them.

Chronic Pneumonitis of Infancy (CPI)

First described by Katzenstein et al.[25] in 1995, CPI is characterized by marked alveolar septal thickening, hyperplasia of type 2 pneumocytes and an alveolar exudate containing macrophages and eosinophilic debris. Although inflammatory cells are not commonly seen, Katzenstein et al. felt that this histologic picture best reflected slowly resolving pneumonia in immature lungs. Children with CPI present early in life; symptoms may begin as early as 2 weeks of age and virtually all infants with CPI have symptoms by 1 year of age. Presenting symptoms are non-specific and typical for a child with chronic lung disease: cough, respiratory distress, and failure to thrive. Outcome was not good in the original cohort. Of 8 patients described 4 died, 1 underwent lung transplantation, and 3 had residual severe respiratory impairment. Non-surgical therapy included corticosteroids and hydroxychloroquine, neither of which produced dramatic results.

More recently, the marked type 2 pneumocyte hyperplasia seen in CPI has led some to question if it is a form of congenital SP-C dysfunction and not the result of an infectious disease. This is supported by the familial nature of the illness in 2 of the 8 originally described cases.

Cellular Interstitial Pneumonia (CIP)

CIP presents with respiratory distress, tachypnea, "Velcro-like" crackles on examination, and hypoxemia. Schroeder et al.[26] noted that symptoms generally present in the first few days of life. In fact, our experience has been that children with CIP may be initially diagnosed as having transient tachypnea of the newborn only to have that diagnosis rescinded when it becomes apparent that the tachypnea is not at all transient.

Chest radiographs show a bilateral, diffuse interstitial pattern and CT scans confirm these finding (Figure 12-5). We have found this presentation so uniform and compelling that we move quickly to lung biopsy to confirm

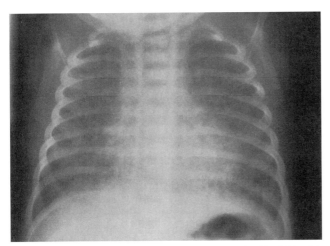

Figure 12-5   Chest radiograph from a 1-month-old child with cellular interstitial pneumonia (CIP). There is a diffuse increase in interstitial markings without focal infiltrates.

the diagnosis in children presenting in this manner. Obviously, other causes of tachypnea and cough in the newborn such as cystic fibrosis, aspiration, tracheoesophageal fistula, and neonatal infection must be ruled out before proceeding to biopsy.

Lung biopsies in children with CIP show a diffuse interstitial process occupying the intra-alveolar septa (Figure 12-6). The infiltrate is comprised mostly of histiocytes but lymphocytes are also present. Spindle-shaped histiocytes in the interstitium are common. Generally, there is no increase in collagen and no fibrosis, and type 2 pneumocytes are not hyperplastic; this is in marked contrast to findings in CPI.

The prognosis in CIP is quite good. Children with this process respond to oral corticosteroids and/or hydroxychloroquine and we have even had success with inhaled corticosteroids in one case (unpublished). Because of the small number of known cases and reports of the use of non-randomized, anecdotal therapy regimens it is unclear whether the primary therapy for CIP should be steroids, hydroxychloroquine or supportive care awaiting spontaneous resolution of the disease. Although there is no definitive therapy, most pediatric pulmonologists do treat these infants with anti-inflammatory drugs and most children show improvement over the first few years of life.

Pulmonary Interstitial Glycogenosis (PIG)

A variant of neonatal ILD called pulmonary interstitial glycogenosis (PIG) has been described by Canakis et al.[27]. There is much in common between PIG and CIP including presentation very early in life, interstitial changes on chest radiographs, and expansion of the interstitium with spindle-shaped histiocytes. Canakis et al. also found glycogen in cells in the interalveolar septa (Figure 12-7). Since this is not normally present in these cells, the authors postulated a developmental abnormality in differentiation of mesenchymal cells. The light microscopic and clinical findings are very similar when comparing PIG and CIP. However, since Schroeder et al. did not look for glycogen in biopsies from their patients with CIP it is unknown whether these two entities are one-and-the-same or are two separate diseases. It is not surprising that the children with PIG showed the same good response to corticosteroids and hydroxychloroquine as seen in CIP. Further studies on both existing and newly diagnosed cases of CIP and PIG will need to be done to determine whether these are two distinct classes of ILD or two descriptions of one entity.

Persistent Tachypnea of Infancy (PTI)

Another of the milder forms of ILD in infants is persistent tachypnea of infancy (PTI)[28]. Patients with PTI do

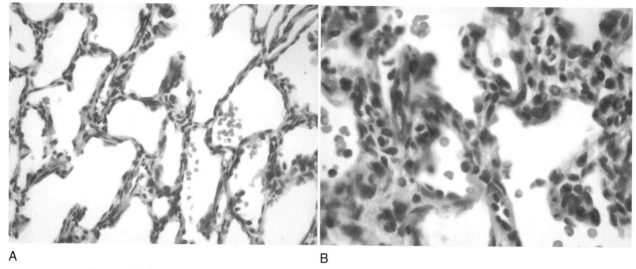

Figure 12-6 Histology of CIP. (**A**) Hypercellularity of alveolar walls is evident. (**B**) Higher magnification demonstrates the presence of histiocytes and spindle-shaped cells in the alveolar septa (hematoxylin and eosin).

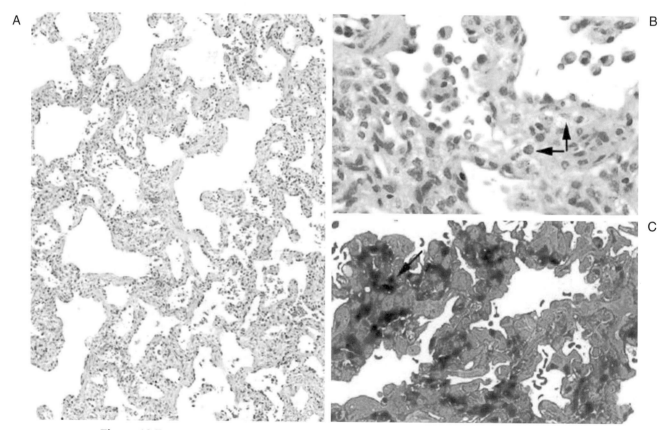

Figure 12-7 Histologic picture of pulmonary interstitial glycogenosis from a 3-month-old infant. (**A**) Diffuse interstitial thickening. (**B**) Higher-magnification view of interalveolar septa. Arrows demonstrate round and spindle-shaped cells with pale cytoplasm. (**C**) Periodic acid–Schiff stain shows massive amounts of glycogen (arrow). (Reproduced with permission from Canakis AM, et al. Pulmonary interstitial glycogenosis. Am J Respir Crit Care Med 165:1557–1565, 2002.)

not have significant cough but do have marked tachypnea, retractions, crackles, and hypoxemia presenting in the first year of life. Hyperinflation and increased interstitial markings are seen on chest X-ray films. Lung biopsy demonstrates mild increase in airway smooth muscle, increased alveolar macrophages, and increased epithelial cells within the distal airways, which are neuroendocrine in origin. Children with this disorder do not have a striking response to corticosteroid therapy but do show mild improvement over time. Supplemental oxygen may be required for months to years.

Follicular Bronchiolitis (FB)

Follicular bronchiolitis is another milder form of ILD, which has been described in adults and children[29,30]. FB presents similarly to CIP and PTI with tachypnea, crackles, and diffuse interstitial findings on chest imaging studies. Histologically, FB is characterized by lymphoid proliferation resulting in hyperplastic follicles of bronchus-associated lymphoid tissue that compress the small intrathoracic airways. FB generally presents in the first 2 months of life and then slowly resolves over the next 2-4 years, although older children may be left with mild obstructive disease. FB does not appear to be responsive to steroid therapy.

Lymphocytic Interstitial Pneumonia (LIP)

LIP in childhood is most frequently seen in combination with HIV/AIDS[17]. LIP was seen commonly in the 1980s prior to the advent of highly active anti-retroviral therapy (HAART) for children with HIV infections. Histologically, LIP in children is essentially the same as in adults. The hallmark of LIP is a monotonous polyclonal lymphocytic infiltration of the interalveolar septa. The incidence of LIP is markedly lower in the era of HAART therapy for HIV infection, but LIP must still be considered in the differential diagnoses of unexplained respiratory disease in a child with AIDS. Other viruses can lead to a lymphocytic infiltration of alveolar walls and case reports exist of infants and young children with EBV-associated LIP[31]. Figure 12-8 shows the histologic changes seen in a teenage girl with LIP caused by EBV infection. This child presented with a sub-acute history of fever, night sweats, and increasing shortness of breath. Therapy with corticosteroids (without anti-viral agents) proved beneficial.

Surfactant Protein Diseases

Although they comprise a relatively small percentage of the entire surfactant moiety, surfactant proteins B and C (SP-B, SP-C) play a vital role in the spreading, adsorption, and stability of surfactant[19,20]. These small proteins

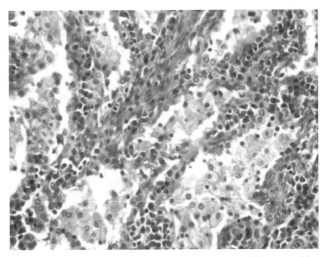

Figure 12-8 Lymphoid interstitial pneumonia (LIP) caused by Epstein–Barr virus infection. The interstitium is expanded and filled with lymphocytes and occasional plasma cells. Normal lung architecture is completely lost. Lymphocyte marker studies showed polyclonality, typical of LIP and inconsistent with tumor.

(SP-B is 79 amino acids long and SP-C is 33-34 amino acids long) are necessary for normal surfactant function and consequent alveolar integrity. Lack of pulmonary surfactant due to prematurity, aspiration, lung injury, or mutations in surfactant genes causes respiratory failure.

Knock-out mice lacking the SP-B gene develop respiratory failure immediately after birth. Analogously, there are reports of infants homozygous for a mutation in SP-B production who have respiratory failure unresponsive to standard therapies including exogenous surfactant administration. Infants with these mutations present in respiratory distress in the first 24–48 hours of life with clinical findings consistent with surfactant deficiency. SP-B deficiency is generally inherited as an autosomal recessive mutation and carriers of one mutation do not have clinically apparent lung disease. Although complete SP-B deficiency is associated with respiratory failure and death in the newborn period, uncommon mutations which cause a partial deficiency have been associated with chronic ILD in childhood[21]. Histologically such disorders may show accumulation of extracellular proteins, epithelial cell dysplasia, and pulmonary fibrosis.

SP-C is a very highly hydrophobic protein and accounts for about 4% of surfactant by weight. It enhances the spreading and stability of surfactant phospholipids. It may also play a role in routing, processing, and trafficking of other proteins. Light and electron microscopy from patients with SP-C deficiency shows atypia and hyperplasia of alveolar type 2 cells with numerous abnormal lamellar bodies and thickened alveoli. An inflammatory hypercellularity consisting of lymphocytes, plasma cells and peribronchial lymphoid aggregates may be seen. Therapy for SP-C deficiency is not standardized at present.

There have been reports of success with both oral steroids and hydroxychloroquine in adults and children with SP-C deficiency.

Mutations in the SP-C gene have been linked to familial forms of ILD[22-24]. Interestingly, adults and children in these kindreds have carried a variety of diagnoses, not necessarily consistent within one family. The fact that people with abnormalities in SP-C production have variously been said to have UIP, DIP, NSIP, LIP, and CIP leads to the obvious question: Are surfactant protein deficiencies the common cause of many "idiopathic" ILDs? Amin et al.[22] reported a kindred with SP-C deficiency including three affected members said to have NSIP, IPF, and LIP. In this study, the investigators looked at surfactant proteins in bronchoalveolar lavage (BAL) fluid and used older adults with IPF as a control group. Although all three family members had low levels of SP-C in BAL fluid, the IPF patients in the control group all had normal amounts of surfactant proteins in BAL fluid. Clearly, then, SP-C deficiency does not account for all cases of ILD. However, the idea that many forms of ILD currently considered disparate may in fact be related at a molecular level is tantalizing.

Diagnosis and Treatment of ILD

Children with ILD present with a constellation of signs and symptoms generally including shortness of breath, dyspnea with exercise (which in the very young infant may mean dyspnea with feeding), hypoxemia, tachypnea, retractions, and crackles on auscultation (Table 12-2). The majority of children with idiopathic ILD present in the first year of life[4,32] and in these infantile forms tachypnea is the most common presenting symptom with crackles the most common auscultatory finding. Babies with ILD often have low pulse oximetry, too, but in milder cases normoxia can be maintained at rest. Since the amount of time the red blood cell spends in the pulmonary capillary is crucial for oxygenation in interstitial diseases, anything that increases red cell transit time (i.e., increased cardiac output) can unmask hypoxemia that is not evident at rest (Figure 12-9). In our clinic we often have older children walk or run up and down a corridor and monitor pulse oximetry during exercise. Infants have pulse oximetry monitored while feeding.

The crackles in children with ILD tend to be diffuse, fine and "Velcro-like" in nature. Any child with tachypnea and crackles should be suspected of having ILD although cystic fibrosis, aspiration due to swallowing dysfunction or gastroesophageal reflux disease, and cardiac disease are more common causes of these symptoms. A chest roentgenogram should be obtained in order to look for increased interstitial markings. Plain chest X-ray films are not as sensitive as CT scans; a normal chest radiograph does not rule out the diagnosis of ILD. A CT scan of the chest should be obtained in any child for whom the diagnosis is suspected. In virtually all cases where interstitial disease is seen on the CT scan a lung biopsy will be needed to make an accurate diagnosis. It is important to get an adequate sample of tissue for all the tests that may need to be performed, including electron microscopy, standard light microscopy stains, stains for fibrin and collagen, and stains for hemosiderin and lipid-laden macrophages, exhaustive microbiology studies, and flow cytometry. Thus, the small sample obtained by

Table 12-2 Clinical Presentation of ILD	
Cough	77%
Dyspnea	71%
Exercise intolerance	65%
Crackles	60%
Tachypnea	54%
Onset of symptoms in first year of life	50%
Retractions	46%
Frequent respiratory tract infections	44%
Wheeze	40%
Failure to thrive	35%
Clubbing	29%
Cyanosis	19%

(From Fan and Langston[4] and Fan et al.[5])

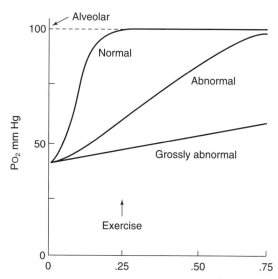

Figure 12-9   Oxygenation of blood as it passes through a pulmonary capillary when diffusion is normal or abnormal. When blood spends a full 0.75 seconds in the capillary PO_2 may be normal even if diffusion is decreased by an interstitial disease. However, under conditions that increase cardiac output (exercise), blood PO_2 cannot reach normal levels in the diseased lung. Normal PO_2 cannot be achieved even at rest in the grossly abnormal lung. (Reproduced with permission from West JB. Respiratory physiology, the essentials. Philadelphia: Lippincott, Williams & Wilkins, 2000.)

transbronchial biopsy is not adequate and open or thoracoscopic biopsy is necessary. Making a specific diagnosis has therapeutic and diagnostic implications and should be pursued vigorously. Of particular importance is ruling out non-idiopathic and treatable causes of ILD such as infection, aspiration, or rheumatoid disease. Blood tests for defects in the surfactant protein genes are available on a research basis. Even with a biopsy, however, a large percentage of cases cannot be neatly placed into one of the previously mentioned ILD categories.

Treatment of idiopathic ILD depends in part on which form of the disease one is dealing with. CIP responds well to steroids and hydroxychloroquine, but FB does not. LIP may require therapy with steroids and acyclovir if secondary to EBV infection. Surfactant protein deficiencies do not have specific therapies at present. Corticosteroids (2 mg/kg/day initially) remain the mainstay of therapy for many of the ILDs. Unfortunately, therapy may need to be continued for prolonged periods of time (months or more) leading to undesirable side effects. Intravenous pulse therapy with methylprednisolone is an alternative way to treat ILD. High doses of steroids are given at monthly intervals, generally 10–30 mg/kg up to a maximum of 1 g, for at least 3 months. After this initial therapy, pulses can be used intermittently for flares of the disease or continued monthly as needed. Pulse therapy has the advantage of limiting steroid-related side effects but requires monthly intravenous infusions for 3 days. Placement of an indwelling central catheter for children needing long-term therapy allows for home therapy.

Hydroxychloroquine (10 mg/kg/day) alone or in combination with steroids has significant efficacy for some children with ILD and can act as a steroid sparing agent. Hydroxychloroquine can cause retinal problems and children receiving it must have periodic ophthalmologic examinations. As opposed to adult ILDs, therapy with steroids or hydroxychloroquine, singly or in combination, can lead to excellent outcome in infants with ILD[32]. Other drugs used in the therapy of ILD include cyclophosphamide, azathioprine, and methotrexate.

Secondary Forms of ILD

A variety of other diseases and chemical exposures (including medications) can lead to lung disease consisting of interstitial changes and abnormalities in gas exchange. A full discussion of these diseases is beyond the scope of this chapter, but a partial list of diseases and chemical agents which can cause ILD are included in Tables 12-3 and 12-4. The non-pulmonary diseases most commonly associated with ILD are inflammatory in nature (e.g., vasculitis, rheumatoid diseases, inflammatory bowel disease) or cardiac diseases which lead to pulmonary venous engorgement. In addition, many

Table 12-3   Causes of Secondary Interstitial Lung Diseases

Collagen vascular diseases
   Systemic lupus erythematosus
   Juvenile rheumatoid arthritis
   Sjögren syndrome
Vasculitis
   Pulmonary renal syndromes
     Wegener's granulomatosis
     Systemic lupus erythematosus
     Goodpasture syndrome
Cardiovascular disorders
   Total or partial anomalous pulmonary venous return
   Cor triatriatum
   Hereditary hemorrhagic telangiectasia
Inflammatory bowel disease
Aspiration syndromes
   Swallowing dysfunction
   Gastroesophageal reflux disease
   Tracheo-esophageal fistula
   Lipid aspiration (lipoid pneumonia)
Infections
   Epstein–Barr virus
   HIV
   Mycoplasma
   Immunoglobulin G-subclass deficiency
Other
   Dust/sand inhalation (chronic)
   Neurofibromatosis
   Sarcoidosis
   Tuberous sclerosis

drugs can cause ILD although relatively few are used in otherwise well children.

Cardiac disease that causes pulmonary vascular problems represents up to 9% of children originally felt to have ILD[33]. Occlusion of return of pulmonary blood flow to the left atrium leads to pulmonary venous congestion and interstitial changes. The most common cause of this problem is total or partial anomalous pulmonary venous return. Cor triatriatum, in which there is a fibromuscular membrane which subdivides the left atrium into a

Table 12-4   Partial List of Drugs Reported to Cause ILD

Amiodarone	Gold
Actinomycin D	Methotrexate
Bleomycin	Mitomycin
Busulfan	Nitrofuantoin
Cephalosporins	Penicillamine
Chlorambucil	Phenytoin
Cyclophosphamide	Sulfamethoxazole
Docetaxel	Sulfasalazine

posterosuperior chamber that receives blood from the pulmonary veins and an anteroinferior chamber which is the true left atrium, also leads to increased pulmonary vascular pressures and interstitial changes[34]. Cor triatriatum should be considered in any child with unexplained tachypnea. Diffuse pulmonary vascular malformations such as hereditary hemorrhagic telangiectasia may also mimic ILD.

Inflammatory bowel disease can be seen in association with BOOP or granulomatous lung disease[35,36]. The vasculitides which cause pulmonary-renal syndrome (Goodpasture syndrome, Wegener's granulomatosis, systemic lupus erythematosus [SLE]) often present with acute pulmonary hemorrhage[37]. However, the earliest lung changes can consist of interstitial granuloma formation and a picture clinically indistinguishable from some forms of ILDs.

Finally, chronic aspiration and infection can lead to ILD-like changes in the pulmonary parenchyma. Children suspected of having ILD should be evaluated for cystic fibrosis, swallowing dysfunction, gastroesophageal reflux disease, and immune defects prior to undergoing lung biopsy[38].

SUMMARY

Interstitial lung disease is an uncommon problem in pediatrics. There are a large number of sub-classes of ILD; the current classification schemes are cumbersome and at times confusing with inconsistent use of adult and pediatric categories. Because these diseases are rare and ill-defined, tissue diagnosis is necessary in most cases. Although the early literature portrayed these diseases as having poor prognosis, more recent studies demonstrate that in some forms of ILD the outlook is quite good with therapy and occasionally even without therapy.

MAJOR POINTS

1. Pediatric interstitial lung diseases consist of a diffuse group of diseases which are distinct from the adult forms of ILD.
2. Any child with tachypnea, crackles, and hypoxemia should be evaluated for ILD.
3. The prognosis in pediatric ILD is better than in the adult form of the disease.
4. Therapy consists of supportive care and anti-inflammatory drugs.
5. Surfactant protein defects may underlie many of the ILDs.

REFERENCES

1. Katzenstein ALA, Myers JL. Idiopathic pulmonary fibrosis: clinical relevance of pathologic classification. Am J Respir Crit Care Med 157:1301-1315, 1998.
2. Gross TJ, Hunninghake GW. Idiopathic pulmonary fibrosis. N Engl J Med 345:517-525, 2001.
3. King TE Jr., et al. Idiopathic pulmonary fibrosis: diagnosis and treatment. Am J Respir Crit Care Med 161:646-664, 2000.
4. Fan LL, Langston C. Chronic interstitial lung disease in children. Pediatr Pulmonol 16:184-196, 1993.
5. Fan LL, et al. Clinical spectrum of chronic interstitial lung disease in children. J Pediatr 121:867-872, 1992.
6. Dinwiddie R, Sharief N, Crawford O. Idiopathic interstitial pneumonitis in children: a national survey in the United Kingdom and Ireland. Pediatr Pulmonol 34:23-29, 2002.
7. Fan LL, Langston C. Pediatric interstitial lung disease: children are not small adults. Am J Respir Crit Care Med 165:1466-1467, 2002.
8. Langston C, Fan LL. The spectrum of interstitial lung disease in childhood. Pediatr Pulmonol Suppl 23:70-71, 2001.
9. Langston C, Fan LL. Diffuse interstitial lung disease in infants. Pediatr Pulmonol Suppl 23:74-76, 2001.
10. Fan LL, et al. Evaluation of a diagnostic approach to pediatric interstitial lung disease. Pediatrics 101:82-85, 1998.
11. Nicholson AG. Classification of idiopathic interstitial pneumonias: making sense of the alphabet soup. Histopathology 41:381-391, 2002.
12. Liebow AA. Definition and classification of interstitial pneumonias in human pathology. Prog Respir Res 8:1-31, 1975.
13. Olson J, Colby TV, Elliott CG. Hamman-Rich syndrome revisited. Mayo Clin Proc 65:1538-1548, 1990.
14. Ziesche R, et al. A preliminary study of long term treatment with interferon gamma-1b and low dose prednisolone in patients with idiopathic pulmonary fibrosis. N Engl J Med 341:1264-1269, 1999.
15. Askin FB. Back to the future: the Hamman-Rich syndrome and acute interstitial pneumonia. Mayo Clin Proc 65:1624-1626, 1990.
16. Katzenstein ALA, Fiorelli RF. Nonspecific interstitial pneumonia/fibrosis: histologic features and clinical significance. Am J Surg Pathol 18:136-147, 1994.
17. Swigris JJ, et al. Lymphoid interstitial pneumonia: a narrative review. Chest 122:2150-2164, 2002.
18. Nicholson AG, et al. The value of classifying interstitial pneumonia in childhood according to defined histologic patterns. Histopathology 33:203-211, 1998.
19. Whitsett JA. Genetic basis of familial interstitial lung disease: misfolding or function of surfactant protein C. Am J Respir Crit Care Med 165:1201-1204, 2002.
20. Whitsett JA, Weaver TE. Hydrophobic surfactant proteins in lung function and disease. N Engl J Med 347:2141-2148, 2002.

21. Nogee, LM, et al. Allelic heterogeneity in hereditary surfactant B (SP-B) deficiency. Am J Respir Crit Care Med 161:973–981, 2000.

22. Amin RS, et al. Surfactant protein deficiency in familial interstitial lung disease. J Pediatr 139:85–92, 2001.

23. Nogee LM, et al. A mutation in the surfactant protein C gene associated with familial interstitial lung disease. N Engl J Med 344:573–579, 2001.

24. Thomas AQ, et al. Heterozygosity for a surfactant protein-C gene mutation associated with usual interstitial pneumonitis in one kindred. Am J Respir Crit Care Med 165:1322–1328, 2002.

25. Katzenstein ALA, et al. Chronic pneumonitis of infancy. Am J Surg Pathol 19:439–447, 1995.

26. Schroeder SA, Shannon DC, Mark EJ. Cellular interstitial pneumonitis in infants: a clinicopathologic study. Chest 101:1065–1069, 1992.

27. Canakis AM, et al. Pulmonary interstitial glycogenosis. Am J Respir Crit Care Med 165:1557–1565, 2002.

28. Deterding RR, et al. Persistent tachypnea of infancy (PTI)—a new entity. Pediatr Pulmonol Suppl 23:72–73, 2001.

29. Kinane TB, et al. Follicular bronchitis in the pediatric population. Chest 104:1183–1186, 1993.

30. Howling SJ, et al. Follicular bronchiolitis: thin-section CT and histologic findings. Radiology 212:637–642, 1999.

31. Mueller GA, Pickoff AS. Pediatric lymphocytic interstitial pneumonitis in an HIV-negative child with pulmonary Epstein–Barr virus infection. Pediatr Pulmonol 36:447–449, 2003.

32. Dinwidie R, Sharief N, Crawford O. Idiopathic interstitial pneumonitis in children: a national survey in the United Kingdom and Ireland. Pediatr Pulmonol 34:23–29, 2002.

33. Sondheimer HM, et al. Pulmonary vascular disorders masquerading as interstitial lung disease. Pediatr Pulmonol 20:284–288, 1995.

34. Howowitz MD, et al. Cor triatriatum in adults. Am Hear J 126:472–474, 1993.

35. Camus P, et al. The lung in inflammatory bowel disease. Medicine 72:151–183, 1993.

36. Al-Binali AM, et al. Granulomatous pulmonary disease in a child: an unusual presentation of Crohn's disease. Pediatr Pulmonol 36:76–80, 2003.

37. O'Sullivan BP, Erickson LA, Niles JL. Case records of the Massachusetts General Hospital: Case 30-2002. N Engl J Med 347:1009–1017, 2002.

38. Popa V, Colby TV, Reich SB. Pulmonary interstitial disease in Ig deficiency. Chest 122:1594–1603, 2002.

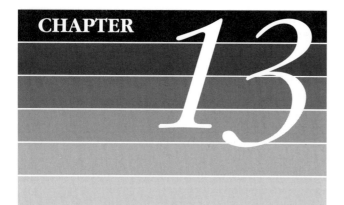

CHAPTER 13

Pulmonary Complications of Neuromuscular Disease

JULIAN L. ALLEN, M.D.

Pulmonary complications are common in pediatric neuromuscular diseases, and represent the leading cause of death in many of them. These complications are preventable and treatable, however, and aggressive diagnosis and treatment can in many cases increase life expectancy. Pulmonary complications often arise from final pathways common to neuromuscular diseases as a whole, although certain complications are unique to various disorders. This chapter will summarize the major characteristics of neuromuscular diseases likely to lead to pulmonary disorders, discuss the physiology and pathophysiology of how such pulmonary complications arise, and discuss an approach to their evaluation, prevention and treatment.

COMMON NEUROMUSCULAR DISEASES OF CHILDHOOD AND ADOLESCENCE

Upper Versus Lower Motor Neuron Disease

Neuromuscular disorders can broadly be divided into diseases that affect the muscle, the lower motor neuron, and the upper motor neuron (Figure 13-1). Diseases that affect the muscle and the lower motor neuron usually lead to flaccid and hypotonic muscles (with certain exceptions, e.g., myotonic dystrophy) and diminished deep tendon reflexes. Diseases that affect the upper motor neuron usually lead to hypertonic muscles and hyperactive deep tendon reflexes due to release of inhibitory impulses from the upper motor neuron. Both disorders lead to muscle weakness on voluntary contraction.

Lower Motor Neuron Diseases

Muscular Dystrophies

Muscular dystrophies are characterized by progressive muscular weakness starting in infancy or childhood. Duchenne muscular dystrophy (MD) is the second most frequent lethal genetic disorder in humans, has an incidence of 1:3500 male births, with a carrier frequency of 1 in 2000, and is inherited as an X-linked recessive disease. New mutations in the dystrophin gene account for 30% of cases. Boys with Duchenne MD typically present as toddlers with mild muscle weakness, waddling, and frequent falling. They gradually lose motor milestones so that by the time they are in elementary school they often need braces and by middle school, progress to needing wheelchairs. Pseudohypertrophy, especially of the calf

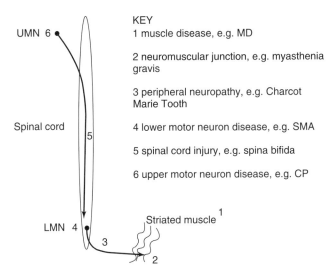

Figure 13-1 Upper motor neuron (UMN) and lower motor neuron (LMN) diseases: site of lesion.

muscles, and an elevated CPK are highly suggestive of this disorder. Mean age of death is 20 years, usually from progressive cardiac or respiratory disease. Duchenne MD is a multisystem disorder, causing a skeletal myopathy, encephalopathy with behavioral disorders and cognitive defects, cardiomyopathy, and dysfunction of the smooth muscle of the vessels and gastrointestinal tract. The disease is caused by mutations in the dystrophin gene at the Xp21 locus. Diagnosis can be made by muscle biopsy or DNA mutation analysis. Becker MD presents in a similar fashion to Duchenne MD, and is caused by a different deletion of the same gene, but is generally milder and presents later. While the mean age at which patients with Duchenne MD become wheelchair-dependent is 11 years, patients with Becker MD remain ambulatory until age 16 years. Treatment with prednisone may delay the age at which these patients become wheelchair-dependent.

Table 13-1 lists the other various common muscular dystrophies. Limb girdle MD can present as an autosomal dominant, an autosomal recessive or an X-linked disorder. Myotonic dystrophy is characterized by distal weakness, inability to relax muscle contractions, and premature aging and anesthetic deaths. Its mode of inheritance is autosomal dominant. Congenital myotonic dystrophy presents in a biphasic fashion, characterized by poor suck and respiratory effort, but transient improvement after the neonatal period. Other congenital myopathies include nemaline myopathy, central core disease and centronuclear myopathy. Nemaline myopathy is characterized by variable onset and severity, ptosis, bulbar weakness, sleep hypoventilation, and autosomal dominant or recessive inheritance. Central core disease can present with malignant hyperthermia.

Myasthenia Gravis

Myasthenia gravis presents in an acquired, immune-mediated form, with circulating antibodies to the acetylcholine receptor on striated muscle. A congenital myasthenic syndrome also exists, caused by maternal antibodies. Myasthenic disorders are characterized by ptosis, ophthalmoparesis, bulbar weakness causing aspiration, and limb girdle weakness. They may be episodic.

Table 13-1 Common Muscular Dystrophies of Childhood
Duchenne muscular dystrophy
Becker muscular dystrophy
Fascioscapulohumeral dystrophy
Limb girdle muscular dystrophy
Congenital muscular dystrophy
Emery–Dreyfuss muscular dystrophy
Myotonic dystrophy

Diagnostic characteristics include increasing fatigue with repetitive stimulation and improved strength with edrophonium (tensilon). Treatment includes immune suppression and thymectomy.

Charcot Marie Tooth Disease

Charcot Marie Tooth disease presents with a distal neuropathy, characteristically affecting the peroneal nerve, and resulting in pes cavus and foot drop. Bulbar neuropathy can rarely occur. Characteristic changes are seen on the electromyogram (EMG) and nerve conduction velocity studies.

Spinal Muscular Atrophy

Spinal muscular atrophy is the most common fatal neuromuscular disease of infancy with an incidence of 1:18,000 to 25,000. It is inherited as an autosomal recessive disorder, and its gene has been localized to chromosome 5q11-q13. Two candidate genes have been cloned: the survival motor neuron genes SMN1 and SMN2, and the neuronal apoptosis inhibitory protein (NAIP) gene. SMA is a genetic disease of the anterior horn cell causing degeneration of the alpha motor neuron. Diagnosis is commonly made by muscle biopsy and EMG; CPK levels are normal. The most common form, Type I SMA (Werdnig–Hoffman disease) has its onset before 6 months of age. Infants present with floppiness, weak cry, and feeding and breathing problems; they cannot sit and often they are noted to have diminished fetal movements in utero. Type I SMA is rapidly progressive, and infants usually die in the first 2 years of life without ventilatory support of some kind. Type III SMA (Kugelberg–Welander disease) presents later in life, frequently in the second or third year, and is more slowly progressive, with patients frequently able to walk and to live beyond the third decade. These children present with gait disturbances, scoliosis and muscle fasciculations. Type II SMA has an intermediate course between Types I and III; patients can sit but not walk alone, and with medical intervention frequently survive to the second or third decade.

Combined Upper and Lower Motor Neuron Diseases

Spinal cord lesions can cause upper motor neuron injury to the nerves passing through the long tracts at the level of the lesion, and lower motor neuron injury at the level of the injury itself.

Spina Bifida

Spina bifida with meningomyelocele is a congenital disorder which can affect any spinal level. It is one of the most common developmental disorders of the central nervous system, with an incidence of 0.2–0.4/1000 live births. It most commonly affects the lumbosacral spine, and can be associated with Arnold–Chiari malformation of the brainstem. The higher the level of spinal involvement, the more likely it is to affect the muscles of respiration. Urinary retention and constipation in these patients can cause significant abdominal distension and worsen a pulmonary restrictive defect by pushing up on the diaphragms.

Spinal Cord Injury

Spinal cord injury resulting from trauma that causes vertebral fractures, crush or compression injuries can occur at any level. Lesions from C3 to C5, resulting in tetraplegia, affect diaphragmatic function by interrupting phrenic nerve traffic and also affect the intercostal muscles whose innervation is below the level of the lesion (T1–T12). Lesions between T1 and T12 result in progressively less severe respiratory muscle weakness, as the lesion level is lowered and the motor injury converts from tetraplegia to paraplegia. These patients can have impaired cough mechanisms, however, since the innervation of the expiratory abdominal muscles arises from T5 to L1. Lesions below T12, resulting in paraplegia, have little effect on the respiratory muscles or those involved in the cough reflex.

Upper Motor Neuron Diseases

Cerebral Palsy

Cerebral palsy results from a wide range of neonatal brain insults. It is more common in infants born prematurely with complicated neonatal courses, and can be a consequence of periventricular leukomalacia or intraventricular hemorrhage, especially of the more severe varieties (grades III and IV). Occasionally it is seen in children without obvious neonatal brain injury. While the muscles are weak, they may be hypertonic and hyper-reflexic. However, many of the pulmonary complications are similar to those of diseases due to lower motor neuron disease, and result from weak ineffective cough and uncoordinated swallowing mechanisms leading to aspiration.

THE RESPIRATORY MUSCLES AND CHEST WALL: NORMAL FUNCTION

Diaphragm

The diaphragm's action as a piston that decreases intrapleural pressure is its best-known mechanism. Two other mechanisms assist the diaphragm in its inspiratory action. The area of apposition of the diaphragm against the inner chest wall (Figure 13-2) places its fibers in a vertical orientation, which, when acting on the downward-declinated lower ribs, lifts them up and out in what is termed the "bucket handle effect." In addition, a significant portion of the abdomen actually lies within the rib cage; the positive intra-abdominal pressure during inspiration thus helps expand the lower rib cage. These latter

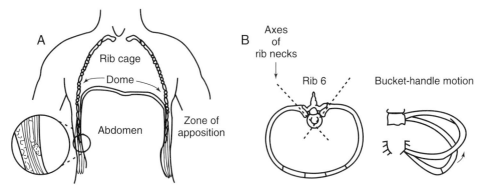

Figure 13-2   Functional anatomy of the rib cage. (**A**) Zone of apposition. (Reproduced with permission from: DeTroyer A, Estenne M. Clin Chest Med 9:175-193, 1988.) (**B**) Bucket-handle effect. (Reproduced with permission from DeTroyer A, Loring SH. Action of the respiratory muscles. In: Macklem PT, Mead J, editors: Handbook of physiology: the respiratory system. Mechanics of breathing, sect 3, vol III, part 2, p 453. Bethesda, MD: American Physiological Society, 1986.)

two mechanisms are less effective in young infants and in children and adults with obstructive lung disease, in whom the diaphragms are relatively flat resulting in a diminished area of apposition.

Intercostal Muscles

The intercostal muscles are aided in their inspiratory and expiratory actions by the direction of orientation of their fibers. If their fibers were oriented vertically, they would exert equal inspiratory and expiratory actions, depending on the point of fixation of the top and bottom ribs. The diagonal orientation of the fibers allows for preferential inspiratory and expiratory activity, depending on the torque developed on the upper and lower ribs between which they are inserted. The external intercostal muscles therefore exert a primarily inspiratory action whereas the internal intercostals exert primarily an expiratory action on the rib cage. Since normally inspiration is active and expiration is passive, the latter are usually active only during active expiration, such as in exercise or obstructive lung disease.

Abdominal Muscles

Contraction of the rectus abdominis and abdominal obliques increases intra-abdominal pressure and raises the diaphragm, thus assisting with expiration. These muscles, too, are usually only active during exercise or in patients with obstructive airway disease. They also serve to preserve the radius of curvature of the diaphragm in patients with flattened diaphragms due to obstructive airway disease and air trapping. Thus, they aid the diaphragm's inspiratory action by increasing the area of apposition (see above).

Upper Airway Muscles

Although not often considered muscles of respiration, the upper airway muscles contract phasically with inspiration, preventing upper airway collapse. This mechanism is dysfunctional in some patients with neuromuscular disease due to upper airway muscle weakness. They can have upper airway obstruction when asleep, or during both sleep and wakefulness. In young healthy infants, partial adduction of the vocal cords (glottic braking) is often used to slow expiration, thereby maintaining end-expiratory lung volume. When this mechanism is lost in infants with neuromuscular disease, low end-expiratory lung volume can result in reduced pulmonary oxygen stores and atelectasis.

Swallow Function

Numerous motor neuron groups are involved in the protection of the airway from aspiration during swallowing. Food materials have the potential to go in four directions during swallowing: back out the mouth, out the nose, into the airway and into the esophagus. Since the latter pathway is the only appropriate one, the function of these various motor neuron groups is to disable the other three pathways, and enable a successful swallow. A swallow is initiated by a voluntary action (oral phase), but once initiated is completed entirely by reflex mechanisms (pharyngeal and esophageal phases). During swallowing initiation, food is swept backward by the tongue. This action prevents egress of food through the mouth by apposition of the tongue against the palate. The soft palate is elevated, preventing nasopharyngeal aspiration. The trachea is elevated against the epiglottis, preventing aspiration into the airway. (This action is impaired in patients with a tracheostomy, in whom the position of the trachea is relatively fixed.) Finally, the pharyngeal constrictors dilate, opening the esophagus to accept the food bolus, thereby initiating the primary esophageal peristaltic wave. Weakness, spasticity or incoordination of any of the motor neuron groups involved in swallowing can predispose patients with neuromuscular disease to aspiration and aspiration pneumonia.

Cough Mechanism

The cough reflex starts with stimulation of irritant receptors with afferents in the vagus nerve (cranial nerve X). Following inspiration to near total lung capacity, closure of the glottis and contraction of the abdominal wall muscles, the glottis is suddenly opened resulting in upward movement of the diaphragm and expulsion of air at velocities of up to 600 miles per hour (950 km/h). The abdominal muscles involved in developing the driving pressures necessary for cough include the external oblique (efferent nerves T7–T12), the internal oblique (T7–L1), and the rectus abdominis (T6–T12). Weakness of the abdominal muscles can significantly reduce the effectiveness of the cough in clearing the airway of foreign particles.

Chest Wall Function

Compliance

Compliance is that mechanical property that relates a structure's pressure to its volume; the greater the change in pressure for a given change in volume, the stiffer (more elastic, or less compliant) that structure is said to be. Both the lungs and the chest wall have their own elastic properties, and together these determine the elastic properties of the respiratory system (Figure 13-3). There is a normal range for both lung and chest wall compliance: if the lungs and chest wall are too stiff, they require excess energy demands to perform the work of breathing. If the chest wall is too compliant, chest wall motion will be inefficient when negative intrathoracic pressure causes inspiratory paradoxical inward chest wall movement. This can result in energy inefficiencies as well. Abnormally high chest wall compliance can also lead to reductions in end-expiratory lung volume (Figure 13-3).

Chest Wall Motion

Observation of chest wall motion can provide clues about underlying lung and chest wall function. Normal chest wall motion is *synchronous*, that is, the rib cage and abdomen both move outward during inspiration and inward during expiration. Respiratory inductive plethysmography can provide a quantitative assessment of respiratory timing mechanics. Two inductance bands are placed on the torso, one around the rib cage and one around the abdomen. Motions of the compartments are

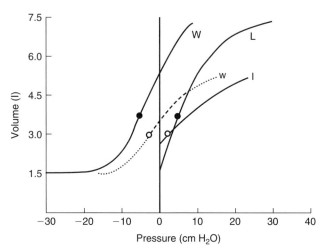

Figure 13-3 Respiratory system pressure–volume (PV) curves in the normal subject (continuous line) and the patient with neuromuscular disease (broken lines). Pressure is on the x-axis and volume on the y-axis. The slope of each curve at a given lung volume represents the compliance at that volume. Passive end-expiratory lung volume is represented by the point at which outward chest wall recoil is equal and opposite to inward lung recoil (filled circles in normal subject, open circles in patients with neuromuscular disease). L, normal lung curve; W, normal chest wall curve; l, neuromuscular lung curve; w, neuromuscular chest wall curve. (Reproduced with permission from DeTroyer A, Estenne M. The respiratory system in neuromuscular disorders. In Roussos C, editor. The thorax. Lung biology in health and disease, pp 2177–2212. New York: Marcel Dekker, 1995.)

translated into an electrical current with output to a recorder. One convenient way to measure timing relationships between the two compartments is to plot rib cage versus abdominal motion in an x-y plot (Figure 13-4). Normal synchronous motion is represented by a straight line with a positive slope, asynchronous motion by various degrees of "looping" and paradoxical motion by a straight line with a negative slope.

THE RESPIRATORY MUSCLES AND CHEST WALL IN NEUROMUSCULAR DISEASE

Strength

Patients with neuromuscular disease routinely have varying degrees of respiratory muscle weakness. The consequences of inspiratory respiratory muscle weakness are wide-ranging. One effect, low tidal volume breathing, can predispose to atelectasis, decreased vital capacity, and a decreased tidal volume to dead space ratio resulting in carbon dioxide retention. It is often characterized by a rapid respiratory rate. Reduced inspiratory muscle strength can also predispose to respiratory muscle fatigue. Decreased expiratory muscle

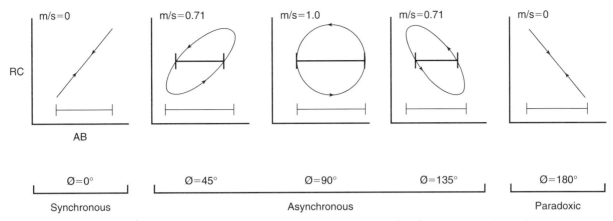

Figure 13-4 Lissajous figures of rib cage (RC) versus abdominal wall (AB) motion. Increasing phase angle, $\varnothing$, is an index of increasing thoraco-abdominal asynchrony. For phase angles $0° < \varnothing < 90°$, $\sin \varnothing = $ m/s; for $90° < \varnothing < 180°$, $\varnothing = 180 - \mu$, where $\sin \mu = $ m/s. (Reproduced with permission from Allen JL, Wolfson MR, McDowell K, Shaffer TH. Am Rev Respir Dis 141:337-342, 1990.)

strength reduces the ability to cough effectively, and is responsible for major morbidity due to inability to remove airway secretions. Respiratory muscle strength can be assessed by measuring the pressure that the respiratory muscles are able to generate against an occlusion. Normal values of inspiratory and expiratory muscle pressures have been published for both children and adults. Maximal pressure is also dependent on lung volume, as it can be affected by the length–tension curve of the respiratory muscles as well as the inward or outward elastic recoil of the chest wall. Normal values for maximal inspiratory pressures in both children and adults range from 80–120 cm H_2O; normal values for maximal expiratory pressure can exceed 200 cm H_2O.

Fatigue

Fatigue is defined as the inability to sustain a given muscle task after repeated exertions. Patients with neuromuscular weakness are more likely to develop respiratory muscle fatigue because the force the muscles generate during breathing is a greater percentage of the maximal force they are able to generate. Muscle fatigue can ultimately lead to task failure, which in the case of the respiratory muscles, leads to respiratory failure. This can occur acutely, e.g., in the setting of an aspiration pneumonia, or more insidiously, in which case the failing respiratory muscles may need to be supported by some form of non-invasive or invasive chronic ventilation. The development of respiratory failure ultimately occurs when there is an imbalance between the load against which the respiratory muscles must act, including elastic and resistive components, and the ability of the respiratory pump to overcome the load (Figure 13-5).

Chest Wall in Neuromuscular Disease

Chest Wall Motion

Observation of chest wall motion (Figure 13-6) can provide valuable clues to the site and cause of respiratory muscle weakness. Diaphragmatic weakness results in passive upward motion of the diaphragm as the now dominant intercostal muscles develop negative intrathoracic pressure; this results in outward chest wall and inward abdominal motion during inspiration. Intercostal muscle weakness with sparing of the diaphragm, such as that seen in patients with spinal cord injuries below C3-5, is characterized by inward rib cage and outward abdominal wall motion during inspiration, as the rib cage is sucked inward by the negative intrapleural pressure developed by the contracting diaphragm.

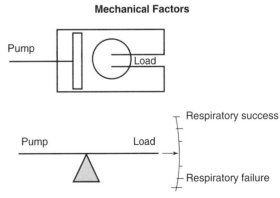

Figure 13-5 The ability of the respiratory pump to exceed the mechanical load of the respiratory system determines whether respiratory "success" or failure ensues. (Reproduced with permission from Allen JL. Monaldi Arch Chest Dis 51:230-235, 1996.)

Chest wall motion: site of weakness

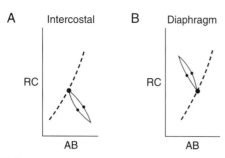

Figure 13-6 Konno–Mead figures in patients with neuromuscular disease during breathing at rest. The filled circle represents end-expiration. (**A**) Intercostal weakness. As the abdominal wall (AB) moves out, the rib cage (RC) is drawn inward. (**B**) Diaphragmatic paralysis. As the rib cage expands the diaphragm moves passively upwards and the abdominal wall is drawn inwards.

Chest Wall Compliance

Infants with neuromuscular disease often have paradoxical inward chest wall motion during inspiration, as their highly compliant rib cage with diminished intercostal muscle tone responds to negative intrathoracic pressure. High chest wall compliance can also lead to diminished end-expiratory lung volume, as the outward chest wall recoil is less able to withstand the inward lung recoil. This, in addition to the effects of low tidal volumes mentioned above, can lead to atelectasis and reduced oxygen stores.

Studies have shown that chest wall compliance, while high in infancy, is reduced in adults with neuromuscular disease. This may be due to the long-term effects of low tidal volume breathing in these patients, leading to contractures of the costo-vertebral joints.

Scoliosis

Neuromuscular imbalance of the paraspinal muscles often leads to scoliosis in patients with neuromuscular disorders. Such scoliosis, when severe (greater than 40° or so), can add to the effects of the underlying neuromuscular disease in diminishing vital capacity and total lung capacity.

Upper Airway Obstruction

Several factors predispose patients with neuromuscular disease to sleep-disordered breathing; one of them is the development of upper airway obstruction. This can occur in the setting of obesity characteristic of certain muscle disorders such as Duchenne MD. However, patients with neuromuscular disease are at an increased risk of upper airway obstruction during sleep even in the absence of obesity. The negative intrapharyngeal pressures generated by the Bernoulli effects of flow through the upper airway will collapse the pharynx and hypopharynx if the upper airway muscles are too weak to resist this collapsing force. Negative pressure ventilation (tank or cuirass) in patients who require assisted ventilation due to respiratory failure exacerbates this mechanism by increasing the flows (and Bernoulli forces) through the upper airway.

Swallowing Dysfunction

Since the motor neurons largely responsible for the timing and sequence of the swallow reflex lie in the brainstem, swallow dysfunction is usually seen in patients with lesions affecting the brainstem or descending upper motor neurons that form synapses with these brainstem motor neurons. Evaluation and treatment of swallowing dysfunction are discussed below.

Cough

Since the afferent nerves of the cough reflex pass through the brainstem and the efferent nerves descend to the level of T6 through L1, lesions in the brainstem or affecting the descending pathways or spinal levels from T6 to L1 can diminish the effectiveness of cough. The further caudal the lesion is, the less the deleterious effect will be. Treatment of inadequate cough reflex is discussed below.

EVALUATION OF THE PATIENT WITH NEUROMUSCULAR DISEASE

History

The history should focus on aspects of the underlying illness that would lead to respiratory complications. Ascertain the length of time the patient has been affected by neuromuscular disease and its severity; functional scores such as the Vignos score[1] are helpful. Ask about recurrent pneumonias or episodic pulmonary congestion suggesting aspiration. Ask about the quality of the patient's cough—strong or weak. Symptoms such as snoring, which suggest upper airway obstruction, should be sought. Ascertain whether the patient uses home oxygen, nocturnal ventilatory support or cough-assist devices such as manually assisted cough techniques or the mechanical in/ex-sufflator. Family history should be obtained to help assess the nature of the underlying neurologic condition, and to ascertain predisposition to airway hyper-reactivity apart from that which is related to aspiration. An immunization history should be obtained—ask about the influenza vaccine and in young infants, passive respiratory syncytial virus (RSV) immunization. A careful nutritional history should be obtained, including use of nasogastric or gastrostomy tube feedings. Ask about choking or gagging with feeding, and nasopharyngeal aspiration. Gastroesophageal reflux is more common among patients with neuromuscular disease and can predispose to pulmonary aspiration as well. History of scoliosis and its progression and treatment should be obtained.

Physical Examination

In addition to the routine physical examination, there are several special areas to which particular attention should be paid. A careful nutritional assessment to include height, weight, and body mass index (BMI) percentiles should be performed. Adequacy of the gag reflex should be ascertained as an index of airway protective mechanisms against aspiration. The patient should be asked to cough voluntarily, so that assessment of the cough quality and strength can be made. Respiratory assessment should include, in addition to thorough auscultation of the lungs, observation of chest wall motion, which can provide clues to the site of respiratory muscle weakness (intercostals versus diaphragmatic, see "Chest Wall Motion," above). Presence and degree of scoliosis should be noted. A careful neurologic assessment, including cranial nerve examination, peripheral muscle strength (Table 13-2), sensory level, which can give clues to level of spinal cord injuries, and deep tendon reflexes, should be performed. Assessment of facial skin breakdown should be made if the patient is being treated with non-invasive positive pressure ventilation through a nasal mask.

Chest Radiograph

The chest radiograph (Figure 13-7) should be evaluated for evidence of chronic aspiration. The degree of scoliosis should be ascertained. The position of the diaphragm should be noted as well as the symmetry of the hemidiaphragms. If diaphragmatic paralysis is suspected, fluoroscopy is helpful in its demonstration.

Pulmonary Function Testing (Table 13-3)

Respiratory muscle weakness causes decreases in vital capacity. Total lung capacity is reduced as well, so the effect

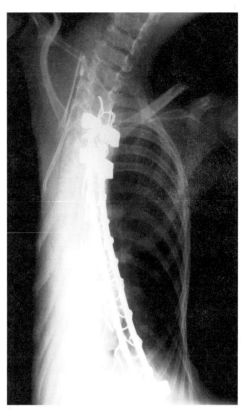

Figure 13-7   Chest radiograph of a patient with neuromuscular disease. Note the chronic "bell-shaped" chest, the atelectasis of the right lung due to an aspiration event, and the scoliosis partially corrected by surgery.

is a classic "restrictive" defect on lung function testing. The defect is usually apparent at both extremes of the vital capacity; not only is total lung capacity reduced but also residual volume can be elevated, due to inability of the weak expiratory muscles to distort the chest wall down to a normal residual volume. The decrease in vital capacity is proportional to the reduction in respiratory muscle strength and therefore to severity of neuromuscular weakness (Figure 13-8). As patients with progressive neuromuscular diseases deteriorate, e.g., in Duchenne MD, there is a progressive loss of vital capacity (Figure 13-9). Appropriate corrections of predicted values

Table 13-2	Peripheral Muscle Strength
0	No flicker of muscle activity
1+	Flicker
2+	Able to move with gravity removed (horizontal plane)
3+	Moves against gravity
4+	Weakness
5+	Full muscle strength

Table 13-3	Pulmonary Function Tests in Neuromuscular Disease
TLC	↓
VC	↓
RV	↓, NL, or ↑
RV/TLC	↑
FEV_1	↓
MMEF	↓
FEV_1/VC	NL

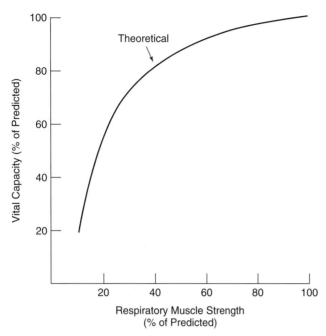

Figure 13-8 Decrease in vital capacity in patients with neuromuscular disease. The decreases are proportional to the decrease in maximal respiratory pressures. (From DeTroyer A, Borenstein S, Cordier R. Analysis of lung volume restriction in patients with respiratory muscle weakness. Thorax 35:603–610, 1980.)

for patients with scoliosis must be made; otherwise results expressed as percent predicted value may be overestimated. In patients with severe scoliosis, the arm span is often used instead of the height in arriving at the correct predicted lung function value.

Flows are also reduced in patients with neuromuscular disease, but this does not usually signify airflow obstruction. Flows are reduced because flow is a volume moved per unit time, and flows are usually reduced proportionally to the reduction in lung volume. For this reason, the FEV_1/VC ratio is usually normal, and this ratio remains the single best discriminator between restrictive and obstructive lung disease in a patient with a low vital capacity. Likewise, the flow–volume curve of a patient with neuromuscular disease usually has a close to normal shape, though restricted in size, as opposed to the typical "scooped" flow–volume curve of a patient with obstructive disease (Figure 13-10). Near residual volume, flows may abruptly drop from the descending limb of the curve, a phenomenon that has been termed "falling off" the curve. It is indicative of a sudden decrease in flow as residual volume is reached and the expiratory muscles can no longer distort the chest wall to a lower lung volume.

Tests of maximal inspiratory and expiratory strength are very helpful in assessing likelihood of respiratory problems and fatigue. Normal values have been discussed above in the section on the respiratory muscles and chest wall in neuromuscular disease. Patients are asked to inhale and exhale maximally through a mouthpiece that is occluded, and the resulting pressure is measured. Technical difficulties can arise in patients in whom oral muscle weakness is so severe that they are not able to form an adequate seal around the mouthpiece of the pressure-testing equipment. In such patients, nasal sniff pressure measurement can be a useful alternative in laboratories experienced in its measurement.

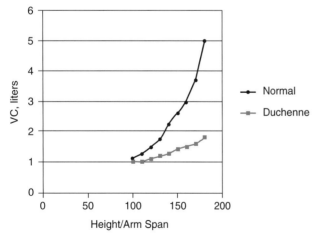

Figure 13-9 Vital capacity (VC) in patients with neuromuscular disease. The increase in VC with growth is reduced compared with normal. (Modified from Jenkins JG, Bohn D, Edmonds JF, Levison H, Barker GA. Evaluation of pulmonary function in muscular dystrophy patients requiring spinal surgery. Crit Care Med 10:645–649, 1982.)

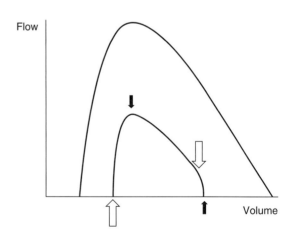

Figure 13-10 Typical changes in the flow volume curve in a patient with neuromuscular disease. The arrows point out the reduced total lung capacity (⇧), peak flow (⬇), elevated residual volume (⬆) and abrupt reduction of flows at residual volume (⇩).

Special Studies

Arterial Blood Gas, Oxygen Saturation, End-Tidal CO$_2$

Respiratory pump failure is characterized by carbon dioxide retention as minute ventilation decreases. The degree of carbon dioxide elimination can be assessed by several means. Arterial blood gases remain the gold standard, and can be performed with minimal discomfort with appropriate use of EMLA cream and subcutaneous lidocaine. They also give information about pH and overall acid–base balance as well as pO$_2$. In patients with hypoventilation due to neuromuscular disease, but without significant pulmonary pathology, the pO$_2$ is usually reduced in proportion to the elevation of CO$_2$, resulting in a normal alveolar–arterial (A–a) gradient for oxygen. While measurement of oxygen saturation by pulse oximetry yields accurate results in most circumstances, slight reductions in pO$_2$ from normal will not be detected. However, since clinically significant differences are probably more important, pulse oximetry remains a very useful tool. End-tidal CO$_2$ measurement is useful primarily in patients who are supported by some form of mechanical ventilation, and in whom trends of CO$_2$ are of interest following interventions or changes in ventilatory support. A set of serum electrolytes, and specifically a serum bicarbonate, reflecting renal compensation, provides a very useful average indicator of whether CO$_2$ retention is occurring. Practically speaking, this and home pulse oximetry provide very effective tools for monitoring a neuromuscular disease patient's gas exchange and overall respiratory pump function.

Nocturnal Polysomnography

Patients with neuromuscular disease are prone to the development of nocturnal hypoxemia for several reasons. Upper airway obstruction has been discussed above and tends to be magnified during sleep when upper airway control is not as active as during wakefulness. In addition, patients with neuromuscular disease can develop nocturnal hypoxemia in the absence of daytime hypoxemia and in the absence of upper airway obstruction. This is in part due to nocturnal hypoventilation when the low tidal volume present during daytime breathing is exaggerated. It also results from a decrease in end-expiratory lung volume due to loss of intercostal muscle tone. If end-expiratory lung volume drops below the lung volume at which there is closure of small airways, the result will be areas of low ventilation/perfusion and consequent hypoxemia. This can occur in asymptomatic patients, so it is best to periodically assess patients with advanced neuromuscular disease with polysomnography. One approach[2] is to obtain polysomnograms every year in patient whose vital capacity is greater than 60% and whose maximum inspiratory and expiratory

pressures (MIPs and MEPs) are greater than 60 cm H$_2$O, and every 6 months in patient whose vital capacity is less than 60% and/or MIP/MEP less than 60 cm H$_2$O.

Swallow Function Studies

Swallow function studies are an essential part of the evaluation of patients with suspected aspiration. A radiologist in conjunction with a speech therapist well versed in the evaluation of disorders of deglutition should perform these studies. At least three different textures—thin liquid, thick liquid, and solids—should be offered, and the barium study should be assessed for nasopharyngeal aspiration, pooling of contrast in the valecula, or frank aspiration below the vocal cords. If aspiration is observed, rapid clearance by an effective cough mechanism should be sought. Aspiration of oral secretions can also be demonstrated by nuclear medicine "salivagrams," in which a small amount of tracer is introduced into the mouth (Figure 13-11).

Respiratory Inductive Plethysmography

Respiratory inductive plethysmography has been used to quantitate the degree of asynchrony between rib cage and abdominal motion. It can give valuable clues as to whether respiratory muscle weakness is primarily intercostal or diaphragmatic, when timed to the phase of the respiratory cycle (Figure 13-6). It can also be used to noninvasively gauge frequency and tidal volume in infants.

Tests of Respiratory Muscle Fatigue

Tests of respiratory muscle fatigue are not in widespread use but their use is being investigated in the evaluation of patients in whom chronic non-invasive or invasive mechanical ventilation is being considered. The tension time index compares the average pressure generated by the diaphragm during inspiration to the maximal pressure the diaphragm is able to develop, and provides a useful predictor of the likelihood of respiratory fatigue. In patients with neuromuscular disease, muscle weakness resulting in low maximal pressures will increase this term in spite of normal pressures developed during the breath, thus predicting that fatigue will be more likely in patients with neuromuscular disease even in the absence of intrinsic lung disease.

PREVENTION AND TREATMENT OF RESPIRATORY COMPLICATIONS OF NEUROMUSCULAR DISEASE

General Supportive

Nutrition

Nutritional assessment and treatment is paramount in patients with neuromuscular disorders. Undernutrition is common, for various reasons. As patients with neuromuscular disease deteriorate, there may be reduced oral intake due to uncoordinated swallow, esophagitis due to

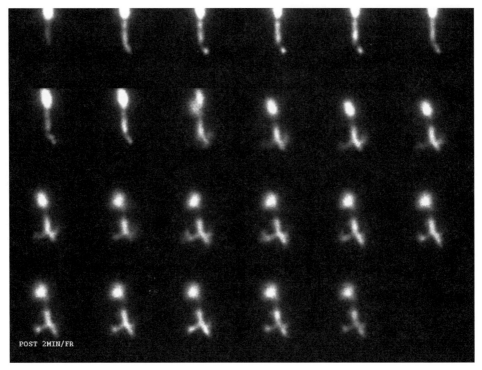

Figure 13-11 Nuclear medicine salivagram demonstrating frank aspiration into the tracheo-bronchial tree during a swallowing effort.

uncontrolled gastroesophageal reflux, and anorexia due to advanced underlying illness. Recurrent pulmonary infections and chest wall stiffness can lead to increased caloric expenditure by increasing the basal metabolic rate and work of breathing. Patients or caretakers sometimes voluntarily reduce caloric intake in an effort to assist patients with activities of daily living under the impression that weight loss may reduce the work that the muscles of locomotion and posture must perform. In addition, in patients who are wheelchair-bound, parents and caretakers may intentionally limit weight gain in order to facilitate transfers from bed to chair, home to car, etc.

Obesity is a characteristic of certain neuromuscular disorders (e.g. Duchenne MD) and can lead to difficulty in ambulation as well as obstructive sleep apnea, described above.

A complete nutritional history should include current diet, types of early and later feeds, nutritional and vitamin/mineral supplements, appetite, food allergies, chewing and swallowing problems, and type, quantity and schedule of gastrostomy tube feedings if applicable, including water supplements. If malnutrition is a concern, a 3-day calorie count should be performed. Careful serial measurements of growth curves including height, weight, head circumference, and BMI should be performed. Since the BMI depends on both a weight and a height measurement, this index may be overestimated in patients with severe scoliosis; potentially the use of arm span rather than height may correct for this. The usefulness of anthropometric measurements such as skin fold thickness are unknown; measures such as midarm circumference as an assessment of nutritional status are probably misleading in patients with primary muscle disorders.

Assessment should be made of vitamin and mineral status. Careful attention to calcium intake and overall bone health is also important; scoliosis will worsen if osteoporosis is a complicating feature; dual energy X-ray absorptiometry (DXA) scans are indicated if osteoporosis is suspected.

There is controversy about optimal nutritional status in patients with neuromuscular disease. Although it may be unrealistic to expect that a patient with muscle wasting be 50th percentile for corrected BMI, an attempt should be made to arrive at an ideal BMI and make sure that it is maintained over time. It should be remembered that muscle wasting may be due to malnutrition as well as the underlying neuromuscular disorder, and every attempt should be made to maintain optimal nutrition in these patients in order that their weakness not be exacerbated by poor nutritional status. High calorie (e.g., 24–27 calorie per ounce) formulas may be used in infancy, and nutritionally complete formulas such as Pediasure and Ensure, or supplements such as Scandishakes and Boost, may be used in older children and young adults. If caloric intake is inadequate as assessed by a 3-day diet record, and if it cannot be improved upon, continuous nasogastric or gastrostomy tube feedings at night may be employed; this reduces, but does not eliminate, the risk of aspiration due to gastroesophageal reflux. In patients in whom aspiration during swallowing is an unacceptable risk, all feedings may be switched over to bolus gastrostomy tube feeds during the day.

Constipation should be aggressively evaluated and treated. Severe constipation can cause abdominal distension, push up on the diaphragms and cause an increased restrictive pulmonary process. We have seen severe constipation precipitate respiratory failure in patients with severe restrictive disease from underlying neuromuscular problems. Its presence may be detected by history, physical examination and flat plate of the abdomen.

In obese patients, judicious use of caloric restricted diets is indicated.

Vaccines

In addition to routine childhood immunizations, infants with neuromuscular disorders should be considered for RSV prophylaxis if they have pulmonary complications. This should be continued for at least the first 2 years of life. Routine influenza vaccinations should be given yearly unless contra-indicated. Although most patients do not have specific immune deficiencies, pneumococcal vaccines such as pneumovax and Prevnar should be considered, since the consequences of a pneumococcal pneumonia can be devastating in this patient group.

Team Approach To Care

No patient requires interdisciplinary and multidisciplinary care more than the patient with a chronic neuromuscular disorder (Table 13-4). In addition to the care of a primary care physician, the input of a pediatric neurologist, orthopedist, and pulmonologist is ideal. Appropriate subspecialty trained nurse practitioners play an invaluable role in the day-to-day management. In addition, cardiology consultation will be necessary in patients with complicating cardiomyopathies as part of their underlying disorders. In spinal-cord-injured patients, or others with problems related to sacral motor

Table 13-4	Team Approach to Care of the Patient with Neuromuscular Disease

Neurologist
Pulmonologist
Cardiologist
Orthopedist
Nutritionist
Nurse practitioner
Case manager
Social worker
Physical therapist
Occupational therapist
Speech therapist

neurons, the input of a urologist, and perhaps renal specialist, is necessary. Physical therapists are crucial for creating a program designed to maintain mobility in otherwise under-used joints and in teaching chest physiotherapy. Speech therapists will be helpful in the assessment and treatment of swallowing dysfunction, and occupational therapists play an invaluable role in assisting with the many activities of daily living. The importance of a nutritionist has been stressed above. A social worker and case manager will assist with dealing with financial and insurance issues, and with the myriad psychosocial problems facing these children and families. The challenge is providing these multiple services in a single setting; many hospitals have multidisciplinary clinics where nearly all the above input can be achieved within the constraints of a half-day or day-long visit. This is particularly important for patients requiring daytime chronic ventilatory assistance, in whom mobility may be impaired.

Swallowing Disorders and Aspiration

The importance of swallowing function in preventing aspiration pneumonias has been discussed above. Once swallowing dysfunction has been diagnosed, the most important decision is whether it is safe to continue oral feedings. Speech therapists expert in the diagnosis and management of swallowing dysfunction should be consulted; they will assess what texture(s) of foods allow for the most successful swallowing in a given patient. Many times, patients who aspirate thin liquids will be able to protect their airway while swallowing thick liquids or solids. Patients who do not exhibit frank aspiration, but who are at an aspiration risk by virtue of pooling of food in their hypopharynx or valecula, can be taught techniques such as "dry swallows," in which repeated swallowing efforts are made after the initial swallow of a food bolus in an effort to clear pooled food particles.

Prevention of Aspiration

Prevention of aspiration is paramount, and relies on home chest physiotherapy and cough assistance. Abdominally assisted coughing, use of a mechanical in/exsufflator device, percussion vest and/or intrapulmonary percussive ventilation are very effective. Oropharyngeal secretions should be suctioned *before* the application of these devices to the airway.

Pneumonia and Atelectasis

Pneumonia and atelectasis should be considered medical emergencies in patients with advanced neuromuscular disease; they often necessitate hospitalization even though the patient "looks well." There are two reasons for this: first, patients with neuromuscular disorders may not display classic signs of respiratory distress such as suprasternal, subcostal and intercostal retractions, since the development of the negative intrapleural pressures necessary to produce retractions requires sufficient respiratory muscle strength to lower pleural pressure. Thus in patients with neuromuscular disease, alternate clinical assessments such as respiratory rate, heart rate, sensorium, pulse oximetry and, if necessary, arterial blood gases should be employed. Second, although patients with neuromuscular disease and an intercurrent respiratory illness who have a new area of atelectasis on chest radiograph often initially look well in the emergency department, they are experiencing a deterioration in their ability to clear secretions which is often progressive; it is not uncommon to have such patients sent home, only to be admitted several days later with a worsening chest radiograph. Prompt admission for aggressive antibiotic therapy, chest physiotherapy and bronchodilators, and treatment with cough-assist devices can often pre-empt a prolonged hospital course.

Respiratory Muscle Function

Strength: Role of Rest and Training

There is controversy over whether weak muscles should be rested or trained. In patients with neuromuscular disease, however, there is evidence that favors

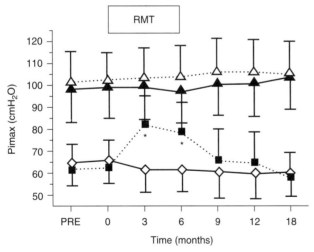

Figure 13-12 Effects of resistive loaded training on respiratory muscle strength in normal subjects (filled triangles), normal controls (open triangles), subjects with neuromuscular disease (filled squares), and controls with neuromuscular disease (open diamonds). In this study, only those patients with neuromuscular disease who underwent respiratory muscle training (RMT) demonstrated a significant increase in respiratory muscle strength during the training period (asterisks). (Reproduced with permission from Gozal D, Thiriet P. Respiratory muscle training in neuromuscular disease: long-term effects on strength and load perception. Med Sci Sports Exerc 31:1522–1527, 1999.)

both approaches. Respiratory muscle training has been evaluated in several studies. In general, while no changes in vital capacity have been seen, several studies report improvements in maximal respiratory pressures generated by the respiratory muscles (Figure 13-12). This can be accompanied by a decreased respiratory load perception. However, both improvements revert to baseline when respiratory muscle training is discontinued. Respiratory muscle rest is discussed in the next section.

Fatigue

Efforts to delay the onset of existing respiratory muscle fatigue or to reduce existing fatigue can be thought of as restoring the balance between the respiratory pump and the respiratory load. These efforts are aimed at increasing the ability of the pump and alleviating the load (Figure 13-13).

Interventions that help decrease the elastic and resistive loads against which the respiratory muscles must operate include those that reduce chest wall rigidity by increasing range of motion (deep breathing exercises, incentive spirometry, mechanical in/exsufflator devices and possibly assisted ventilation, either invasive or noninvasive). In addition, any measures that improve pulmonary toilet, mobilize secretions and reduce atelectasis (chest physiotherapy, mechanical in/exsufflator devices, bronchodilators), also decrease airways resistance and improve compliance and should be a part of each patient's daily routine. Frequency (daily, BID, TID, QID or prn) should be dictated by the clinical picture.

Chronic assisted ventilation can help increase the endurance of the respiratory pump by reducing fatigue. Over-reliance on mechanical ventilation has the theoretical disadvantage of contributing to respiratory muscle atrophy, so judgment must be used in how many hours a day assisted ventilation is provided, and should probably be the minimal number of hours necessary to avoid fatigue. Unfortunately, there are currently no proven

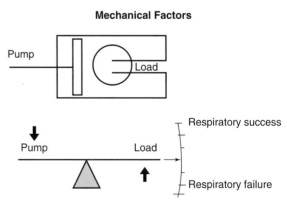

Figure 13-13 Techniques to reduce respiratory muscle fatigue either decrease the respiratory load or increase the ability of the pump.

ways to reliably assess respiratory muscle fatigue or its treatment in this setting. Complications of non-invasive ventilation can include upper airway obstruction in patients treated with negative pressure cuirass or tank ventilators (as described above) and facial skin breakdown in patients ventilated non-invasively through a nasal mask. Meticulous attention to nasal skin care at pressure points, use of alternate (at least two) mask designs in a given patient, and reducing the tightness of the seal around the nose by allowing small amounts of air leak may help avoid this complication. We prefer the use of nasal masks to full-face masks, especially in the home setting, to reduce the risk of aspiration. In patients in whom 24-hour ventilation is necessary, tracheostomy and mechanical ventilation allows more head mobility, communication and overall comfort compared with mask ventilation. Use of speaking valves in patients with tracheotomies, even in those patients who are ventilated, allows for vastly improved vocalization and speech as long as there is sufficient leak to allow for expiration around the tracheostomy tube. There are many ways to choose ventilator settings which will accomplish goals of maintaining adequate end-expiratory lung volume (PEEP), adequate lung and chest wall expansion (peak pressure or tidal volume adjustments), degree of respiratory muscle rest achieved (pressure support and ventilator rate), and near-normal blood gases (all of the above plus F_IO_2). Ventilators the size of laptop computers are now available which can be attached to a wheelchair and provide the ventilator-dependent patient with optimal mobility.

MAJOR POINTS

1. Neuromuscular disorders that result in pulmonary complications can include diseases affecting any site along the neuromuscular axis, including the upper motor neuron, the lower motor neuron, the neuromuscular junction and the muscle itself.
2. Normal neuromuscular function is essential (1) in performing the pump function of respiration, (2) in maintaining upper airway patency during inspiration, (3) in protecting the airway from aspiration by the presence of a normal swallow

---

MAJOR POINTS—Cont'd

mechanism, and (4) (once this mechanism is broached) in clearing aspirated secretions by an effective cough.
3. Abnormalities of the above functions in patients with neuromuscular disease result, respectively, in (1) respiratory muscle fatigue and failure, (2) upper airway obstruction, especially during sleep, (3) swallowing dysfunction, and (4) weak cough leading to recurrent atelectasis and pneumonia.
4. The pulmonary evaluation of patients with neuromuscular disease has many components and may include, in addition to a specialized physical examination, imaging studies, tests of lung function, respiratory muscle strength and fatigue, gas exchange, polysomnography, and swallowing function studies.
5. Many newer supportive therapies exist to prevent and treat pulmonary complications of neuromuscular diseases. These include aggressive optimization of nutritional status, and interdisciplinary programs designed to prevent aspiration using swallowing training, and to prevent atelectasis and pneumonia using assisted cough techniques and chest physiotherapy. Additionally, the judicious use of non-invasive ventilation can support fatigued respiratory muscles and help prevent chronic respiratory failure.

REFERENCES

1. Archibald KC, Vignos PJ. A study of contractures in muscular dystrophy. Arch Phys Med Rehabil 39:150–157, 1959.
2. Gozal D. Pulmonary manifestations of neuromuscular disease with special reference to Duchenne muscular dystrophy and spinal muscular atrophy. Pediatr Pulmonol 29:141, 2000.

SUGGESTED READING

Allen JL. Respiratory function in children with neuromuscular disease. Monaldi Arch Chest Dis 51:230, 1996.

Schramm CM. Current concepts of respiratory complications of neuromuscular disease in children. Curr Opin Pediatr 12:203, 2000.

CHAPTER 1

Respiratory Failure in Children

DANIEL J. WEINER, M.D.

INTRODUCTION AND DEFINITION

Respiratory failure occurs when the respiratory system can no longer adequately transfer oxygen into or carbon dioxide from the blood. "Adequate" transfer is somewhat subjective, and there are thus no strict criteria that define respiratory failure. In adults, a $pO_2 < 60$ torr while breathing supplemental oxygen ($FiO_2 > 0.6$), or $pCO_2 > 50$ torr are frequently used as guidelines, but these values are arbitrary and should be used with caution. Some children may be clinically stable despite this hypoxemia or

hypercarbia, and treatments should be tailored to the child and not to these laboratory values.

Respiratory failure can be "acute" or "chronic," and these terms, too, are ill defined. One use of the terms addresses whether the disease process itself is insidious in onset (weeks to months or longer, such as might be caused by muscular dystrophy) or rapid in onset (minutes to hours, such as might be caused by a toxic inhalation), while others use the term to describe the duration of assisted ventilation. For purposes of this review, "acute" or "chronic" respiratory failure will describe the duration of the disease process.

One cause of acute respiratory failure arises from the acute respiratory distress syndrome (ARDS). This was originally termed the adult respiratory distress syndrome, first described in 1967[1], although the original case series included one pediatric patient, and the illness may be seen in patients of all ages. It may be caused by numerous pulmonary insults. Criteria for ARDS include:

- Predisposing illness
- Respiratory distress and hypoxemia refractory to supplemental oxygen
- Bilateral pulmonary infiltrates
- Absence of cardiac failure

Here, "hypoxemia" is usually defined as the ratio $PaO_2/FiO_2 < 200$, and "absence of cardiac failure" is usually defined as a pulmonary capillary wedge pressure < 18 cm H_2O. A less stringent definition ($PaO_2/FiO_2 < 300$) has been used to describe "acute lung injury"[2].

Inconsistent application of these diagnostic criteria makes studying the epidemiology of ARDS, as well as optimal management, very challenging. It is estimated that 1-4% of all admissions to pediatric critical care units are due to ARDS. Mortality has remained high (40-60%) despite many advances in critical care, and is higher if multiple organ dysfunction is present. Despite the heterogeneous nature of ARDS, it is nonetheless considered a prototype disease for studying respiratory failure.

There are many other causes of acute respiratory failure (see below). At high risk are patients with chronic respiratory insufficiency (e.g., due to neuromuscular weakness) who may have further deterioration with intercurrent infections, aspiration of secretions, or for other reasons. These patients may be said to have acute-on-chronic respiratory failure.

In this chapter, we will examine the causes, pathophysiology, and management of respiratory failure in children.

ETIOLOGIES

Respiratory failure can be caused by defects anywhere along the pathway that results in normal respiration. These can be grouped into three main areas: the central nervous system (CNS, responsible for respiratory drive), the chest wall and respiratory muscles (responsible for generating the force to inspire), and the lung (responsible for gas exchange). A partial list of disorders in each of these areas is given in Table 14-1.

PATHOPHYSIOLOGY

To understand the derangements that occur in respiratory failure, we must first consider the normal processes of gas exchange. We will separately consider ventilation (the movement of air, responsible for elimination of CO_2) and oxygenation. Indeed, respiratory failure is sometimes further described as "hypoxemic" or

---

Table 14-1 Causes of Respiratory Failure

(a) CNS Causes
- Congenital central hypoventilation syndrome
- Brainstem malformations (e.g., Dandy–Walker cyst, Arnold–Chiari)
- Medication effects (e.g., narcotics)
- Infections (e.g., meningitis)

(b) Pump Causes
- Muscular dystrophy (e.g., Duchenne, Becker)
- Spinal muscular atrophy (e.g., Werdnig-Hoffman)
- Demyelinating diseases (e.g. Guillain–Barré)
- Disorders of the neuromuscular junction (e.g., myasthenia gravis, medications)
- Chest wall disorders (e.g., scoliosis, Jeune syndrome)

(c) Lung Causes
- Infections (e.g., pneumonia, bronchiolitis, bronchiectasis)
- Inflammatory airway obstruction (e.g., asthma, inhalational injury)
- Vascular disorders (e.g., veno-occlusive disease, pulmonary hypertension)
- Congenital lung anomalies (pulmonary hypoplasia, cystic adenomatoid malformation, diaphragmatic hernia)

"hypercapneic" respiratory failure, although frequently these two processes are disordered in the same patient.

Ventilation

The volume of gas that enters and leaves the lungs with each breath is termed the *tidal volume* (Vt); physiologic tidal volumes are approximately 5–7 ml/kg. *Minute ventilation* ($\dot{V}E$) is the amount of gas entering and leaving the lungs per minute, and is calculated by multiplying the tidal volume by the respiratory rate. A portion of the tidal volume resides in the conducting airways where no gas exchange occurs (the anatomic dead space). Similarly, no gas exchange occurs in the tubing connecting the ventilator to the patient; this, too, can be thought of as dead space (Vd). *Alveolar ventilation* ($\dot{V}A$) refers to the amount of gas that is available for gas exchange, which is defined as RR × (tidal volume – dead space volume). The most convenient way to gauge alveolar ventilation is to measure the arterial partial pressure of CO_2; increases in alveolar ventilation decrease $PaCO_2$: $\dot{V}A = k \times (\dot{V}CO_2/pCO_2)$ where $\dot{V}CO_2$ is CO_2 production.

In patients with lung disease, some portions of the lung, despite the presence of alveoli, do not participate in gas exchange for one reason or another. This volume of lung is termed the *alveolar dead space*. When taken together with the anatomic dead space, the sum is termed the *physiologic dead space* (Figure 14-1). This can be measured using Bohr's method, which is based on the principle that all exhaled CO_2 comes from the alveoli rather than the anatomic dead space: $V_D/V_T = (P_ACO_2 - P_ECO_2)/P_ACO_2$, where P_ACO_2 is the partial pressure of CO_2 in the alveolus, and P_ECO_2 is the partial pressure of CO_2 in the mixed exhaled gas. Measuring the alveolar partial pressure is difficult, but in normal subjects it is nearly identical to the arterial partial pressure of CO_2 ($PaCO_2$). Therefore, by measuring the $PaCO_2$ and mixed expired CO_2 (this requires collection of exhaled gas in a bag), we can estimate the *ratio* of physiologic dead space volume to tidal volume. This is normally 0.2–0.3 but may rise significantly in disease states.

Increased dead space is one cause of hypercapnea in patients because for a given minute ventilation, as dead space ventilation increases, alveolar ventilation decreases. Other causes include hypoventilation (most common), or increased CO_2 production (such as occurs in malignant hyperthermia or sepsis). Hypoventilation results from a variety of abnormalities in respiratory drive, or inadequate generation of respiratory muscle force (Table 14-1a, b).

Oxygenation

The partial pressure of oxygen in the alveolus (P_AO_2) can be predicted from *the alveolar gas equation*:

$$P_AO_2 = PiO_2 - (PaCO_2/R) = [(P_B - P_{H_2O}) \times FiO_2 - (PaCO_2/R)]$$

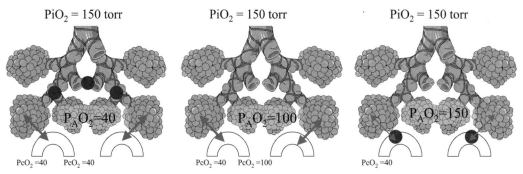

Figure 14-1 Dead space and alveolar ventilation in normal (left) or diseased states. Vd/Vt in the normal situation is approximately 0.3. A pulmonary embolus is depicted in the center panel, and obstructive airway disease in the right panel. The heavy black bars denote anatomic dead space; the shaded circles denote alveolar dead space. When dead space is increased, the minute ventilation must increase dramatically to maintain alveolar ventilation.

where P_B is barometric pressure, P_{H_2O} is the partial pressure due to water vapor, P_AO_2 is the alveolar partial pressure of oxygen, PiO_2 is the inspired partial pressure of oxygen, R is the respiratory quotient, and FiO_2 is the inspired fraction of oxygen. From this one can see that the amount of oxygen in the alveolus is maximally determined by barometric pressure and the fraction of oxygen in the air; this maximum is decreased by CO_2 production; the respiratory quotient, R, is a measure of the metabolic rate of the tissues (CO_2 production/O_2 consumption). At sea level, barometric pressure is 760 torr, and the partial pressure due to water vapor is 47 torr; the fraction of oxygen in air is 21% (most of the rest being nitrogen). Therefore, the partial pressure of oxygen in inspired air is $(760 − 47) × 0.21$, or 150 torr. The *A-a gradient* is calculated as the difference between the alveolar oxygen tension (from the alveolar gas equation) and the arterial oxygen tension (from a blood gas measurement). The A-a gradient can be useful in identifying the cause of hypoxemia.

From the alveolar gas equation, two of the several causes of hypoxemia can be demonstrated. At high altitude, barometric pressure is much lower, reducing PiO_2. Additionally, an elevated pCO_2 due to obstructive lung disease or hypoventilation will increase the $PaCO_2$/R ratio, decreasing P_AO_2. The other causes of hypoxemia are shunt, ventilation–perfusion ($\dot{V}/\dot{Q}$) mismatch (the most common), and diffusion block (rare in pediatrics). These will be dealt with in more detail later.

By examining the alveolar gas equation, it is apparent that a normal pCO_2 cannot be presumed from a normal pO_2 (or more practically clinically, from a normal oxyhemoglobin saturation), especially when the patient is receiving supplemental oxygen. A patient receiving no supplemental oxygen (21%) could have a normal SpO_2 (95%) and pO_2 (~80 torr), and the pCO_2 could be at most 55 torr. However, a patient whose FiO_2 is 30% could have the same measures of oxygenation and yet have a pCO_2 of 107 torr! The clinician should not be falsely reassured about the adequacy of ventilation by a normal saturation in a patient with respiratory distress.

Gas Transport to the Periphery

Oxygen is carried in the blood in two forms: dissolved and bound to hemoglobin. The dissolved amount (0.003 ml O_2/100 ml blood/mmHg PO_2) contributes only a small amount to the total content of oxygen in the blood. In contrast, 1.36 ml of oxygen can combine with each gram of hemoglobin. The percentage of hemoglobin that is bound to oxygen is termed the *oxyhemoglobin saturation* and may be affected by temperature, pH, pCO_2, and structural changes in the hemoglobin molecules. The relationship between arterial oxygen tension and oxygen saturation is described by the oxyhemoglobin dissociation curve (Figure 14-2).

The curve has a flat portion where the saturation is minimally affected by changes in pO_2, and a steep portion where tissues can withdraw large amounts of oxygen (i.e., large change in saturation) for small decreases in capillary pO_2. The curve shifts to the right (i.e., has a

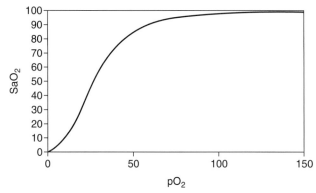

Figure 14-2 The oxyhemoglobin dissociation curve. Note the sigmoidal shape of the curve, with a steep segment (where most unloading of oxygen occurs) and flatter portions (where little change in saturation occurs despite large changes in pO_2).

lower saturation for the same PaO_2) for increases in temperature, acidity (Bohr effect), and 2,3-diphosphoglycerol (2,3-DPG) concentration. Muscle that is exercising, for instance, usually has an increased temperature due to increased blood flow. It also has increased acidity because of lactate production, and these effects act in concert on oxygen binding to facilitate providing extra oxygen to the muscle. Banked blood usually has very low amounts of 2,3-DPG; this deficiency increases the avidity of the hemoglobin for oxygen, impairing delivery to the tissues.

The *oxygen content* of arterial blood (CaO_2) then can be calculated by adding the dissolved and bound amounts of oxygen in the blood:

$$CaO_2 = (0.003 \text{ ml/torr} \times PaO_2 \text{ torr}) + (1.36 \text{ ml/g} \times Hb \text{ g} \times \% \text{ saturation}) = \text{ml } O_2/\text{dl blood}$$

It can be seen from this equation that most oxygen is bound to hemoglobin; oxygen content is related to oxygen saturation in a linear fashion. Notice that the oxygen content can be increased by increasing the PaO_2 or saturation, or by increasing the hemoglobin. Both methods are sometimes used in the care of patients with hypoxemic respiratory failure. **Oxygen delivery** (to the tissues) is calculated by multiplying the oxygen content by the cardiac output (CO). Transfusions may increase the oxygen content, but they may also decrease CO by increasing blood viscosity. The net effect, then, could be a decrease in oxygen delivery to the tissues if the decrease in cardiac output is greater than the increase in CaO_2 after transfusion.

Carbon dioxide can be transported in three forms: dissolved (5%), as carbamino compounds (5%), and as bicarbonate ion (90%). In the erythrocyte and in the presence of carbonic anhydrase, CO_2 combines with water to produce carbonic acid, which then dissociates into bicarbonate and a proton:

$$CO_2 + H_2O \Leftrightarrow H_2CO_3 \Leftrightarrow H^+ + HCO_3^-$$

Some of these protons can combine with oxygenated hemoglobin, allowing for unloading of oxygen and loading of CO_2; this process facilitates the necessary gas transport at the tissue level and is known as the **Haldane effect**. In the pulmonary capillary, oxygen can displace protons from hemoglobin, which can then combine with bicarbonate, generating CO_2 to be exhaled.

$\dot{V}/\dot{Q}$ Relationships

Effective delivery of oxygen to the body's cells requires a precise balance between ventilation of lung units and blood flow to those units. Imbalances in these relationships, termed *ventilation-perfusion* ($\dot{V}_A/\dot{Q}$) *ratios*, are the most common cause of hypoxemia in patients. There are two extremes of $\dot{V}_A/\dot{Q}$ imbalance: *shunt* and *dead space*. Shunt refers to situations where there is blood flow ($\dot{Q} > 0$) that comes into contact with

non-ventilated lung units ($\dot{V}_A = 0$) or does not come into contact with the lung at all; in these situations, $\dot{V}_A/\dot{Q} = 0$. Shunts can be "irreversible" or "fixed" such as intracardiac shunts or intrapulmonary shunts (e.g., arteriovenous malformations). They are designated "irreversible" or "fixed" because they do not respond to hyperoxia. "Reversible" shunts are really areas of very low $\dot{V}_A/\dot{Q}$ which will respond to hyperoxia (see below). Dead space refers to situations where airflow ($\dot{V}_A > 0$) comes into contact with non-perfused lung units ($\dot{Q} = 0$), such as occurs in a pulmonary embolus. The blood gas abnormality resulting from shunt is hypoxemia, while that resulting from increased dead space is hypercarbia. In between the two extremes, varying degrees of $\dot{V}_A/\dot{Q}$ mismatch can exist.

Any disease process that alters ventilation or perfusion will likely result in some imbalance in $\dot{V}_A/\dot{Q}$ ratios. For example, acute airway obstruction or lobar atelectasis decreases ventilation to lung units. Autoregulation of pulmonary blood flow reduces but does not completely eliminate perfusion of these regions. Furthermore, the redirected blood will pass by other alveoli whose ventilation will not be adequate for the increased perfusion. Both phenomena result in regions with a decreased $\dot{V}_A/\dot{Q}$ ratio. The oxygen and CO_2 tensions in the alveolus and end-capillary blood will approach that of mixed venous blood (Figure 14-3).

In contrast, a pulmonary embolism ablates blood flow to certain regions without affecting ventilation, increasing the $\dot{V}_A/\dot{Q}$ ratio. The oxygen and CO_2 tensions in the affected alveolus will approach those in the inspired gas.

Quantifying $\dot{V}_A/\dot{Q}$ relationships is very difficult. The simplest estimation of imbalances in $\dot{V}_A/\dot{Q}$ can be obtained by calculation of the A–a gradient. This gradient is usually very small (<15 torr), but will be elevated if there is a block in diffusion, $\dot{V}_A/\dot{Q}$ imbalance, or shunt. Note that in the other respiratory causes of hypoxemia (low inspired oxygen tension or hypoventilation), the alveolar pO_2 and arterial pO_2 will both be equally depressed, resulting in a normal A–a gradient. More complicated techniques to measure $\dot{V}_A/\dot{Q}$ ratios (i.e., multiple inert gas exhalation technique, MIGET) can describe the distribution of $\dot{V}_A/\dot{Q}$ relationships in the lung, but are not readily clinically available.

As discussed above, hypoxemia due to "irreversible" (e.g., intracardiac) shunts cannot be corrected with supplemental oxygen. Consider a two-compartment lung, one compartment with normal $\dot{V}_A/\dot{Q}$ relationships and the other compartment with perfusion but no ventilation (shunt). The "normal" compartment has an oxygen saturation of 98% and pO_2 of 110 torr, but the "shunt" compartment has a saturation of 75% and pO_2 of 40 torr (i.e., similar to values in mixed venous blood). Although overly simplistic, let us also assume that the two units receive equal amounts of blood flow. At first glance, one might

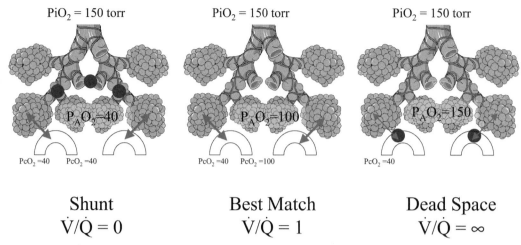

Figure 14-3   Matching of ventilation and perfusion in normal (center) or disease (left, right) conditions. In conditions of shunt (left), the partial pressures of oxygen in the alveolus and pulmonary capillary pressures will equilibrate to values near that of mixed venous blood. In conditions of dead space (right), the partial pressures of oxygen in the inspired gas and the alveolus will equilibrate.

assume that the pO_2 of the blood mixed from these two compartments would be the average of the tensions of the two compartments ($110 + 40/2 = 75$ torr). When measured, however, the pO_2 of the mixed blood is found to be only 53 torr! This demonstrates that the mixed blood pO_2 is determined by the mixing of the oxygen *contents* of the individual compartments (Figure 14-4). This is in part because the poorly saturated, shunted blood readily picks up oxygen from the better-saturated blood, reducing the pO_2 of the mixed blood. It is also due to the fact that the oxyhemoglobin dissociation curve (and the oxygen content curve) is not linear, but rather sigmoidal. To confirm this, we can calculate the oxygen content of the "normal" unit [$(1.36 \times 0.98 \times 15) + (0.003 \times 110)$] and the "shunt" unit [$(1.36 \times 0.75 \times 15) + (0.003 \times 40)$], assuming a value for hemoglobin of 15 gm/dl. The two contents

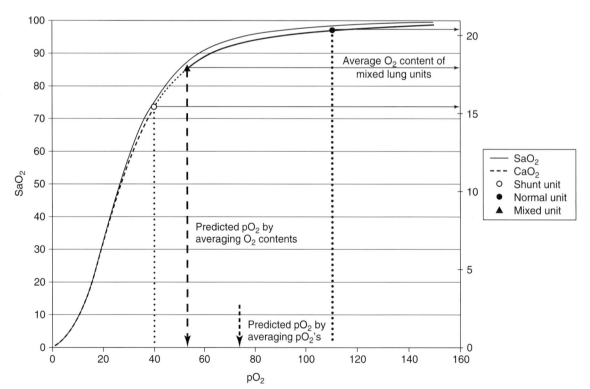

Figure 14-4   Oxyhemoglobin saturation and oxygen content as a function of the partial pressure of oxygen.

(20.3 ml/dl and 15.4 ml/dl) are then averaged to be 17.8 ml/dl; this corresponds to a pO_2 of 53 torr.

Now imagine that 100% oxygen is administered to this lung. The "shunt" region, by definition, does not receive any more oxygen. The "normal" unit now has a pO_2 of 663 torr and a saturation of 100%. The oxygen content of the blood, however, has changed minimally as this lung unit was already on the flat upper part of the oxygen dissociation curve. The saturation has only increased 2% and the dissolved pO_2 increase is negligible (1.66 ml/dl). The average of the two contents is then $[(1.34 \times 1.0 \times 15) + (0.003 \times 663)] + [(1.34 \times 0.75 \times 15) + (0.003 \times 40)]/2 = (22.1 + 15.1)/2 = 18.7$ ml/dl; this corresponds to a saturation of 91% and pO_2 of ~64 torr, not the 352 torr which would be predicted from averaging pO_2 values.

When treating patients with hypoxemia refractory to supplemental oxygen, disease processes that cause shunting must be considered and treated. Hypoxemia can also be due to a "reversible" shunt related to $\dot{V}_A/\dot{Q}$ mismatch. This hypoxemia can be improved with administration of supplemental oxygen, because "reversible" shunts represent areas of low (but not zero) $\dot{V}_A/\dot{Q}$. These lung units sit on the steep portion of the oxygen dissociation curve. Since they receive some (but not normal) ventilation, supplemental oxygen will increase their oxygen tension, which may be enough to move the lung unit onto the flat portion of the oxygen dissociation curve and attain a normal saturation and therefore higher oxygen content.

Fick's law can be used to estimate the "shunt fraction". This law assumes that the oxygen content of the blood leaving the heart is the sum of oxygen from the pulmonary capillaries (non-shunted) and from shunted regions (either within the lung or extrapulmonary). Mathematically,

$$\dot{Q}t \times CaO_2 = \dot{Q}c \times CcO_2 + \dot{Q}s \times C\bar{v}O_2$$

This equation can be rearranged to calculate the "shunt fraction," $\dot{Q}s/\dot{Q}t = (CcO_2 - CaO_2)/(CcO_2 - CvO_2)$, where $\dot{Q}s$ is the shunted blood flow, $\dot{Q}t$ is the total blood flow, CcO_2 is the pulmonary capillary blood oxygen content, CaO_2 is the arterial blood oxygen content, and $C\bar{v}O_2$ is the mixed venous blood oxygen content.

Taken together, the measurements of dead space, shunt fraction, and A–a gradients for O_2 and CO_2 can give meaningful insight into the maldistribution of ventilation and perfusion, and help identify the cause(s) of respiratory failure (Table 14-2).

DIAGNOSIS AND MONITORING OF PATIENTS WITH RESPIRATORY FAILURE

Blood Gases

Measurement of gas tensions in arterial blood (ABG) have long been the standard for monitoring patients at risk for or already in respiratory failure. They provide information about oxygenation, ventilation, and the acid–base status which reflects pulmonary and renal homeostasis. Blood gas analyzers *measure* pH, pO_2, and pCO_2; the reported saturation is calculated from the pO_2 and the oxyhemoglobin saturation curve, and the reported HCO_3^- is calculated from the pH, pCO_2, and Hb using a nomogram. Obtaining ABGs can be painful for the patient, but there is usually adequate time to apply topical anesthetics. Alternatives such as sampling capillary (CBG) or venous (VBG) blood are frequently employed. CBGs obtained from a warmed extremity are a closer representation of arterial pCO_2 and pH than are VBGs, which frequently represent local tissue acid–base status; neither alternative is particularly accurate for assessment of arterial pO_2. Proper collection and handling of the specimen is important; excess heparin in the collection syringe may alter the pH of the collected blood, while air bubbles will equilibrate the patient's pO_2 and pCO_2 with room air (150 torr and 0 torr, respectively). Samples should be processed rapidly or placed on ice to decrease ongoing metabolism of oxygen within the sample. A systematic approach should be utilized in interpreting blood gas values. The observed pO_2, SaO_2 and CO_2 must be interpreted in the context of the FiO_2 and the patient's respiratory rate. A complete description of blood gas interpretation is beyond the scope of this chapter, but several excellent reviews are referenced[3,4].

Table 14-2 Causes of Hypoxemia				
	A–a O_2 Gradient	A–a CO_2 Gradient	Increased pO_2 with Increased FiO_2	$\dot{Q}s/\dot{Q}t$
$\dot{V}/\dot{Q}$ mismatch, low $\dot{V}/\dot{Q}$	↑	Normal	Yes	↑
$\dot{V}/\dot{Q}$ mismatch, high $\dot{V}/\dot{Q}$	Normal	↑	Yes	Normal
Hypoventilation	Normal	Normal	Yes	Normal
Shunt (irreversible)	↑	Normal	No	↑
Diffusion block	↑	Normal	+/−	↑
Low inspired FiO_2	Normal	Normal	Yes	Normal

Pulse Oximetry and Capnography

The advent of non-invasive pulse oximetry (SpO_2) has made feasible the continuous monitoring of oxygenation in patients with respiratory failure. This allows much more rapid detection of changes in clinical status than do intermittent measurements of blood gases. The technique is based on light absorption by oxygenated and reduced hemoglobin at two different (visible and infrared) wavelengths. It should be noted that this technique is subject to several sources of error. Carboxyhemoglobin absorbs visible light in a way similar to oxygenated hemoglobin, and can cause artificially high SpO_2 measurements in patients with carbon monoxide poisoning. In contrast, methemoglobin absorbs visible light in a way similar to reduced hemoglobin, frequently resulting in artificially low measured SpO_2 (approximately 85–88%). Additionally, the oximeter signal depends on detection of a pulsatile waveform, and poor perfusion or edema may interfere with readings. Patient motion is the most common cause of artifactual readings, and comparison of the pulse rate recorded by the oximeter and that from electrocardiographic monitoring provides one method of determining the accuracy of the reading. With these caveats, continuous pulse oximetry is extremely useful for monitoring of patients in respiratory failure.

As previously noted, normal oximetry values do not assure normal ventilation. Exhaled gas can be analyzed for CO_2 concentration (usually also by infrared light absorption), and the waveform can be displayed continuously, by a capnograph. The normal capnogram demonstrates a flat initial portion (from dead space with no CO_2), followed by a rapid and sharp increase in exhaled CO_2 (as alveolar gas begins to empty), and a subsequent plateau as alveoli empty during exhalation (Figure 14-5). In the healthy lung, the concentration of CO_2 at the end of a breath ($ETCO_2$) closely approximates

arterial pCO_2. In disease states, however, capnography can render inaccurate measurements. Increased dead space may dilute alveolar CO_2 with gas devoid of CO_2, and the $ETCO_2$ could underestimate arterial CO_2. Similarly, exhaled gas that does not reach the sensor (e.g., due to leak) will result in an artifactually low $ETCO_2$. Absence of a plateau in the capnogram suggests the presence of airway obstruction (Figure 14-5). Because of these possible errors, as well as the technical difficulties in measurement of humidified gases, the $ETCO_2$ should be correlated with measurement of CO_2 in blood. Additionally, the interpretation of the $ETCO_2$ value will be facilitated by the capnogram waveform, as described above.

Imaging

As mentioned earlier, the presence of bilateral pulmonary infiltrates is one of the diagnostic criteria for ARDS. In the early stages (0–24 hours) of ARDS, the chest radiograph may appear normal or reflect mild interstitial edema. As the disease progresses, there will be progressive atelectasis, interstitial edema, and ground-glass opacification of the airspaces. In the later stages, air bronchograms and more dense consolidations appear. The standard chest radiograph can help detect complicating factors or alternative diagnoses such as cardiogenic pulmonary edema as well as pneumothorax, or improper positioning of endotracheal tubes or central catheters. The resolution of radiographic changes in ARDS may be quite slow, and the benefit of daily radiographs in the ICU setting has not been well demonstrated.

Computed tomography (CT) studies obtained in patients with ARDS surprisingly have demonstrated that the disease is not as homogeneous as would be suspected from the plain radiograph. Indeed, the dependent portions of the lung are significantly more densely opacified than the non-dependent regions. This observation of a gravity-dependent gradient of disease was important in considering the use of prone positioning in the treatment of ARDS (Figure 14-6). CT has also been used to study the effects of other treatments such as positive end-expiratory pressure (PEEP) and liquid ventilation in ARDS.

Pulmonary Function Measurements

Measurements of pulmonary function in patients with respiratory failure can guide therapy, particularly in adjusting ventilator support. In children receiving mechanical ventilation, bedside measurements of lung mechanics (e.g., respiratory system compliance, resistance) can allow rational adjustments of distending pressures or other ventilator settings, as well as providing objective data regarding response to therapy (i.e., bronchodilators, diuretics) and assessments of disease course. Bedside estimates of compliance and resistance can be made by measuring changes in pressure (usually between peak

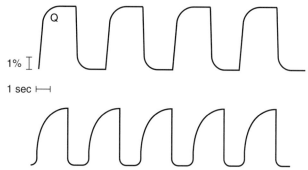

Figure 14-5 Capnogram tracings. The normal capnogram (top tracing) has a rectangular wave pattern, exhibiting a rapid ascending slope, an almost 90° angle to the alveolar plateau, the end-tidal peak, and a vertical descending slope. In the presence of obstructive disease (bottom tracing), the capnogram loses its rectangular shape and is sometimes described as a "shark fin."

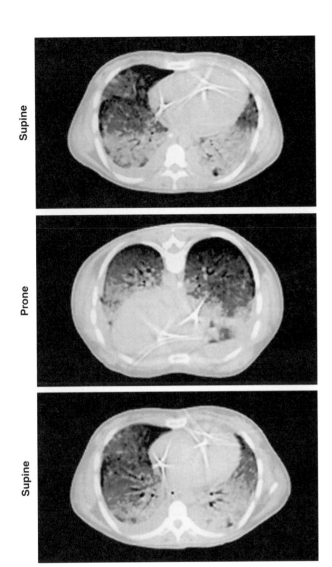

Figure 14-6 CT images of ARDS in supine (upper panel), prone (middle panel), and return to supine position (lower panel). Note how gravity-dependent densities shift from dorsal to ventral within minutes when the patient is turned prone. (From Gattioni, et al. Am J Respir Crit Care Med 164:1701–1711, 2001.)

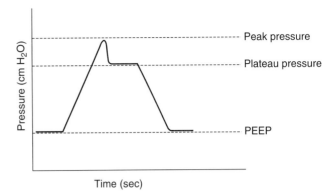

Figure 14-7 Airway pressures used to measure lung mechanics.

inspiratory pressure, PIP, and the end-expiratory pressure, PEEP, or the plateau pressure, Pplat) and changes in volume (exhaled tidal volume) (Figure 14-7). Specifically, compliance is calculated as the change in volume (Vt) divided by the change in pressure (Pplat – PEEP), and resistance as change in pressure (PIP – Pplat) divided by flow (Vt/inspiratory time).

Measurement of the plateau pressure requires an end-inspiratory hold, a technique available on many commercial ventilators. The patient must also be relaxed and allowed to exhale passively. Some newer ventilators measure breath-by-breath dynamic compliance and resistance. Graphic displays of pressure–volume or flow–volume curves can provide additional information about pulmonary mechanics[5], and can provide rapid feedback to the clinician making ventilator adjustments.

MANAGEMENT

When Eli'sha came into the house, he saw the child lying dead on his bed. So he went in and shut the door upon the two of them, and prayed to the Lord. Then he went up and lay upon the child, putting his mouth upon his mouth, his eyes upon his eyes, and his hands upon his hands; and as he stretched himself upon him, the flesh of the child became warm. Then he got up again, and walked once to and fro in the house, and went up, and stretched himself upon him; the child sneezed seven times, and the child opened his eyes.

Kings II 4:32

This may be one of the earliest recorded reports of "assisted ventilation" or resuscitation in a pediatric patient. In the following section, we will consider more commonly used treatments for pediatric patients with respiratory failure. The goals of most ventilation strategies are to normalize gas exchange while minimizing lung injury or cardiovascular compromise.

Conventional Therapies

Positive-Pressure Ventilation

The majority of patients with acute respiratory failure are treated with positive-pressure ventilation through an endotracheal tube. There are numerous different ventilator modes and styles[6], and a full discussion of them is beyond the scope of this text. However, there are some underlying principles that are common to most modes: the clinician usually sets a ventilator rate, end-expiratory pressure (PEEP), and inspired fraction of oxygen; the amount of gas delivered by the ventilator can be *limited* by pressure or volume, and the duration of inspiration can by *cycled* by time or flow. For example, in pressure-limited (sometimes called "pressure controlled") ventilation, the clinician chooses a peak inspiratory pressure that limits the magnitude of inspiratory pressure delivered over the breath, and the tidal volume of that breath

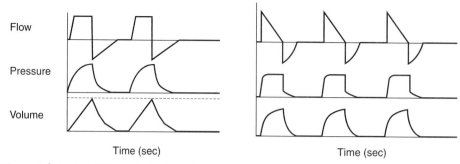

Figure 14-8   Left: Volume-limited ventilation. Note the square wave flow pattern. Right: Pressure-controlled ventilation. Note the decelerating flow pattern.

will vary depending on the lung compliance and resistance at the time. In volume-limited (sometimes called "volume controlled") ventilation, the clinician chooses a tidal volume that limits the delivered breath, and the peak inspiratory pressure used to achieve that volume will vary depending on the lung compliance and resistance (Figure 14-8).

For each of these strategies, the ventilator can be set to deliver a complete breath for each effort initiated by the patient (*assist-control*) or to cycle based only on the set rate (*control* mode, where the patient cannot breathe spontaneously between mandatory breaths, or *intermittent mandatory ventilation*, where spontaneous breaths are permitted). Most recent ventilators attempt to synchronize the mandated breaths with the efforts of the patient (*synchronized intermittent mandatory ventilation*), to avoid the uncomfortable delivery of a breath when the patient wishes to exhale (Figure 14-9).

In addition, many ventilators offer *pressure support* where patient-initiated efforts trigger delivery of flow up to a preset pressure level, which the patient can terminate. In contrast to assist-control ventilation, pressure support ventilation affords partial, not complete support for patient-triggered breaths. In fact, if pressure support is used as the sole mode of support, the patient controls

most aspects of the ventilation. For this reason, it is felt to be a "comfortable" mode for the patient.

Positive end-expiratory pressure (PEEP) can help minimize airway collapse and maintain lung volume. This latter function of PEEP may improve lung compliance, and allow for ventilation with lower peak pressures. It also increases the mean airway pressure, which can improve oxygenation by improving ventilation–perfusion matching. Central airway collapse (i.e., due to tracheomalacia or bronchomalacia) may be overcome by PEEP. However, excess PEEP could overdistend the lung, decreasing compliance.

Positive-pressure ventilation, while life-sustaining, also has adverse physiologic consequences. By increasing alveolar pressure, it may decrease blood flow to intra-alveolar capillaries, resulting in ventilation–perfusion mismatch. High intrathoracic pressures (related to PIP or PEEP) have the potential to decrease venous return to the heart. Additionally, very high transmural pressures could cause rupture of some lung tissue resulting in pneumothorax.

It is usually not possible to decide a priori which ventilator or mode will be optimal for a patient with a given disease, and frequent bedside assessments are the best guide. With whatever mode of ventilation is chosen, many adjustments in the acute setting are usually needed. These should be guided by assessment of

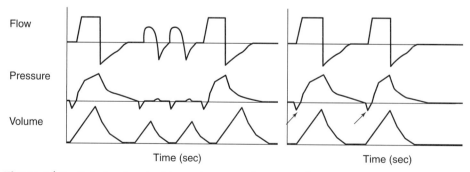

Figure 14-9   *Left*: Synchronized intermittent mandatory ventilation. Note the larger, mandated breaths and the smaller, spontaneous breaths. *Right*: Assist-controlled ventilation. Note the negative pressure (initiated by the patient, arrows), triggering the assisted breath.

patient comfort and synchrony with the ventilator, blood gas determinations, non-invasive monitoring (SpO_2, $ETCO_2$), and in some cases, measurements of lung mechanics. For example, worsening hypercarbia can be addressed by increasing minute ventilation by increasing either the ventilator rate or tidal volume. Worsening hypoxemia can be addressed by increasing inspired fraction of oxygen or mean airway pressure.

Ventilator-induced lung injury (from "volutrauma", i.e., overdistension of the lung, or "barotrauma", i.e., high pressures in the airway) can be minimized by strategies to minimize transmural pressures. Additionally, attention to peak airway pressures and mean airway pressures is necessary. Indeed, it is now accepted practice to allow for some degree of hypercarbia, rather than attempting to achieve eucapnea, if a normal pCO_2 can only be obtained through the use of high airway pressures. This "permissive hypercapnea" strategy recognizes the need to balance normalization of blood gases against the potential to cause airway and lung injury. Overdistension of the lung can be recognized from the pressure–volume curve (displayed by many hospital ventilators).

For patients with chronic respiratory failure, several ventilators are available for home use. Some of these are fairly simple (i.e., providing only volume-limited ventilation), while others provide many of the same modes as hospital ventilators (Table 14-3).

Home ventilators can be powered by a portable battery, further enhancing patient mobility. Monitoring in the home setting is usually accomplished by pulse oximetry, and sometimes capnography. Care of the home ventilator patient requires a team approach, which necessitates participation by nurses, respiratory therapists, physicians, and most importantly trained family caregivers[7].

Non-invasive Positive-Pressure Ventilation

Non-invasive positive-pressure ventilation (NIPPV) is typically provided via a nasal interface (masks or prongs, Figure 14-10), and delivers flow in a pressure-support pattern.

The most commonly used style is termed bi-level positive airway pressure (B_LPAP), in which the clinician chooses an inspiratory positive airway pressure (IPAP) and expiratory positive airway pressure (EPAP); the ventilator cycles between these two pressures. The inspiratory flow from the ventilator (to reach IPAP) is usually triggered by the patient, and terminated when the inspiratory flow rate has decreased to a predetermined percentage of initial flow rate. A "back-up" rate can be set if there are concerns about patient ability to trigger the ventilator, or abnormalities in respiratory drive. Newer B_LPAP generators include features that allow time-cycled termination of the breath, and a "ramp" function which slowly increases the inspiratory pressures over a period of 15–30 minutes to allow patients to accommodate to the pressures.

NIPPV has been used more commonly for chronic respiratory failure, especially in patients who require support for only a portion of the day or for patients who refuse endotracheal intubation[8]. More recently, NIPPV has also been used for acute respiratory failure with good success[9]. It obviates the need for an artificial airway, thus enhancing patient communication and possibly decreasing the risk of infectious complications. Complications of NIPPV can be related to the mask/interface, and include skin or nasal irritation; any persistent area of facial erythema is worrisome and requires measures to prevent ulcer formation. Anxiety can develop, resulting from a feeling of claustrophobia from the mask, high air flow rates, or ineffective ventilation. Air leakage through the mouth can result in ineffective ventilation, and leakage around the interface can cause irritation of the eyes. Gastric distension can occur, as the airflow is not directed solely to the airway, but to the esophagus as well. If this is severe, it can be treated with nasogastric tube decompression. Close monitoring for these complications is warranted in the care of patients receiving NIPPV.

Inhaled Nitric Oxide

Previously called "endothelial-derived relaxing factor", nitric oxide (NO) mediates (amongst other things) vascular smooth muscle relaxation via cGMP-dependent

Table 14-3 Ventilators Used in the Home Setting					
	Pressure-control	Volume-control	Pressure Support	CPAP	Continuous Flow
LTV (Pulmonetics)	✓	✓	✓	✓	✓
T-Bird (Bird Ventilators)		✓	✓	✓	✓
LP-10 (Puritan Bennett)		✓			
PLV-100 (Respironics)		✓			
HT-50 (Newport)	✓	✓	✓	✓	✓

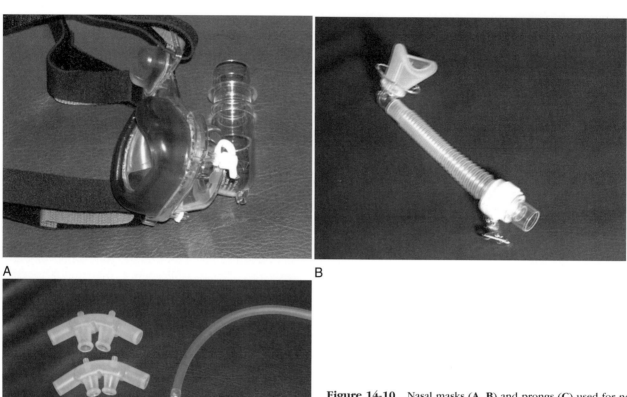

Figure 14-10 Nasal masks (**A**, **B**) and prongs (**C**) used for non-invasive positive-pressure ventilation.

protein kinases. The discovery that a gas could act as an endogenous messenger resulted in the Nobel Prize being awarded to Drs. Robert Furchgott, Louis Ignarro, and Ferid Murad in 1998, and nitric oxide was named "Molecule of the Year" by the journal *Science* in 1992. NO is produced by the pulmonary vascular endothelium by nitric oxide synthetases (NOS), which can be constitutive or inducible, from L-arginine. It has been well demonstrated that inhaled nitric oxide (iNO) decreases pulmonary artery pressure, and because it is rapidly (seconds) inactivated upon binding hemoglobin, it has minimal effects on peripheral vascular tone. Additionally, when the molecule is administered by inhalation, it will be preferentially delivered to areas with good ventilation, thus preserving hypoxic vasoconstriction in areas that are poorly ventilated and possibly improving ventilation–perfusion matching in areas that are well ventilated. It has been used with good results in neonates with persistent

pulmonary hypertension of the newborn, demonstrating improvement in oxygenation and reduced need for extracorporeal membrane oxygenation (ECMO). iNO (Innomax, INO Therapeutics) was approved by the U.S. Food and Drug Administration (FDA) in 1999 for use in neonatal hypoxemic respiratory failure. As with many therapies, there is less clear evidence that iNO benefits older patients with respiratory failure. Indeed, in a randomized, double-blinded trial of 385 adults with ARDS, there was no effect of iNO on mortality or ventilator-free days. Patients with ARDS in whom pulmonary hypertension is a predominant pathophysiologic mechanism are more likely to benefit from iNO. The therapy is not without potential complications; oxidation of NO produces methemoglobin, as well as free radical species including superoxide and peroxynitrite, which can be cytotoxic. Because of these toxicities, care and monitoring of patients receiving iNO includes carefully measuring delivered gas concentrations, scavenging exhaled gases for nitrogen dioxide, and measuring serum methemoglobin levels.

Extracorporeal Membrane Oxygenation

The techniques that underlie the use of extracorporeal membrane oxygenation (ECMO; also known as extracorporeal life support, ECLS) were developed in the early 1950s by cardiothoracic surgeons, and extended to patients outside of the operating room in the early 1970s[10-12]. The main principle is that the gas exchange functions of the lung (oxygenation and ventilation) can be provided by an artificial membrane in place of the alveolar-capillary membrane. While this support is provided extracorporeally, many of the detrimental pulmonary effects of mechanical ventilation can be minimized. The goal of this strategy is to support the patient while allowing the underlying disease (pneumonia, sepsis, persistent pulmonary hypertension, meconium aspiration) to improve.

It can be sometimes difficult to balance the risks of ECMO (see below) against the potential benefits, and choosing the optimal time to initiate this therapy is not straightforward. Commonly, neonatal patients with an oxygenation index (OI = Mean airway pressure $\times$ FiO$_2$/PaO$_2$), greater than 40 are considered candidates due to their high risk of mortality with conventional therapy. Premature infants (<34 weeks) are typically excluded due to the risk of intracranial hemorrhage; less premature but growth-retarded infants (<2 kg) may not be able to accommodate the ECMO intravascular catheters. Most physicians would consider irreversible lung disease (severe pulmonary hypoplasia or fibrotic processes) or terminal disease (metastatic cancer) to be contraindications, but the literature contains reports of all these types of patients being treated with ECMO.

ECMO can be achieved by two main configurations—veno-arterial (V-A) and veno-venous (V-V) bypass—although the general methods are quite similar (Figure 14-11). For both, blood is drained from the patient via a large central vein (typically the internal jugular vein or, in larger patients, a femoral vein); drainage occurs by gravity to a reservoir (bladder). The blood is pumped from the bladder into the membrane "lung" using a roller pump that will de-activate if the bladder is empty; in this way, venous return controls the input into the circuit. The "lung" (usually composed of silicone) allows for diffusion of oxygen (in) and carbon dioxide (out), the rates of which are dependent on the flow rate of blood through the lung and the partial pressures of the gas on the other side of the membrane ("sweep gas"). Carbon dioxide transfer is so efficient that CO$_2$ usually needs to be added to the gas mixture. After the blood has passed through the lung, it is re-warmed and returned to the patient. In V-A ECMO, the route is typically via the right carotid artery; thus the majority of the flow in this configuration bypasses the

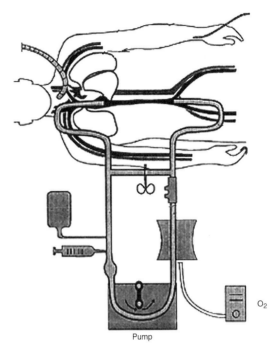

Figure 14-11   Circuit configuration for veno-venous extracorporeal membrane oxygenation (ECMO). Venous blood is drained from the right femoral vein, oxygenated, and pumped back to the right atrium. (From Zwischenberger JB, Steinhorn RH, Bartlett RH. ECMO: extracorporeal cardiopulmonary support in critical care, 2nd edition, p 24. Ann Arbor, MI: Extracorporeal Life Support Organization [ELSO], 2000.).

heart and so does not require normal cardiac output; it is therefore preferred in situations of severe cardiac dysfunction. It should also be noted that most blood also bypasses the lungs, and the effects of the lungs being relatively unperfused have not been well studied. A short length of "bridge" tubing connects the venous (from the patient) and arterial (to the patient) portions of the circuit, allowing for intermittent periods when the patient can be temporarily separated from the circuit (during the weaning process, or for maintenance of the tubing). In V-V bypass, the return of the oxygenated blood occurs through a second lumen of the catheter providing the venous drainage, and is deposited in the right atrium. Thus, in V-V bypass, there is a certain amount of "recirculation" of oxygenated blood from the circuit that is re-drained via the venous catheter, complicating interpretation of oxygen delivery. Additionally, the flow through the circuit is dependent on native cardiac output. As the patient's underlying disease improves, the flow through the ECMO circuit can be gradually decreased, aiming towards decannulation from bypass.

Both V-A and V-V ECMO presently require systemic anticoagulation to prevent clotting in the circuit (heparin bonded circuits are in development), and this represents one potential source of ECMO complications.

Monitoring of the anticoagulation status at the bedside usually occurs hourly, and adjustments in the rate of heparin infusion can be made. Indeed, surgery can be safely accomplished while the patient receives ECMO support, albeit with increased attention to anticoagulation status. Nonetheless, potential for intracranial bleeding limits the applicability of this technique in premature infants. Other potential complications include infection, circuit failure/rupture, and fluid retention. The vessels used for bypass are ligated when the patient is decannulated, and this results in impairment of venous drainage (VV, jugular vein) and/or arterial supply (VA, carotid artery) to the ipsilateral side of the brain.

Caring for patients on ECMO requires a dedicated multidisciplinary team, including but not limited to nurses, respiratory therapists, neonatal or pediatric intensivists, and surgeons. Patients require continuous monitoring and frequent laboratory studies, medications, and adjustments. The resources involved in providing this care to an individual patient, and in maintaining such a program, are extensive.

In neonatal patients, it is clear that use of ECMO has substantially improved the survival of infants with persistent pulmonary hypertension of the newborn and meconium aspiration syndrome. As ECMO centers have gained experience over the years, the indications for use of ECMO have been broadened, and it has become more difficult to assess the results. Similarly, in pediatric patients, the causes of respiratory failure are quite varied, complicating an analysis of benefits. There are several studies attempting to address the developmental outcomes of infants treated with this therapy, and it seems that most infants survive without handicaps markedly different from those of other graduates of the NICU.

Non-traditional Therapies

With the exception of negative-pressure ventilation, use of the following therapies has been restricted to ARDS.

Prone Positioning

Since the early 1970s, it has been recognized that the lung disease in ARDS is non-homogeneous, and that there is a gravity-dependent gradient of opacification (worse in the dependent regions). Studies using chest CT demonstrated that this distribution shifted when patients were placed prone, resulting in better aeration and perfusion of the posterior (and larger) portions of the lung, and subsequent better oxygenation. This was confirmed in several small clinical studies in adults, and there are only limited supporting data in pediatric patients[13,14]. Complications from prone positioning appear to be uncommon, but can include transient oxyhemoglobin desaturations or increased secretions, vomiting, hypotension, and displacement of catheters or endotracheal tubes. Which patients will benefit most from this technique, and how often and for how long to position patients prone, are unanswered questions.

Negative-Pressure Ventilation

As in positive-pressure ventilation, flow of air into the lungs is dependent upon a pressure gradient between the mouth and the alveoli. In negative-pressure ventilation (NPV), this gradient can be achieved by lowering the body surface pressure below atmospheric pressure. This requires an interface between the negative-pressure generator and the patient, and can be a tank (e.g., the "iron lung" of the 1950s poliovirus epidemic), body suit/poncho, or cuirass/shell (Figure 14-12).

One advantage of this mode of ventilation is that it does not require an endotracheal tube, and therefore the patient is able to speak and eat. Additionally, the negative intrathoracic pressure enhances venous return (in contrast to possible impairment of venous return with positive-pressure ventilators). Most negative-pressure ventilators, however, are not portable. In addition, upper airway collapse may be exacerbated. The ventilators tend to be time-cycled, pressure-limited, but many of the newer ventilators have modes of ventilation that are

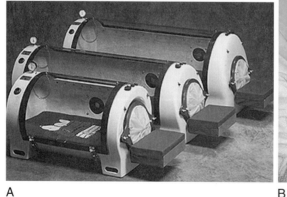
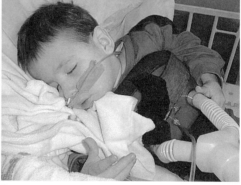

A   B

Figure 14-12 Negative-pressure ventilators. (**A**) The tank (www.porta-lung.com) and (**B**) cuirass interfaces are depicted both are connected to the negative-pressure generator (not shown). (Part **B** courtesy of Professor Anne Thomson, Radcliffe Hospital, Oxford, UK.)

similar to their positive-pressure counterparts, including CNEP (continuous negative expiratory pressure), intermittent mandatory ventilation, and assist-control (using a nasal cannula to sense patient effort). This mode of ventilation may be particularly useful for patients with chronic respiratory failure who require continuous ventilation but who wish to avoid tracheostomy, or for patients who find the facial interfaces for non-invasive positive-pressure ventilation uncomfortable.

High-Frequency Oscillatory Ventilation

High-frequency ventilation (HFOV) has the potential to recruit lung units with the use of high mean airway pressure while limiting ventilator injury by using extremely small tidal volumes and lower peak inspiratory pressures. In this way, the lungs are ventilated on the steeper (more compliant) portion of the pressure–volume curve. In fact, the tidal volumes that would be achieved by these pressure swings are smaller than the anatomic dead space. Gas exchange, therefore, occurs by means other than those typical for traditional ventilation, and includes molecular diffusion and pendulluft (gas mixing that occurs within the lung). In this mode of ventilation, the modifiable parameters are Paw (mean airway pressure), oscillating frequency (usually 5–10 Hz, or 300–600 breaths/minute), FiO_2, and pressure amplitude (usually set to result in visible chest wall shaking). Some institutions utilize aggressive re-recruitment maneuvers (rapid increases in Paw) to achieve maximum effectiveness of HFOV. However, disconnecting the patient from the ventilator for suctioning, transport, etc., can result in loss of recruited lung units. Additionally, spontaneous breathing during this type of ventilation is ineffective, and patients are usually paralyzed and deeply sedated.

A randomized trial comparing HFOV and conventional ventilation in 70 pediatric patients with ARDS[15] demonstrated no differences in important clinical outcomes (e.g., mortality). In a post-hoc analysis, there was a lower mortality in the subgroup of patients treated only with HFOV. In most institutions, HFOV is used as a rescue therapy for pediatric patients rather than as a primary mode of treatment.

Liquid Ventilation

Liquid ventilation aims to achieve gas exchange in the lung via inhalation of an inert fluid (e.g., a perfluorochemical) in place of the gases normally filling the lung. Perfluorochemicals have a very high density (approximately twice that of water), low viscosity, low surface tension, and a very high solubility for oxygen and carbon dioxide. There are several potential advantages to this strategy. First, the liquid-filled lung has no air–liquid interfaces; this dramatically reduces surface tension and improves lung compliance. Secondly, perfluorochemicals distribute more evenly than gas in the diseased lung,

thus potentially allowing for widespread drug delivery. This distribution effect also allows the liquid to recruit atelectatic lung units, improving ventilation–perfusion matching. Additionally, because they are nearly completely immiscible with most other liquids, perfluorochemicals may enhance removal of airway debris, which floats to the top of the perfluorochemical. This effect has been noted in infants treated for meconium aspiration and a child with hydrocarbon aspiration[16]. Liquid ventilation has been attempted using either completely liquid-filled lungs (total liquid ventilation) or partially filled lungs in combination with standard gas ventilation (also known as PAGE, or perfluorochemical assisted gas exchange). In partial liquid ventilation (PLV), the lungs are typically inflated with a volume of perfluorochemical equivalent to the functional residual capacity, or about 30 ml/kg.

In one preliminary study of partial liquid ventilation in premature infants with respiratory distress syndrome, oxygenation and lung compliance improved[17]. In an uncontrolled phase II study in adults with ARDS, PLV-treated patients demonstrated a decreased mortality compared with patients treated with conventional gas ventilation. However, a recently completed phase II-III trial with 311 adult ARDS patients at 56 centers in the United States, Canada, and Europe (Alliance Pharmaceuticals), failed to demonstrate any improvement in mortality or ventilator-free days. In this study, the control group had a very low mortality (15%), which may be due to newer strategies for traditional gas ventilation. At present, liquid ventilation must be considered strictly experimental.

The Recovery Phase

In some situations, as the acute lung injury resolves, withdrawal of ventilatory support may become possible. Strategies include incremental reductions in ventilator pressures or rate and daily attempts to discontinue ventilator support ("sprints"). The choice of weaning strategy depends, in part, on the cause of the acute lung injury. The optimal manner in which a patient is liberated from support remains controversial[18,19]. Some children with chronic respiratory failure that improves (e.g., the older child with bronchopulmonary dysplasia) may also be candidates for liberation from mechanical ventilation. In these situations, too, there is great variability in how to accomplish this goal. At the author's institution, frequent telephone assessments are made with information provided by parents or home caregivers. This information (which includes growth measurements, assessments of stamina for play or therapies as well as oxygenation and ventilation, and tolerance of "sprints") guides decisions about moving forward in the process of liberation.

SUMMARY

Children may experience respiratory failure from diverse causes that can affect respiratory drive, respiratory muscles, or gas exchange units. A wide spectrum of therapies (including positive-pressure ventilation, negative-pressure ventilation, and non-invasive ventilation) are routinely involved in the management of respiratory failure. Other therapies (ECMO, nitric oxide, liquid ventilation) are reserved for cases where standard therapies have failed. The overall goal of management is to maintain gas exchange and oxygen delivery while minimizing iatrogenic lung injury as the underlying cause of the respiratory failure is treated. Chronic ventilation is increasingly used in the home setting for children with chronic respiratory failure. It is to be hoped that research in all these areas will result in continued improvements in survival and pulmonary and developmental outcomes.

MAJOR POINTS

1. Normal transport of oxygen and carbon dioxide requires careful matching of ventilation and perfusion.
2. Respiratory failure can occur from a multitude of causes involving all aspects of the respiratory system, including the respiratory drive center, chest wall, respiratory muscles, and gas exchange units.
3. Treatment goals for acute respiratory failure include supporting organ function while recovery from the underlying injury occurs.
4. Optimal ventilator strategy cannot be determined a priori, and requires frequent reassessment and monitoring of the patient.
5. Chronic respiratory failure may be treated in the home setting using a multidisciplinary team approach.

REFERENCES

1. Ashbaugh DG, Bigelow DB, Petty TL, Levine BE. Acute respiratory distress in adults. Lancet II:319-323, 1967.

2. Bernard GR, Artigas A, Brigham KL, Carlet J, Falke K, Hudson L, Lamy M, LeGall JR, Morris A, Spragg R. Report of the American-European consensus conference on ARDS: definitions, mechanisms, relevant outcomes and clinical trial coordination. The Consensus Committee. Intensive Care Med 20:225-232, 1994.

3. Williams AJ. ABC of oxygen: assessing and interpreting arterial blood gases and acid-base balance [review]. Br Med J 317:1213-1216, 1998.

4. Shapiro BA. Arterial blood gas monitoring [review]. Crit Care Clin 4:479-492, 1988.

5. Sinha S, Nicks J, Donn S. Graphic analysis of pulmonary mechanics in neonates receiving assisted ventilation. Arch Dis Child Fetal Neonatal Ed 75:F213-F218, 1996.

6. Tobin MJ. Advances in mechanical ventilation. N Engl J Med 344:1986-1996, 2001.

7. Panitch H, Downes J, Kennedy J, Kolb S, Parra M, Peacock J, Thompson M. Guidelines for home care of children with chronic respiratory insufficiency. Pediatr Pulmonol 21:52-56, 1996.

8. Meduri GU, Fox RC, Abou-Shala N, Leeper KV, Wunderink RG. Noninvasive mechanical ventilation via face mask in patients with acute respiratory failure who refused endotracheal intubation. Crit Care Med 22:1584-1590, 1994.

9. Corbetta L, Ballerin L, Putinati S, Potena A Efficacy of non-invasive positive pressure ventilation by facial and nasal mask in hypercapnic acute respiratory failure: experience in a respiratory ward under usual care. Monaldi Arch Chest Dis 52:421-428, 1997.

10. Bartlett RH, Fong SW, Woldanski C, Hung E, Styler D, MacArthur C. Hematologic responses to prolonged extracorporeal circulation (ECC) with microporous membrane devices. Trans Am Soc Artif Intern Organs 21:250-257, 1975.

11. Hill JD, O'Brien TG, Murray JJ, Dontigny L, Bramson ML, Osborn JJ, Gerbode F Prolonged extracorporeal oxygenation for acute post-traumatic respiratory failure (shock-lung syndrome). Use of the Bramson membrane lung. N Engl J Med 286:629, 1972.

12. Hill JD, De Leval MR, Fallat RJ, Bramson ML, Eberhart RC, Schulte HD, Osborn JJ, Barber R, Gerbode F. Acute respiratory insufficiency. Treatment with prolonged extracorporeal oxygenation. J Thorac Cardiovasc Surg 64:551-562, 1972.

13. Numa AH, Hammer J, Newth CJ. Effect of prone and supine positions on functional residual capacity, oxygenation, and respiratory mechanics in ventilated infants and children. Am J Respir Crit Care Med 156:1185-1189, 1997.

14. Curley MA, Thompson JE, Arnold JH. The effects of early and repeated prone positioning in pediatric patients with acute lung injury. Chest 118:156-163, 2000.

15. Arnold JH, Hanson JH, Toro-Figuero LO, Gutierrez J, Berens RJ, Anglin DL. Prospective, randomized comparison of high-frequency oscillatory ventilation and conventional mechanical ventilation in pediatric respiratory failure. Crit Care Med 22:1530-1539, 1994.

16. Pranikoff T, Gauger PG, Hirschl RB. Partial liquid ventilation in a child on extracorporeal life support. Asaio J 42:317-320, 1996.

17. Leach CL, Greenspan JS, Rubenstein SD, Shaffer TH, Wolfson MR, Jackson JC, DeLemos R, Fuhrman BP. Partial liquid ventilation with perflubron in premature infants with severe respiratory distress syndrome. The LiquiVent Study Group. N Engl J Med 335:761-767, 1996.

18. Hess DR. Liberation from mechanical ventilation: weaning the patient or weaning old-fashioned ideas? Crit Care Med 30:2154-2155, 2002.

19. Scheinhorn DJ, Chao DC, Stearn-Hassenpflug M Liberation from prolonged mechanical ventilation. Crit Care Clin 18:569-595, 2002.

CHAPTER 15

Viral Infections of the Respiratory Tract

MICHAEL R. BYE, M.D.

Croup
Acute Bronchitis, or Upper Respiratory Illness
   with Persistent Cough
Bronchiolitis
Pneumonia
Acute Asthma Exacerbation

Viruses cause the overwhelming majority of infections of the respiratory tract in children. In some cases it may be difficult to differentiate between bacterial and viral disease, but most of the time viruses are causing the infection. This chapter will start at the larynx and work down through the airways to the lung parenchyma. The infections to be discussed include croup, bronchitis, bronchiolitis, and pneumonia. Although asthma is not a viral disease, acute asthma attacks are often triggered by viral infections. There is therefore a brief discussion of asthma at the end of this chapter. With each of the infections, the common etiologies, the pathophysiology, and an approach to therapy will be reviewed.

CROUP

Croup is typically a viral infection of the upper airways. Croup is also known as laryngotracheobronchitis, suggesting the wide segments of the airway that may be involved. Croup is most commonly caused by parainfluenza, and less frequently by respiratory syncytial virus (RSV). Other, even less common causes include adenovirus and rhinovirus. In the era before immunization for *Haemophilus influenzae* type b, it was often important to differentiate between acute croup and epiglottitis. With the increasing immunization against that bacterium, bacterial epiglottitis, which can be a life-threatening illness, has become very uncommon. Although croup may occur at virtually any age, it typically occurs between the ages of 6 months and 3 years. Because parainfluenza

and RSV cause the majority of cases of croup, most cases of croup occur in the fall through winter months. In the Northeast United States there are occasional summer outbreaks of parainfluenza with concomitant outbreaks of croup.

Croup typically begins with simple coryza. After 1–2 days of coryza, the croup symptoms begin. The hallmark of the disease is airway obstruction in the extrathoracic airways, especially the subglottic space. Thus the typical clinical finding is of stridor. This is an inspiratory crowing noise generated by air moving through the narrowed extrathoracic airways. The pathophysiology of croup includes edema and inflammation of the vocal cords and the subglottic space. As the name indicates, this airway inflammation and edema will often spread into the trachea and the bronchi. In some cases the pathology extends into the bronchioles as well. Because there is inflammation and swelling of the vocal cords and the subglottic space, a barky cough may be present, and the cry or voice may be hoarse. For unknown reasons, croup symptoms often begin at night. The symptoms frequently progress for 1–2 days, and remit after 3–7 days. There are usually no sequelae. Since the intrathoracic airways can be involved, wheeze may be present, but crackles are uncommon. Because much of the pathology is above the carina, gas exchange is rarely affected. Patients will therefore often have normal oxygen saturation, unless there is enough obstruction to cause hypoventilation. If the airways distal to the carina are involved, ventilation–perfusion mismatch may occur and hypoxemia is more likely to occur.

Children with spasmodic croup may not have any prodrome, and they usually have recurrent disease. In most cases, despite the recurrence of episodes, an investigation of the airway does not reveal any anatomic abnormalities. These children may have a form of airway reactivity. In such children a combination of corticosteroids and bronchodilators, sometimes in combination with inhaled epinephrine, can be helpful. Such children may subsequently develop the more typical lower airway manifestations of asthma.

At physical examination, the child with croup will often have mild tachypnea. It is advantageous to attempt to maintain laminar flow through the obstructed airway by keeping the child calm and breathing as slowly as possible. Elevated respiratory rates and flow rates will result in more turbulent flow, which will pass through the obstructed airway with more difficulty. Trying to explain this physiology to a 3-year-old is patently absurd. However, children with croup learn to accommodate quickly, and maintain an advantageous respiratory pattern, without having read a physiology textbook. As indicated above, stridor is a prominent finding in acute croup. Stridor may be defined as any inspiratory noise. With croup, it is typically a crowing noise that is purely inspiratory. There may be an exhalatory component if there is sufficient obstruction of the subglottic space or if the obstruction extends into the intrathoracic airways. Examination of the chest wall reveals retractions at the level of the sternum, and often in the suprasternal chest wall. These are caused by use of the accessory muscles of inspiration, and since the obstruction is primarily extrathoracic, the child has difficulties getting air in. Because hyperinflation is uncommon with croup, subcostal retractions are also uncommon. With increasing obstruction, intercostal retractions may occur. As above, wheezes may be heard if the obstruction descends into the intrathoracic airways, or if the subglottic obstruction is fixed and significant. Crackles are uncommon because the pathology rarely progresses into the small airways. The degree of respiratory difficulty is best assessed by the level of comfort of the child, the presence of stridor, and the severity of the retractions. Assessing air entry with a stethoscope is important. If the child's oxygenation is not normal, this is a worrisome sign.

The diagnosis of croup is usually a clinical one. Differentiating croup from epiglottitis is no longer a major issue, as the incidence of *Haemophilus influenzae* type b infection is decreasing markedly. An acute laryngeal foreign body is always a possibility in this age range. However, given the typical clinical scenario, radiographs or endoscopy are not routinely warranted. If radiographs of the neck are obtained, both anteroposterior and lateral films give information about the diagnosis. The most prominent findings occur on the anteroposterior film (Figure 15-1). Normally, if one looks at the subglottic space on the film, the airway is outlined by "square shoulders" as the air column juts out from the vocal cords into the subglottic space (Figure 15-1A). Because in croup the subglottic space is narrowed, the shadow on the film has a "steeplechase" appearance, with a more gradual widening of the airway as one descends into the trachea (Figure 15-1B). The lateral neck film often reveals distension of the hypopharynx, a radiographic demonstration of the air not entering the airway.

Croup is a self-limited disorder. Therefore, therapy is indicated for those children more severely affected. Thus, acute intervention might be indicated for those children with supplemental oxygen requirements, excessive work of breathing which might interfere with adequate nutrition or lead to respiratory fatigue, or those who might otherwise require admission to the hospital.

Mist therapy helps some children with croup. Empirically, both warm mist and cool mist have helped. Therefore an early approach is to bring the child into the bathroom and keep the shower running, developing mist in the room. With small infants, it is important that a parent stay in the bathroom with the infant. Cool mist can simply be provided by night air. Therefore, a second step might be to take the child for a walk around the block, or for a drive in the car with the windows open. Very often, after these two procedures, the child is well enough to fall back to sleep. Despite the utility of mist as an early therapy, if the child is admitted to hospital, placing him or her in a mist tent is often counterproductive. This separates the child from the parent, which increases the anxiety on the part of the child. As a result, the child's respiratory rate will increase, making inspiratory airflow more turbulent. In addition, once the child is in the mist tent, it is difficult to assess the child's chest wall, critical to the sequential assessment of the child with croup.

If the child has a history of asthma, the virus causing croup can also trigger asthma. In those children, bronchodilators are helpful. In patients with recurrent or spasmodic croup, bronchodilators may also help. However, for most children with croup, beta-agonists are not useful. Corticosteroids have been shown to reduce the severity of disease, the length of the disease, and for hospitalized patients to reduce transfers to the intensive care unit. Dexamethasone at 0.6 mg per kilogram is effective by both parenteral and oral routes. One study suggested nebulized budesonide 2 mg to be effective. Lower oral doses of dexamethasone, including 0.3 mg per kilogram and 0.15 mg per kilogram, have also been successful. However, the number of patients enrolled in the studies has been low. Given the relative lack of toxicity, a current recommendation might be to use the higher dose of dexamethasone, given orally. Although dexamethasone is the most commonly studied steroid for croup, there is no reason why equivalent doses of prednisone or prednisolone should not be effective.

The child who is dyspneic, has supplemental oxygen requirements, seems fearful or fretful, or has insufficient gas exchange is clearly a candidate for therapy. If admission to hospital is being considered for these or other reasons, therapy should be instituted. The time-honored therapy is inhaled epinephrine. This primarily causes

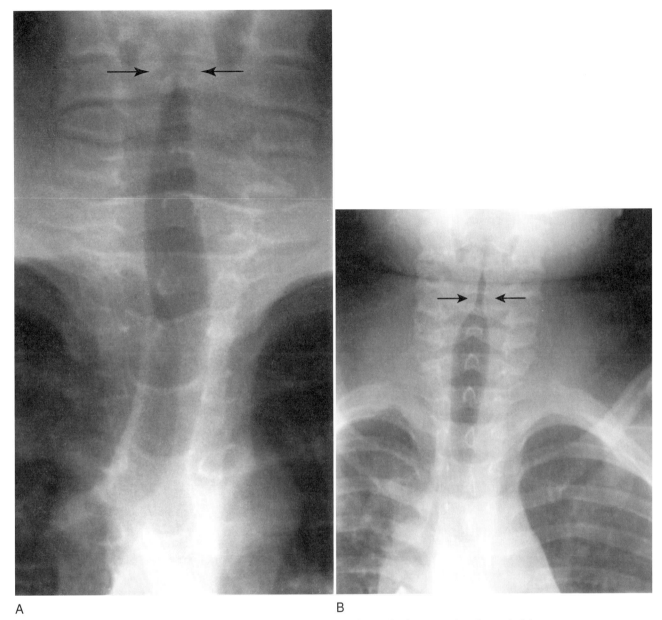

A   B

Figure 15-1 (**A**) Normal anteroposterior view of the neck, demonstrating the typical "square-shouldered" appearance of the subglottic space. (**B**) Anteroposterior view of the neck in a child with acute laryngotracheobronchitis (croup). Note the extended area of narrowing of the air tracheogram in the immediate subglottic space (arrows). (Radiographs courtesy of Avrum N. Pollock, M.D., FRCPC.)

vasoconstriction in the upper airways, and reduces the swelling in the epithelium. It also acts as a bronchodilator, important for those children with pre-existing asthma. Inhaled epinephrine may be given either as the racemic form, which is time-honored; or as levoepinephrine. In either case, the medication should be given through a nebulizer. An over-the-counter form of epinephrine exists as a metered dose inhaler. This could be delivered through a valved holding chamber with mask apparatus. We have used this for some children with spasmodic croup. In these children, the croup is a forme fruste of

asthma, with edema of the upper airway more prominent than usual. This is not for routine cases of croup.

For many years, there was concern about the potential for rebound obstruction after epinephrine, where airway mucosal edema might increase as the vasoconstrictive effects of the drug wore off. However, careful studies have not borne out this phenomenon. These data suggest that if the child does not worsen 1–2 hours after treatment, it is not likely to happen. At that point the decision to admit or send the child home can be based purely on the current clinical status.

Children with increasing oxygen requirements or with deteriorating gas exchange, or in whom progressive respiratory fatigue appears to be occurring, should be transferred to a Pediatric Intensive Care Unit (PICU). An adjunct therapy in the PICU might be institution of inhalation of a mixture of helium and oxygen. Helium, because of its lower density than room air, will move through the narrowed airways more readily. This reduces the work of breathing and improves gas exchange. The risk of this mixture is the limitation of supplemental oxygen that can be given. However, in many cases the improved gas exchange and decreased work of breathing more than compensate for the difficulty in delivering high oxygen concentrations, and the child is able to ventilate and oxygenate adequately. If the respiratory status continues to deteriorate, endotracheal intubation should be considered. The endotracheal tube should be able to bypass the obstructed airway, and allow for better gas exchange and oxygenation, until healing of the airway occurs. The smallest possible endotracheal tube that allows adequate ventilation should be used. Airway intubation should be done in conjunction with, or by, a pediatric intensivist or pediatric anesthesiologist. Using too large an endotracheal tube increases the risk of further damage to the inflamed subglottic space, prolonging the acute damage and increasing the risk of subglottic stenosis after the acute infection has subsided. In most cases, an uncuffed tube should be used, again to reduce mucosal damage and allow healing of the airway wall. The endotracheal tube should be left in place until there is clinical evidence of a leak around the tube, suggesting that the swelling has subsided sufficiently, and that the child should be able to maintain gas exchange and oxygenation. We normally continue systemic corticosteroids until the child has been successfully extubated, and for a few days beyond. Unless there is pre-existing asthma or persisting airway obstruction, we do not routinely use long-term corticosteroids.

ACUTE BRONCHITIS, OR UPPER RESPIRATORY ILLNESS WITH PERSISTENT COUGH

Bronchitis technically refers to inflammation of the airways. It occurs frequently in children, in conjunction with an upper respiratory infection (URI). After the onset of the URI the child will begin to cough, and rhonchi may be heard. Bronchitis in otherwise healthy children is almost never bacterial, and almost never requires antibiotic therapy. The same virus causing the URI usually causes the bronchitis. Symptomatic therapy is usually all that is necessary for bronchitis. There has been no proven benefit to antibiotics, cough suppressants or decongestants. A special note should be made for the child with asthma. When making the diagnosis of bronchitis in the child with asthma, or the diagnosis of asthmatic bronchitis, the therapy should be directed towards the underlying asthma. In most cases asthmatic bronchitis is in fact asthmatic asthma. Once a child has been diagnosed more than two or three times with bronchitis, or has prominent or prolonged chest symptoms with colds, one should strongly consider the diagnosis of asthma.

BRONCHIOLITIS

It has been suggested that over 90% of children will be infected with RSV during the first 2 years of life. In some children, RSV infection will trigger bronchiolitis. Viruses, including RSV, are the most common cause of bronchiolitis. Other viruses which can cause bronchiolitis include parainfluenza and adenovirus. Data show that those children who develop bronchiolitis with RSV infection are likely to have had abnormal lung function before the RSV infection; are likely to have higher histamine content in the airways, and specific IgE towards the RSV; and are likely to have increased levels of pro-inflammatory cytokines in the blood and airways compared with those who experience upper respiratory symptoms. Children who develop bronchiolitis with RSV infection are at greater risk of subsequently developing asthma. This appears to be at least in part because of pre-existing lung abnormalities as well as an abnormal immune response. Bronchiolitis accounts for significant numbers of hospital admissions each year, primarily in children under 2 years of age. There are some children at increased risk of severe disease from RSV infection. These include children with bronchopulmonary dysplasia or other chronic lung disease of infancy; children with cyanotic heart disease, or those with significant pulmonary hypertension; and children born at less than 32 weeks gestation, even without chronic lung disease. Children with human immunodeficiency virus (HIV) infection have been shown to be more likely to develop pneumonia with RSV infection, and to harbor the virus for longer periods than immunocompetent children. Acute severe bronchiolitis has been described in infants with cystic fibrosis, and decades ago this accounted for significant mortality in affected children. However, this has not been a major problem for this population in recent years.

With bronchiolitis, the virus infects the airway epithelium and causes intense edema and an inflammatory reaction, leading to obstruction of the airways. This is manifested in the child by tachypnea, hypoxemia from ventilation–perfusion mismatch, wheezing, crackles, and hyperinflation. The latter may be seen on physical examination or on the radiograph. Fever is often present.

The complications of bronchiolitis include hypoxemia, respiratory failure, dehydration from decreased fluid intake, and apnea. The cause of the apnea is unclear, but it is more likely to occur in young infants who were born prematurely. RSV has a typical season. In the United States it starts around October and lasts 5 months, although it may begin earlier and last longer in some southern states. Occasional summertime epidemics are seen. Children infected with HIV are likely to harbor the virus longer than other children. This can account for sporadic infection as the virus is transmitted to other children.

Bronchiolitis typically starts with rhinorrhea. After 2–3 days, cough and wheeze develop. The cough and wheeze clear in 7–14 days, though they may last up to 3–4 weeks in some children. On examination, the child is typically tachypneic with varying degrees of hypoxemia. The heart rate is usually elevated. The infant may have nasal flaring. Wheezes are a hallmark of the disease, from the intrathoracic airway obstruction. Crackles are heard as the inflammation obstructs the small airways. Subcostal retractions are a manifestation of hyperinflation. Increasing degrees of respiratory difficulty will cause intercostal retractions as well as accessory muscle use. The typical chest radiograph (Figure 15-2) reveals hyperinflation and peribronchial thickening. Areas of atelectasis are not uncommon.

In most cases bronchiolitis is a self-limited illness. The therapy of bronchiolitis has been unrewarding and often debated. Because these children look and sound like children with asthma, they often get the same medications. Most studies show little to no effect from systemic corticosteroids. Several studies looked at inhaled corticosteroids after the acute bronchiolitis subsided, and found no reduction in the frequency of subsequent wheeze. Bronchodilators, especially albuterol, work in some patients. However, most studies show that most patients do not benefit from albuterol or theophylline. Therefore, their routine use is discouraged. Early pathology data showed significant airway edema in infants with bronchiolitis. Therefore, epinephrine was tried as a means of reducing the airway edema through its

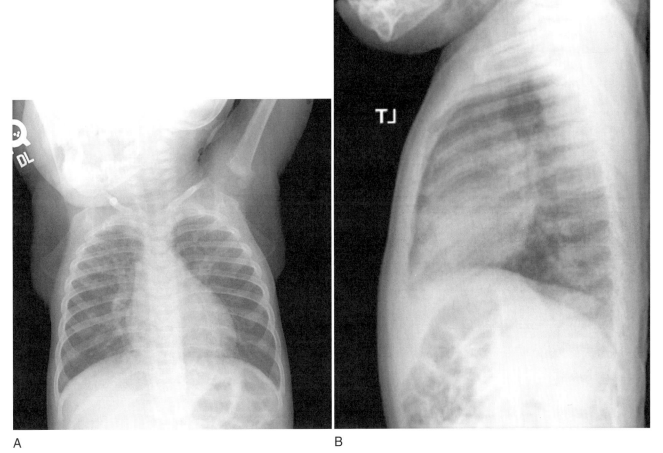

A   B

Figure 15-2 (**A**) Anteroposterior chest radiograph of an infant with bronchiolitis. Note the widened spaces between the ribs reflecting mild hyperinflation, and increased interstitial markings. Bibasilar subsegmental atelectasis is also present. (**B**) Lateral view of the chest. The diaphragm is moderately flattened, again reflecting air trapping and hyperinflation. (Radiographs courtesy of Avrum N. Pollock, M.D., FRCPC.)

α-adrenergic vasoconstriction effect, while simultaneously providing bronchodilatation by its β-adrenergic effects. Recent data, in fact, have suggested that inhaled epinephrine is more effective than albuterol at improving clinical score and shortening hospitalization, with fewer side effects. It is critical to remember, however, that most infants with bronchiolitis improve and heal spontaneously.

Most patients are not helped by medications, which have potential for side effects. One recommendation would be not to give any treatment unless the child absolutely requires therapy. A common definition of requiring therapy could include either hypoxemia necessitating supplemental oxygen, or inability to take adequate fluids by mouth. In these cases, inhaled epinephrine might be helpful. One might try albuterol as well. However, a suggestion has been made that if the albuterol does not help, it should not be repeated. Routine use of corticosteroids for children with bronchiolitis is discouraged. If steroids are used in more severely ill patients, however, the systemic route (PO, IM or IV) has been shown to be more effective than administration by inhalation. Although an excellent adjunct to ill patients with asthma, ipratropium has not been shown to be helpful in children with bronchiolitis. If the child has significant hypoxemia, usually defined as oxygen saturation below 90%, supplemental oxygen should be administered. In addition, if the child were unable to take adequate fluids, intravenous fluids may be necessary. If there is any question about the child's ability to maintain the state of hydration, intravenous fluids should be considered. There are recent data suggesting an increased incidence of gastroesophageal reflux and aspiration during acute bronchiolitis, which resolves when the acute infection has resolved. Recent studies suggest increased amounts of leukotriene in the urine and endotracheal secretions of children with acute bronchiolitis. Clinical trials of leukotriene antagonists are anticipated. Unfortunately, only one of these agents is approved for use in infants, and that approval is down to age 12 months: most ill infants with bronchiolitis are below that age.

Recently attempts have been made at preventing serious RSV disease, defined as a lower respiratory illness requiring hospitalization. The most helpful products have been RSV-specific immunoglobulin (RSV-IVIG), and, more recently, a monoclonal antibody (palivizumab). Studies using the monoclonal antibody have shown a high degree of safety. Furthermore, children at risk, such as those with bronchopulmonary dysplasia, or children born prematurely with lung disease, children born prematurely without lung disease, children with chronic lung disease, and children with congenital heart disease have been shown to experience decreased severity of illness with the monoclonal antibody product. It is important to warn parents that this product does not prevent infection; it only reduces the severity of the acute illness. There are no data as to whether the product reduces the subsequent development of asthma. Nor are there any data available on the drug's effectiveness in other populations. The American Academy of Pediatrics Committee on Infectious Diseases, in its 2000 Red Book, recommends palivizumab for children under 2 years of age with chronic lung disease of infancy who have required medical therapy within 6 months of the RSV season; infants born at 28 weeks gestation or earlier without chronic lung disease, up to 12 months of age; and infants born between 28 and 32 weeks gestation, up to 6 months of age.

PNEUMONIA

Viruses cause the majority of cases of pneumonia in children. Unfortunately, it is often difficult to decide whether a virus or bacterium has caused pneumonia in a particular patient. It is a suspicion of many that focal disease associated with high fever is more likely a bacterial process, and diffuse disease with wheeze is more likely to be viral. However, neither of these is an absolute finding and, as discussed above, this has been difficult to prove because of a lack of a readily accessible gold standard. While there are factors that lead many to suspect one or the other (Table 15-1), these have been difficult to prove. Part of the problem is in defining a gold standard for pneumonia. A definitive diagnosis of pneumonia would require obtaining lung tissue such as from a percutaneous lung puncture. It would be difficult to imagine any institutional review board approving such a study in children.

In most cases, pneumonia develops either as part of, or shortly after, a viral infection. Thus, unlike in adults where pneumococcal pneumonia often has a sudden onset of fever and respiratory symptoms, in children there is usually a prodrome of upper respiratory infection. The child then develops progressive lower respiratory symptoms, including fever, tachypnea, dyspnea, and associated signs and symptoms including malaise, decreased appetite, and lethargy. Chest pain is uncommon unless there is pleural involvement.

On physical examination, the child is often tachypneic and tachycardic with fever. Infants will show nasal flaring in an attempt to increase inspiratory airflow, a manifestation of dyspnea. While cyanosis may be present, oxygen saturation decreases significantly well before this overt manifestation of hypoxemia. Subcostal retractions are a manifestation of hyperinflation, such as seen with diffuse airway disease. Intercostal or supraclavicular retractions indicate progressive dyspnea. With more airways obstruction, the accessory muscles in the neck are used to overcome the increased airway

Table 15-1   Factors Favoring a Diagnosis of Viral or Bacterial Pneumonia

Factor	Viral Pneumonia More Likely	Bacterial Pneumonia More Likely
Prodrome	Prodrome to respiratory distress	Prodrome to febrile illness
Vital signs	More tachypneic; less febrile; more hypoxemic	Less hypoxemic; higher fever
Physical examination	Respiratory distress; wheeze; diffuse crackles; subcostal retractions	Acute febrile illness; focal crackles; egophony; decreased breath sounds
Radiograph	Hyperinflation; peribronchial thickening	Focal infiltrate; effusion

resistance. Examination of the chest may include crackles, wheeze, and areas of decreased airflow. It is important to remember that crackles do not indicate alveolar disease, and are not necessarily indications of infection.

Crackles occur when the small airways are occluded, such as with inflammation, edema, or infectious material within the airways; or inflammation, edema, or fibrosis outside the airways. These airways are thus closed and open as the child progressively inspires, the sound being caused as they snap open. Obviously, many disease processes can cause crackles. Crackles can be part of an asthma attack as the inflammation and edema close those small airways.

The gold standard for diagnosing pneumonia remains the chest radiograph. Obviously, in a child with no pre-existing lung disease who presents with relatively sudden onset of lower respiratory symptoms and has findings including crackles, the diagnosis of pneumonia should be entertained and treated. In that case a radiograph is not necessary. However, with pre-existing lung disease such as asthma, the findings can be ascribed to the underlying disease. In those cases, a radiograph may be helpful. As anyone who has waited for a radiograph can attest, the problem of lag of development of the radiographic findings is overplayed. Similarly, the role of dehydration in masking a radiographic abnormality is overplayed. It has been shown that overhydration during acute pneumonia in dogs worsened the radiograph but did not alter the pattern. If a radiograph is abnormal, the abnormalities will often take up to 2 months to clear. While an elevated white blood cell count and increased numbers of polymorphonuclear cells and/or bands will increase the likelihood of a bacterial process, even under those circumstances most infections are viral. If a child is able to produce sputum, its examination can be rewarding. The finding of polymorphonuclear cells or intracellular organisms strongly suggests an acute bacterial process, and the need for antibiotics. Careful analysis has shown that neither thickness of the sputum nor discoloration correlates with the likelihood of an acute bacterial process.

ACUTE ASTHMA EXACERBATION

By including asthma in this chapter, I by no means imply that asthma is a viral disease. However, the majority of asthma attacks that get children to the emergency room or admitted to hospital are triggered by viral infections. Thus, children with acute asthma attacks will often have fever, as a manifestation of the viral infection triggering the asthma. The physical examination may include wheeze, crackles, and areas of decreased air entry similar to those findings in the child with pneumonia. If the child with an acute asthma attack has a chest radiograph, areas of atelectasis can often be misinterpreted as acute infiltrates. Just managing the underlying asthma, with bronchodilators and corticosteroids, can treat most of these children. Antibiotics are not necessary for the majority of these children.

MAJOR POINTS

1. Croup is almost always a viral infection, and antibiotics are almost never required. Systemic corticosteroids can shorten the course of the disease, and make the symptoms more manageable. Other acute management includes inhaled epinephrine. Treatment with inhaled epinephrine is no longer considered an automatic indication for admission to hospital.

2. Bronchiolitis is virtually always a viral infection. If a child can eat and oxygenate adequately, therapy is probably not necessary. If therapy is indicated, acute albuterol has been shown to provide relief in some children. If albuterol does not help, and the child is still having respiratory difficulty, inhaled epinephrine can be tried. The data on systemic corticosteroids show varying degrees of response.

Continued

MAJOR POINTS—Cont'd

At best, the benefits are meager. One recent meta-analysis of steroids in children admitted to hospital with bronchiolitis showed the steroids to reduce length of stay by 0.4 days; this means almost 10 hours. Nor have steroids been shown to be helpful for the prolonged "postbronchiolitis" cough and wheeze so frequently seen.

3. In children who are nonsmokers without underlying pulmonary disease, bronchitis is usually part of a simple cold. Antibiotics are almost never necessary in these children. If the child has a pattern of recurrent bronchitis, or frequent or prolonged chest symptoms with colds, consideration must be given to the diagnosis of asthma. In such cases, a trial of systemic corticosteroids (prednisone or prednisolone 1-2 mg/kg per day divided BID) and inhaled bronchodilators is often rewarding.

4. The majority of cases of pneumonia in children are caused by a virus. The likelihood of a bacterial process is increased if the child has a high fever, focal findings on examination and radiograph, lack of wheeze, and pleural effusion. If sputum analysis is possible, finding either neutrophils or intracellular organisms suggests a bacterial etiology.

SUGGESTED READING

American Academy of Pediatrics. Respiratory syncytial virus. In Pickering L, editor: 2000 Red Book: Report of the Committee on Infectious Diseases 2000, 25th edition, pp 483-487. Elk Grove Village, IL: American Academy of Pediatrics, 2000.

Berger I, Argaman Z, Schwartz SB, Segal E, Kiderman A, Branski D, Kerem E. Efficacy of corticosteroids in acute bronchiolitis: short-term and long-term follow-up. Pediatr Pulmonol 26:162-166, 1998.

Bye MR. Bronchiolitis and bronchitis. In Burg FD, Ingelfinger J, Polin RA, Gershon AA, editors: Gellis & Kagan's current pediatric therapy, 17th edition, pp 484-485. Philadelphia: Saunders, 2002.

Bye MR. Persistent or recurrent pneumonia. In Schidlow DV, Smith DS, editors: A practical guide to pediatric respiratory diseases, pp 99-103. Philadelphia: Hanley & Belfus, 1994.

Englund JA. Prevention strategies for respiratory syncytial virus: passive and active immunization. J Pediatr 135: 38-44,1999.

Geelhoed GC, Macdonald WBG. Oral and inhaled steroid in croup: a randomized, placebo-controlled trial. Pediatr Pulmonol 20:355-361, 1995.

Geelhoed GC, Macdonald WBG. Oral dexamethasone in the treatment of croup: 0.15 mg/kg versus 0.3 mg/kg versus 0.6 mg/kg. Pediatr Pulmonol 20:362-368, 1995.

Geelhoed GC. Croup. State of the art. Pediatr Pulmonol 23:370-374, 1997.

IMpact-RSV Study Group. Palivizumab, a humanized respiratory syncytial virus monoclonal antibody, reduces hospitalization from respiratory syncytial virus infection in high-risk infants. Pediatrics 102:531-537, 1998.

Johnson DW, Jacobson S, Edney PC, et al. A comparison of nebulized budesonide, intramuscular dexamethasone, and placebo for moderately severe croup. N Engl J Med 339: 498-503, 1998.

Kaditis AG, Wald ER. Viral croup: current diagnosis and treatment. Pediatr Infect Dis J 17:827-834, 1998.

Kellner JD, Ohlsson A, Gadomski AM, Wang EE. Bronchodilators for bronchiolitis. Cochrane Database Syst Rev CD001266, 2000.

Khoshoo V, Edell D. Previously healthy infants may have increased risk of aspiration during respiratory syncytial viral bronchiolitis. Pediatrics 104:1389-1390, 1999.

Loughlin GM. Bronchitis. In Chernick V, Boat T, editors: Kendig's disorders of the respiratory tract in children, 6th edition, p 461. Philadelphia: Saunders, 1998.

Mallory GB Jr., Motoyama EK, Koumbourlis AC, Mutich RL, Nakayama DK. Bronchial reactivity in infants in acute respiratory failure with viral bronchiolitis. Pediatr Pulmonol 6:253-259, 1989.

Martinez FD, Wright AL, Taussig LM, Holberg CJ, Halonen M, Morgan WJ. Asthma and wheezing in the first six years of life. The Group Health Medical Associates. N Engl J Med 332:133-138, 1995.

Rodriguez WJ. Management strategies for respiratory syncytial virus infections in infants. J Pediatr 135:45-50, 1999.

Sanchez I, De Koster J, Powell RE, Wolstein R, Chernick V. Effect of racemic epinephrine and salbutamol on clinical score and pulmonary mechanics in infants with bronchiolitis. J Pediatr 122:145-151, 1993.

Shay DK, Holman RC, Newman RD, Liu LL, Stout JW, Anderson LJ. Bronchiolitis-associated hospitalizations among US children, 1980-1996. JAMA 282:1440-1446, 1999.

Tepper RS, Rosenberg D, Eigen H, Reister T. Bronchodilator responsiveness in infants with bronchiolitis. Pediatr Pulmonol 17:81-85, 1994.

Wong JY, Moon S, Beardsmore C, O'Callaghan C, Simpson H. No objective benefit from steroids inhaled via a spacer in infants recovering from bronchiolitis. Eur Respir J 15: 388-394, 2000.

Index

Page numbers in italic, e.g. *215*, refer to figures. Page numbers in bold, e.g. **191**, denote entries in tables.